W9-CDJ-847

100 Perks
of
Having Cancer

plus

100 Health Tips
for Surviving It!

Florence Strang
& Susan Gonzalez

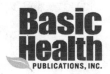
Basic Health
PUBLICATIONS, INC.

The information contained in this book is based upon the research and personal and professional experiences of the authors. It is not intended as a substitute for consulting with your physician or other healthcare provider. Any attempt to diagnose and treat an illness should be done under the direction of a healthcare professional.

The publisher does not advocate the use of any particular healthcare protocol but believes the information in this book should be available to the public. The publisher and authors are not responsible for any adverse effects or consequences resulting from the use of the suggestions, preparations, or procedures discussed in this book. Should the reader have any questions concerning the appropriateness of any procedures or preparation mentioned, the authors and the publisher strongly suggest consulting a professional healthcare advisor.

Basic Health Publications, Inc.
28812 Top of the World Drive
Laguna Beach, CA 92651
949-715-7327 • www.basichealthpub.com

Library of Congress Cataloging-in-Publication Data

Strang, Florence
    100 perks of having cancer : plus 100 health tips for surviving it / Florence Strang and Susan Gonzalez.
        pages cm
    Includes bibliographical references and index.
    ISBN 978-1-59120-356-8
    1. Cancer—Popular works. 2. Self-care, Health—Popular works. I. Gonzalez, Susan II. Title.
    RC263.S73   2013
    616.99'4—dc23

                                                            2013017856

Editor: Carol Killman Rosenberg
Typesetting/Book design: Gary A. Rosenberg
Cover design: Mike Stromberg
Illustrations: Theresa McCracken
Photo for Health Tip #69 and pages 63, 64, 103, 378, and 424: jgubelman photography

Printed in the United States of America

10   9   8   7   6   5   4   3   2   1

Contents

Foreword by Bernie S. Siegel, MD, xi

Introduction, 1

For Patches, who was my constant and loving companion
through many difficult days.
RIP Patches.
—FLORENCE

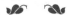

For my dad, who always found a way to
work in his daily 10,000 steps.
—SUSAN

Foreword

I believe this book provides the reader with the resources necessary to help you find your perks, through the various tips and directions it will expose you to. I feel we all need life coaches but rarely have any available to us as we are growing up, so let the authors become your coaches and their perks and tips become the instructions that can turn you into a star performer. No book can change you. You have to read on and show up for practice to be exposed to the wisdom and make the changes that this book makes clear to you to make it happen. You change your life and existence due to the desire and intention that reside within you. They direct you to the wisdom and help you to learn about being a survivor.

I call these difficulties our labor pains. They lead us to rebirth and re-parent ourselves and create a new and meaningful life and body we can love. When the essential teachings of the ages are made clear to us, we can learn before the disaster occurs. It is a lot easier to be strong enough to withstand the difficulties and to not break down so the cancer, or other problem, does not have to be your teacher, new beginning, or wake-up call. My dad said his father's dying when he was twelve was one of the best things that ever happened to him. I was shocked by his statement until he went on to explain that it was what he learned about life from all the difficulties he experienced that made him say that. A rather painful perk, but it made him focus his life on helping others to live.

I have learned that, if the inspiration is within you, then the information that you can derive from this book and its perks and tips can help you to become a survivor. This is not about becoming immortal. We all die someday, but when your body knows you love your life, it does all it can to keep you alive and help you to thrive. The natives know the territory and can help the tourists, who haven't experienced "cancer land," to find their way home. They can expose you to the common themes that survivors portray. I must add that these lessons are for all of us to learn now. You don't need to use cancer as an excuse or to have permission to take care of yourself. From here on, you are to let your heart make up your mind.

You need to know that you are not a statistic and that you can exceed expectations by living the examples expressed in this book. You do not live or die based upon numbers but upon your will to live and the life you are willing to create. If the past was full of wounds, you can abandon it and re-parent yourself and develop a sense of self-love and worth you never received. There are many factors that are perks and improve your chances of being a survivor—from laughter and relationships to pets. When you are grateful for life and find happiness, your body gets the message and your internal chemistry produces healing and growth and increased protection from disease as our immune function is enhanced by those feelings.

Fear does not become an issue when you have faith in yourself, others, and a higher authority. You also become a teacher for your children, family, and friends by displaying survivor behavior. When you learn you become a *respant*, a responsible participant in your life and not a submissive sufferer, or good patient. Also by displaying your wounds, you become a healer for others who know they can share with you and learn from you. Hiding your wounds and denying your needs are not survivor behaviors. Just as the authors reveal, only the wounded healer can truly serve because they have lived the experience and are natives and not tourists.

The mind and body are a unit and must be seen as such. When one is going through treatment for cancer, the body experiences what the mind visualizes. So learn to empower yourself by visualizing the desired response and results. Again like an actor or athlete, you can rehearse and practice and get it right. This also includes your right to say no to what your inner wisdom says is not right for you to do. It means keeping your power and choosing treatments you visualize as gifts and not poisons or mutilations. You can learn to give yourself health days and not sick days by doing what makes you happy. When you act out of love, there are no burdens. The cancer should not force you or motivate you to do anything. It is not in charge. You must be the force and the motivator. You can let your mortality be a factor and be sure you spend your life's time doing what makes you happy, and not what makes others happy and lose your life to their choices and desires. You are to live because of your desires and choices and become a work in progress.

The authors can help guide and coach you as you become a work of art.

And remember to not give the cancer credit for what happens. You did it, and you deserve the credit. When you learn how to handle your fear and worries, you are creating a healing environment. Fear is appropriate when you are in a threatening situation, but when every situation is seen as a threat it becomes self-destructive. Fear lowers immune function and increases stress-hormone levels and makes changes to help you in an acute threatening situation, but when it becomes chronic and long lasting, it reduces your ability to overcome illness. As I mentioned, the faith, hope, love, and laughter are what enhance immune function and lower stress-hormone levels. Again, see this book as you would a script for a play, and incorporate the perks and tips into the role you are playing. Then you rehearse and practice until you get it right. Let this guidebook become your map and the people in your life become your coaches, and be critical of your performance until you become the person you want to be.

Ask yourself to describe what the experience of cancer is like, and if the words you come up with have a negative connotation, eliminate anything else in your life that fits those words, like failure, pressure, confusion, and that fear. My hope is that when you are done reading this book, you will answer that the experience has been a wake-up call, a new beginning, and then you will begin your true and authentic life.

Let me say in closing: Do not focus on waging a war against disease and empowering your enemy, and don't give cancer credit for the changes, because you did it. You responded and did not fear issues of guilt, shame, and blame when the future was uncertain. In the face of uncertainty, it takes courage to move forward and take on the challenge of life and cancer. So work on healing your life, and not defeating the enemy. With the healing of your life, the body is also far more likely to be cured. As Mother Teresa said, "I will not attend an antiwar rally, but if you ever have a peace rally call me." So heal your life and find your inner peace, and your body will respond to the perks and tips it experiences.

—Bernie S. Siegel, MD, author of the classics *Love, Medicine and Miracles: Lessons Learned About Self-Healing from a Surgeon's Experience with Exceptional Patients* and *Peace, Love and Healing: Bodymind Communication & the Path to Self-Healing: An Exploration*

Introduction

Congratulations! You have just taken a major step in empowering yourself with the tools you need to live a healthy and happy life after a cancer diagnosis! It is not often you hear the words "healthy," "happy," and "cancer" used in the same sentence, but we are living proof that it is possible, and we know that you can make it happen, too.

With this book, we will provide some of the answers to your questions, and we'll also help you to develop some new questions that will lead you down your own personal road to wellness. We are delighted that you chose us to be your guides along this road. Please read on for our individual introductions before you get started.

From Florence

When I was diagnosed with stage-3 breast cancer in April 2011, my first thought was: *Stage 3. That must mean 3 out of 10. That's not so bad. At least I'm still in the early stages.* Then I discovered that stage 4 is as bad as it gets. I had some serious cancer to deal with! Over the next year, I endured numerous uncomfortable tests and procedures; three surgeries resulting in the loss of my left breast and associated lymph nodes; four months of chemotherapy; and twenty-five radiation treatments. In many ways, it was the WORST year of my life. In that same year: I met my soul mate and fell in love; I started a blog that would change my life; I fulfilled a lifelong dream of being published; and I turned my passion for garden design into a new business venture. In many ways, it was the BEST year of my life!

While I did not have a choice in getting cancer, I realized early on that I did have a choice in how I was going to face the challenge. Rather than focus on all that cancer has taken away from me, I made it my mission to focus on the many positive changes that have come from facing my mortality. Not only did I make changes in how I care for my body, but I also made healthy changes on the levels of mind and spirit. Cancer forced me to take a journey to my soul, to face my deepest fears, to let go of old resentments, and to fully and unconditionally love myself. That is when the real healing began.

While I joke about my cancer experiences in this book, I assure you that cancer is no laughing matter. My goal is not to make light of this horrible disease, but rather to show that no matter how bad your life circumstances, there are always reasons to smile. If I live another forty years, it would be wonderful if I can reflect back on my year of cancer treatments and say that I lived it with joy, grace, and a positive attitude. If I live only one more year, then it is even more important that I be able to say I lived it that way.

Some credit my positive attitude with saving my life. I disagree. If a positive attitude alone could save you from cancer, I know a lot of people who would be alive today. I believe that it is a SURVIVOR'S ATTITUDE that gives you the best chances of overcoming this disease or any challenge that life throws your way. Having a survivor's attitude means using all of the resources within and around you to face your challenge. A survivor's attitude combines a positive attitude with positive ACTION!

It is my prayer that this book will inspire you to take on your challenges with a survivor's attitude. Through my perks and Susan's health tips, you will be presented with hundreds of possible actions that you can choose from to help you live your life like a survivor. By the end of this book, you should be ready to design your very own survival plan, which addresses the health of your body, mind, and spirit. You are not expected to adopt every suggestion in this book. Just take what resonates with you and leave the rest. May God bless you on your journey.

From Susan

I was lying there looking at the ultrasound screen thinking, *This chick doesn't know what the heck she is doing.* Being a registered nurse and a cardiac sonographer, I was tempted to grab the wand from this incompetent sonographer's hand and find something in my breast other than what was showing on the screen: a blizzard.

The reason there was nothing on the screen was that my tumor was so large it blocked out all the sound waves.

The thought that I had cancer never even entered my mind. I was a cardiac nurse, and I wasn't just "talking the talk," I was "walking the walk," too. Skinless chicken, low-fat yogurt, baked potatoes, and an exercise program had been my routine for the past twenty years. I taught others, those "sick people," how to get healthy. And besides, there was no history of breast cancer anywhere in my family. (I later learned that close to 90 percent of women diagnosed don't have a family history of the disease either.)

So when the ultrasound led to a biopsy, which led to me leaving the office with an oncologist's name in my hand, I felt betrayed. I did everything I was supposed to do. I ate a low-fat diet. I didn't smoke. I breastfed my two daughters. I exercised. I wasn't overweight. How could such a "healthy" person get breast cancer? I set out on a quest to find the answer to just that question. I needed to come up with factors that may have put me at risk, and I also needed to examine my current lifestyle to see if I was doing everything I could do to fight my cancer and prevent its return. That quest proved to be quite a struggle.

As a health professional I knew how to navigate my way through everything: the pathology report, the chemo side effects, and my immunity-boosting injections. But I couldn't seem to weed through all the crap I was running into when it came to finding out how to live a "healthy, cancer-free life." What I did find was that misinformation and hidden agendas did a great job at tangling and twisting the truth. But with persistence, I started to find the useable information I needed to piece together my battle plan. And as I would uncover each nugget of wisdom, I wanted to hold it up and show everyone what I had found. And so, my blog was born. It was just a logical progression that Florence and I would team up to allow me to "show my nuggets" to as many people as possible.

I have one request before you start reading this book. Don't take the word *surviving* in the title of this book literally. As I'm sure you know, no one can give you 100 tips that will 100 percent eliminate your risk of cancer 100 percent of the time. The word *survival* used here means reaching your highest level of health, no matter what else is trying to keep you from it. Whether you're newly diagnosed, living with metastatic disease, or struggling with other conditions like diabetes or heart disease, anyone can benefit from these health tips. Even those who think of themselves as "healthy" will find lots of useful information.

Health is complex. It does not just include the physical. You can't claim to be healthy by only considering your physical strength when you're a mental and spiritual train wreck. These tips cover all the bases. And they're dang easy, too!

Think of these tips as a menu of sorts, not an instruction manual. And just like picking vegetables from a garden, you take what you can eat now, and leave the rest until it looks ripe to you. My hope is that you will come back and revisit the list, because chances are, as you see how easy the tips are and how your choices are positively affecting your life, you'll be ready for a few more.

I don't belong to any advocacy groups and I don't have an agenda, hidden or otherwise. My only "ulterior motive" is to share the knowledge I have accumulated over my twenty-plus years as a registered nurse, and my years since a stage-3 cancer diagnosis, so that maybe others will be helped. Through exchanging and sharing information with others, I would love to create a tangled and twisted web of health and happiness. (Now, that's a place I wouldn't mind being trapped.)

Please feel free to contact me for any reason at susan@MOON-Organics .com.

Before You Get Started

The book you are now holding is not the work of just one author, but two. Flo's perks are a collection of inspiring insights and humorous anecdotes documented over the course of a year as she was undergoing treatments for cancer.

Susan's reader-friendly health tips were written to correspond to Flo's perks, but with the intent to promote the best practices for living a healthy lifestyle. Please keep in mind as you proceed from chapter to chapter that you will be hearing the voice of two distinct writers.

Also, we would like to emphasize that none of the information in this book is meant to override the advice of your doctor. Any change to your daily regimen should be discussed with your personal healthcare professional, especially if you decide to add supplements to your survival plan.

Cancer Made a Blogger Out of Me

*L*ife following a cancer diagnosis is an emotional roller coaster. Like most people when diagnosed with a life-threatening illness, I underwent the typical stages of grieving: denial, anger, bargaining with God, depression, and acceptance. I can almost pinpoint the exact moment that I transitioned from depression to acceptance. It was a beautiful day in October, six months after my initial diagnosis, and my body was under assault from a difficult round of chemotherapy. I was lying in bed, looking through the window as my mother collected the last of the tomatoes from my greenhouse. I was feeling too sick and exhausted to lift my bald head from the pillow. It saddened me that I was not out there with her, enjoying the sunshine and harvesting the fruits of my labor. *It's just not fair*, I thought. *I set those seeds, I grew those plants. I should be the one picking those tomatoes. Cancer sucks.*

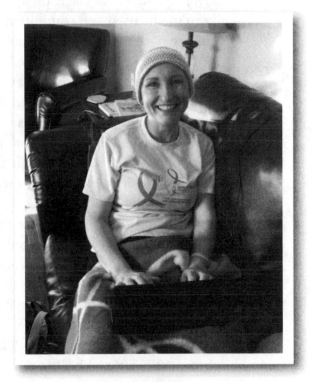

Flo the blogger.

While wallowing in self-pity, I came to an important realization. It suddenly dawned on me that feeling sorry for myself was not going to help me get well. As a psychologist, I knew that positive emotions, such as happiness, joy, and love, help to boost the immune system and enhance healing. Negative emotions, such as anger, bitterness, and depression, on the other hand, have been proven to suppress the immune system. Since I needed a healthy immune system to fight cancer, a positive attitude was vital to my recovery!

I convinced myself that cancer wasn't *that* bad; hey, it even had its perks. For example, since getting cancer, not once did I have to help with the dishes at big family dinners. The thought of that made me smile, and instantly I felt a little better. I then issued myself a challenge: if finding one perk could bring a smile to my face, then I would find 100 perks of having cancer. To keep me focused and committed to my goal, I decided to blog these perks. (Please note that while this book is written in the past tense, all 100 of my perks were written and blogged as I was actively undergoing cancer treatments, over the course of about a year.)

Since I have always enjoyed writing, blogging became a creative outlet for me. It also gave me a sense of purpose. After spending nearly twenty years in the helping profession, a big part of my life was missing when I stopped working for more than a year. Through my blog and the response from my readers, I knew that I was still helping people, if only by making them smile.

Blogging also connected me to so many kindred spirits. Seeing new posts from my fellow cancer bloggers was like getting an e-mail from an old friend. I loved to grab a cuppa and find out what my cyber friends were up to: *What health tips will Susan share in this post? How did Rachel's scan turn out? Who made Marie's Friday Round Up? What shenanigans has Nancy's pig gotten up to this week?* These people became part of my support network as we shared our highs and lows. Blogging has been, for me, one of the most therapeutic perks of having cancer.

It is good to have a creative outlet when you are dealing with cancer. Try blogging, journaling, gardening, painting, or whatever it is that lets your creative juices flow.

HEALTH TIP #1
You Don't Have to Be Picasso to Benefit from Art Therapy

The word *therapy* has such a broad range of connotations, doesn't it? There's cryotherapy, psychotherapy, physical therapy, chemotherapy (of course), and the ever-dreaded maggot therapy—Ew, I'm not making that up—and that's just to name a few.

But there's one kind of therapy that provides you with improved health and, as an added bonus, something you can hang on your wall.

Introducing . . . art therapy.

Art therapy has been around for about forty years, but because it isn't available everywhere, not many know about it. According to the American Art Therapy Association:

> Art therapy is a mental health profession that uses the creative process of art-making to improve and enhance the physical, mental, and emotional well-being of individuals of all ages. Research in the field confirms that the creative process involved in artistic self-expression helps people to become more physically, mentally, and emotionally healthy and functional, resolve conflicts and problems, develop interpersonal skills, manage behavior, reduce stress, handle life adjustments, and achieve insight.

Who wouldn't want to be involved in this?! Research shows that art therapy is extremely helpful in restoring health, specifically for cancer patients who have to deal not only with their physical illness, but also with the emotional and mental issues that go with it.

Here is a charcoal drawing done by a woman with newly diagnosed leukemia:

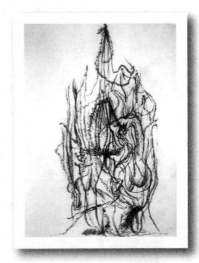

I don't think you need a degree in psychology to interpret what this woman is feeling. The drawing allows her to be able to identify and express what she is feeling without using one word. It also provides her therapist with a tool to use for opening up discussions about her emotions.

Nancy Nainis, MAAT, ATR-BC, is a retired art therapist who conducted research on the benefits of art therapy for cancer patients. Nancy told me, "Art therapy often surprised cancer survivors. They enjoyed the creative process more than expected and experienced reduced pain. Art-making gave a lift to their self-esteem, and many gave the items they produced to care-givers to express their gratitude. For a relatively small investment the rewards were great."

The "art" doesn't have to be a fancy, intricate oil painting. In fact, you don't need any experience with art at all. While painting is an option, there is also clay, sculpture, drawing, mobiles, collages, and jew-elry making.

Consider art therapy along with your chemotherapy and physical therapy to help bring you back to your optimum health.

Therapy implies treatment that leads to healing. With cancer, there's a lot of healing to do. Not everyone is able, for whatever reason, to express the feelings associated with a cancer diagnosis and everything that it encompasses. Art therapy can help with expression and can also help with the healing process necessary to regain physical, mental, and emotional health.

Check with your local hospital or medical center, or your oncologist to find an art therapist near you, or contact the American Art Therapy Association at www.arttherapy.org.

Cancer Helped Me Find My Soul Mate

As fate would have it, at almost exactly the same time that I found my lump, I also found my soul mate. Shawn and I were first introduced online. I immediately confided in him that I had found a lump in my breast, but at that time I was convinced that it was harmless. We spent the next few weeks e-mailing and talking on the phone, getting to know one another and planning to meet in person.

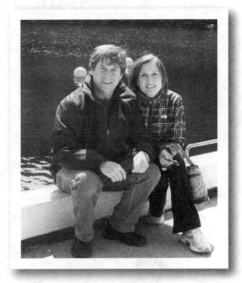

Flo and Shawn, celebrating their three-month anniversary.

When I was officially diagnosed, my hopes of meeting the man of my dreams were dashed. Although we had not met in person, I really liked Shawn. He was funny, honest, hardworking, and handsome to boot! After being divorced for nearly ten years, I thought that he could really be "the one." However, how could I possibly enter into a new relationship when my prognosis for survival was so uncertain?

Reluctantly, I called him in tears to say, "There is no point in us meeting. I just found out that I have breast cancer and I don't know what lies ahead for me."

To my surprise, he replied, "If you are trying to ditch me, it's not going to work. I am coming out there this weekend to take you out to dinner."

As cliché as it might sound, it was love at first sight, and Shawn has been by my side ever since.

How can I be sure that he is really "the one"? Well, who but a soul mate would enter a relationship with a woman who is about to lose a breast, all of her hair, and be catapulted into early menopause by chemo drugs? (I just hoped chemo would leave me with enough estrogen to keep the spark alive!)

Cancer may not help you find your soul mate, but it will certainly let you know if he or she is by your side. If you are still looking for that special someone, don't let cancer hold you back.

HEALTH TIP #2
You Need Estrogen to Make Your Kitty Purr

Ahhhhhhh, estrogen . . . the very essence of a woman. It is the hormone responsible for many things that make a woman a *woman*, such as breast development, libido, and intelligence (*wink*). Men also produce estrogen, but in very small amounts. Hence why they lag behind women in the niceness department (as well as breast size—in most cases).

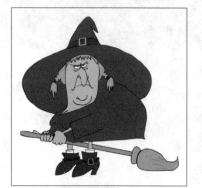

Without estrogen.

One of the purposes of estrogen in women is to make the sex organs ready, willing, and, more important, able to have *enjoyable* sex. Unfortunately, after menopause, even if it is chemo-induced menopause, the "kitty" may become unresponsive. But wait—there is hope!

If you are in your twenties or thirties, without medical complications, you probably don't need extra estrogen as your ovaries and adrenal glands are hard at work producing enough female hormones to keep you feeling healthy and "horny"! However, as estrogen wanes, due to menopause, drugs, or health issues, the following can happen:

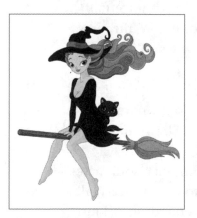

With estrogen.

- increased cholesterol, causing arteries to become clogged and possibly leading to a heart attack

- decreased bone density, possibly causing osteoporosis

- "hot flashes" or incredibly annoying episodes where you feel as if you will spontaneously combust

- sleep disturbances—either insomnia or waking up during the night

- mood swings, including (but not limited to) general bitchiness, homicidal tendencies, and spontaneously crying at Hallmark commercials

- vaginal dryness, and a compulsive tendency to methodically repeat the phrase, "Not tonight, honey; I have a headache."

If you are postmenopausal or have had a hysterectomy that includes an oophorectomy (removal of the ovaries), or if you take medications for estrogen-receptor-positive breast cancer, then I hate to break it to you, but your estrogen has been sucked dry (pardon the pun).

What Is Hormone Replacement Therapy (HRT)?

Not so many years ago, if you went to your doctor with any of the above symptoms, he/she would likely have written a prescription for a hormone replacement therapy (HRT) pill. Most likely it would have been the drug Premarin. Premarin is produced from pregnant mares' urine (hence the name: PREgnant-MAre's-uRINe). I dunno, call me crazy, but I find it hard to believe that ingesting anything from the pee of a horse can be good for the body. (It ranks right up there with the eye of a newt or the spit of a toad to me. Somebody stop me if I am carrying the witch analogy too far.) However, before Premarin, the only option available to women in menopause was to take injections of hormones. Needless to say, when Premarin was released in pill form, women lined up for it.

As with any pharmaceuticals, Premarin was not without side effects. Synthetic hormones, such as Premarin, do not work "in tune" with your body (unless you are a horse) and therefore may produce more problems than they were meant to correct. Some of the risks associated with this drug are cervical cancer, breast cancer, and blood clots. *Hmmmm*, let me think this over; so I go into early menopause because of my breast cancer, then I have to take an HRT that may cause breast cancer. Something just does not add up here.

Mother Nature to the Rescue

Bioidentical hormone replacements are estrogen medications made from plants, namely soy and wild yams (not sweet potatoes), and they mimic, more closely, the actions and mechanisms of your own body's natural hormones. While still a form of HRT, they are a more "natural" way to get your hormones because they are made from substances your body recognizes, like food. However, while bioidenticals may seem like the obvious choice, more studies need to be done to determine their long-term side effects. And like synthetic hormone replacement, those with estrogen-receptor-positive cancers (specific cancer that flourishes in an estrogen-rich environment) won't be candidates for bioidenticals, unfortunately.

I Can't Take Estrogen, So What Do I Do Now?

Okay, then, here is where it gets personal. My only problem was with the kitty. After having a bilateral mastectomy, chemotherapy for stage-3 breast cancer

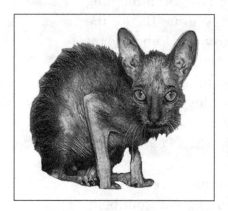

Poor kitty before estrogen cream.

fried my ovaries and I entered the no-estrogen zone. Then, three years later, I was treated to a hysterectomy with an oophorectomy (all girl parts including ovaries removed) because of a benign uterine tumor. This left me void of every part that made me a female of the species . . . no boobs, no ovaries, no uterus. I was officially an android! And understandably, my kitty suffered greatly. (The official medical term is "vulvovaginal atrophy" or "VVA" as us hip-but-shriveled-up gals call it.) Imagine, if you will, going from a plump juicy grape to a five-year-old raisin that has been left out of the box in the scorching sun. . . .

Okay, I'm sure you get the picture. And the worst part was I really thought I just had to "suck it up" and there was nothing I could do about it. But luckily for me (and ole fluffy), I was wrong.

Women with a history of breast cancer, specifically estrogen-receptor-positive breast cancer, should not go near estrogen, or anything that resembles estrogen, because of the increased risk of stirring up those cancer cells that are fed by said hormone. However, here is the good news: It is possible to have your estrogen, and NOT eat it, too. Using estrogen directly on the vaginal tissue is an extremely safe and effective alternative to hormone pills or injections if your kitty is your only issue.

The vaginal wall tissue is like a sponge when it comes to soaking up estrogen preparations. This has a direct effect on the thinning vaginal wall tissue and actually brings it back to life. It changes the appearance, the plumpness, the color, and the ability to lubricate. It really was amazing to see and experience the change. (My spouse thought it was pretty cool, too.)

An *extremely* small amount of the estrogen is absorbed into your body, but based on recent and ongoing research, it is not enough to increase the risk of cancer recurrence, and its safety is currently widely accepted in the medical community.

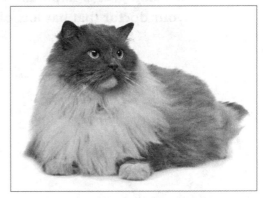

Same kitty after six weeks of vaginal estrogen cream.

I have the cream prepared in a compounding pharmacy using bioidentical estrogen because then I can get the estrogen made with natural ingredients and without all the chemical preservatives that the drug companies use in their preparations. (I don't use paraben preservatives because of their ties to cancer.) A single dose of the cream is inserted into the vagina several times a week for six weeks, then weekly to maintain kitty health.

The result, in my case, was so worth the effort. Not only were things working well in the "customer satisfaction" department, but I also cut my risk of bladder infections dramatically. Bladder infections, or UTIs, are common in postmenopausal women because the tube for the bladder is right next to the vagina. When the vagina and the tissue around it is dry and shrunken, the whole area becomes malformed, leaving a slight opening to the bladder where

> Your hormones may take a beating from treatment, but help is available in the form of safe bioidenticals for certain symptoms.

there should be plump tissue to cover it. This opening allows bacteria to enter the bladder, causing frequent infections. Plumping the tissue closes the path for bacteria and reduces the risk for infection.

If kitty is looking a bit haggard, or you are getting recurrent bladder infections, see your gynecologist to discuss topical bioidentical estrogen therapy to see if it's right for you. You've got nothing to lose but ol' wrinkle-puss.

Note: Be aware that not all compounding pharmacies know what they are doing. It is important that you find a compounding pharmacy from your doctor that has lots of experience with these types of preparations.

Cancer Made Me Really Appreciate the Good Days

I recall lying in bed in full chemo-attack mode fondly reminiscing about my precancer days when I could perform amazing feats like take a shower, walk up the stairs, and make myself a sandwich. Before cancer, I took those little things for granted. After my diagnosis and subsequent treatment, however I would have given anything just to be able to partake in those ordinary, normal activities of daily living.

The thing that helped me through the rough days (and still does) is my favorite mantra: **This, too, shall pass.** I would say to myself, *It will pass, and I will feel good again!* Even on the days when I felt "normal-ish," I could almost hear the Alleluia chorus singing: Alleluia, Alleluia, Alll-eee—luuuuu—IAAAAAA! I could only imagine how grateful I would be when I finally recovered. With months of chemo still ahead, I made a promise to myself that I would never again take another "good day" for granted.

When times get rough, just remember:
This, too, shall pass.

HEALTH TIP #3
Pass Too on the DEET (When Bothered by Bugs)

No one likes to get bitten or pestered by pesky pests, but before you reach for the nearest bottle of bug repellant, consider this: Are chemical bug repellents your best option? Sure they'll keep the bugs away, but at what cost?

Bug repellents are different from insecticides in that repellents don't kill bugs; they just make them stay away from you. The one popular chemical you will find in most repellents is DEET. DEET—short for N,N-diethyl-meta-toluamide—is found in more than 240 different products used to repel mosquitos and other flying insects.

DEET was developed in the United States in 1946 by the U.S. army to be used in the jungles of Africa and Korea. The army was looking for a solution to repel disease-ridden mosquitos, and their chemists found it. They're

not even sure exactly how it works, but the thought is that it has something to do with blocking the scent of certain substances in human sweat and making us invisible to bugs.

DEET is labeled as a "Class III" in the EPA's toxicity classification, which means it is "slightly toxic." (Kinda like being "slightly pregnant"?) It should be noted that this chemical does not just stay on your skin where it is applied. DEET is absorbed into your bloodstream and travels through all of your body's organs—heart, lungs, kidneys, liver, and brain—before it is excreted in your urine.

According to the National Pesticide Information Center:

> Researchers applied technical grade DEET, and DEET formulated in a 15% ethanol solution, to the forearm skin of male human volunteers for an 8-hour exposure period. DEET was absorbed within two hours after application and absorption continued at a constant rate over the 8-hour exposure period.

DEET was approved for public use ten years after the army created it. Since there was no Environmental Protection Agency (EPA) at the time, there were no public safety standards for these types of chemicals. When approval was finally granted in 1998, the approval for use by the public was given only when the EPA considered that public DEET use would be "brief . . . and not long-term." The EPA did not clarify what "brief" use was. Put it on for one hour, and then wash it off? Only use it every third day? It was not really made clear.

DEET melts plastics, polyester, leather, and other materials on contact. (You may want to read that again.) There are cases of sunglasses and GPS screens melting with DEET exposure.

While cancer is not currently a concern in relation to DEET (and neither was asbestos at the time of its early use), DEET has been shown to cause neurotoxicity symptoms in some that include tremors and seizures. There have also been cases of extremely low blood pressure and low heart rates as well with topical application of DEET. Currently, products containing 30 percent DEET or more are banned in Canada and cited as having multiple health risks.

So you don't want to apply the DEET directly to your skin, and you think that using the new "clip on" fan devices would be a better choice? Actually they aren't. Breathing the vapors of metofluthrin, the chemical ingredient in the "fan type" bug repellants, is just as harmful and carries the same risk of seizures and nerve toxicity as the spray-on DEET. But the metofluthrin also carries a cancer risk. It's a small risk, but liver tumors were seen in tested animal populations.

The odd thing is, the directions for these devices say: "Clip the unit to your belt, pants/shorts waistband, purse, or any other convenient location next to you [or] place the unit next to you on a table." But the precautions on the label say: "Harmful if inhaled. Avoid breathing vapors, mist or gas." Confused? Yeah, me, too. If it's clipped to me, I would imagine that I can't help but breathe this stuff in.

On a side note, but certainly worth mentioning, is that many chemicals have been approved for safe use initially by the government only to have the approval reversed when the truth was revealed about its dangers. One brave woman who is often named as the "pioneer of the environmentalist movement" was Rachel Carson. While battling cancer herself, she spent years investigating and uncovering the harsh truth about the cancer-causing pesticide DDT. Her book, *Silent Spring*, and the public outcry it initiated, led the U.S. government to ban DDT in 1972. Rachel ended up dying from cancer, but not without starting a movement of public awareness that has grown into the hundreds of watchdog groups and organizations that stand up to unethical business practices and hopefully keep us a little safer. Unfortunately, because DDT use was so widespread and exists in the soil for hundreds of years, current U.S. food supplies still test positive for this chemical. The point of this side note is: Just because a chemical has been "approved" does not mean it is safe. It is up to you to seek the truth and decide if that product fits with your healthy lifestyle.

Luckily Mother Nature has provided us with some great alternatives to harmful synthetic chemicals. Essential oils like lemon eucalyptus, lemongrass, citronella, and peppermint seem to have the same smell-altering effect for bugs, but with less worry for you. Brands like Burt's Bees and Herbal Armor are two natural brands that use the power of nature to combat bugs. Badger (www.badgerbalm .com) also makes a wonderful organic "Anti-Bug-Balm" using organic citronella, rosemary, lemongrass, and geranium essential oils, with no mineral oil or petroleum products. The downside of all naturals is that you must apply them every hour or two for effectiveness, and there is no guarantee that you won't be allergic or sensitive to one of the natural oils, so always test a small amount of the finished product on your inner wrist to see if you get a reaction.

> You do have choices when it comes to avoiding biting insects. It's just as easy to buy a natural repellant, as it is an unhealthy chemical one.

Making your own bug repellant is very simple. Essential oils (not *fragrance* oils) can be purchased online or from your local health food store. Make sure, if you buy online, that it is from a reputable company that you can trust not to use additives and impurities in your oils. I have trusted Mountain Rose Herbs for years (www.MountainRoseHerbs.com), and I love their fair trade and ethical corporate practices.

Here is a very basic bug repellant recipe: Place 3 ounces of distilled water and 2 ounces of witch hazel extract in a six-ounce spray bottle. All these items are available at most pharmacies. You can get organic witch hazel online. Then add your essential oils as follows:

Add 20 drops *each* of:

- citronella essential oil (*Cymbopogon winterianus*, NOT lamp oil)

- lemon eucalyptus essential oil (*Eucalyptus citriodora*)

Then pick any *two* of these essential oils and add $1/8$ teaspoon (about 10 drops) each to the mixture:

- cedarwood essential oil (*Cedrus atlantica*)

- peppermint essential oil (*Mentha piperita*)

- spearmint essential oil (*Mentha spicata*)

- lavender essential oil (*Lavandula angustifolia*)

Shake the mixture well before each application and spray lightly on exposed areas of skin and to clothing. Avoid getting into eyes or mouth as it may be irritating. Wash your hands after applying to avoid getting it into your eyes. You may need to apply every two hours or so. Use common sense when applying to clothing as it contains oils. (Don't use on leather, suede, or other materials that might stain.)

Again, just because it is a natural product does not mean you can't get a reaction to it. Remember: Poison ivy is natural, too! So test a small amount to see if you are sensitive. There are many more recipes online. Try to find one that works best for your needs.

Unlimited Foot Massages

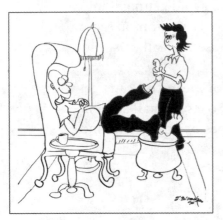

I just love to have my feet massaged. I will admit, though, it is often a challenge to convince my partner/child/sister/friend to do the nasty deed. After being diagnosed with cancer, however, I got foot rubs on demand. I could almost see my loved ones cringe when they asked, "Is there anything I can do for you?" and I'd start to peel off my socks. But hey, I was determined to take advantage of that little perk for as long as I could.

With more than 7,000 nerve endings in the feet, it is little wonder that a massage feels so good! This sensual pleasure can help to alleviate anxiety and bring about a sense of tranquility. According to theories of reflexology, foot massage can release energy blockages, allowing one's life-force energy to flow freely through the body. As with any type of massage, a foot massage also helps with blood circulation. With so many therapeutic benefits, I made foot massage a definite part of my survival plan.

It is important to be extra kind to your body when you have cancer.
Treat yourself to a massage, foot reflexology, or even a hot bath.

HEALTH TIP #4
How to Turn That Foot Massage into a Healthy Pedicure

Common sense says you should be limiting your time at the nail salon to avoid breathing in those toxic fumes and acrylic powders. However, a part of you still wants those soft pampered feet and the total sense of relaxation that you can only get from a pedicure. What's a girl to do?

Get a guilt-free, five-star, healthy pedicure right at home using things you probably already have around your house. This pedicure can be done alone (nice), or with a partner (even nicer), and it costs pennies. (Leaving you with enough money to buy those cute, strappy sandals to show off your feet.)

This pedicure is best done right before bedtime so your feet can get maximum softening time from the oils.

First, gather your necessities. Some of these are optional; so don't worry if you don't have everything.

- Foot basin or other container to soak your feet. You can use the bathtub filled to your ankles as you sit on the side if you want. Adjust the additives for the amount of water you are using. (This isn't science, so you can "eyeball" the amounts of baking soda and sea salt.)

- 1 cup of baking soda

- $1/4$ teaspoon essential oil of peppermint (NOT artificial peppermint food flavoring), found at most health food stores

- 1 avocado, cut in half; remove the flesh (to have for lunch) and save the skins

- $1/2$ cup coarse sea salt and $1/2$ cup Epsom salt, which can be found at any drugstore (or 1 cup coarse sea salt)

- 1 teaspoon honey (a natural exfoliator)

- 3 tablespoons olive or safflower oil; these household salad oils have great beauty value for your skin

- clean cotton socks

- pumice stone: a natural volcanic rock that can be used to scrub callouses smooth

- nail clippers and file

- towels

1. Place your phone in another room and turn off the TV. (This step is *not* optional.) Lay out towels in your work area.

2. Make a scrub in a small bowl by combining $1/2$ cup of coarse sea salt, 1 teaspoon of honey, and 3 tablespoons of oil. Mix well and set aside.

3. Dissolve 1 cup of baking soda and $^{1}/_{2}$ cup of Epsom salt or sea salt in your basin or tub of hot/warm water. The water will sit for a while, so it should be on the hotter side of warm *without feeling uncomfortable.*

4. Add $^{1}/_{4}$ of teaspoon peppermint essential oil to the water and stir. This is optional but gives your feet a clean tingly feeling and is a natural deodorant.

5. Soak your feet in the treated water for 10 to 15 minutes. During this time, you must relax (hence direction #1). This would be a great time to practice your deep breathing or mindful breathing (*see Health Tip #95 for more info*). Visualize world peace . . . or whirled peas . . . or whatever makes you calm and content. (For added relaxation, your partner can massage your shoulders during this time, or you can use a heated shoulder wrap or heating pad on your shoulders and neck.)

6. After soaking, scrub one foot at a time with the pumice stone, paying close attention to rough spots. Run your fingers over the surface of your feet to find callouses and scrub gently to smooth them. Don't try to remove all callouses in one treatment. Repeated treatments give better results, gradually removing dead skin cells until the soft skin is revealed.

7. Take the avocado skin and rub the inside of the skin (where the flesh was) on heels and dry spots. Massage gently for several minutes. Use one half on each foot.

8. Before rinsing the avocado off, take the honey/oil scrub you made earlier and massage into bottoms and tops of feet as well, up your ankle, including your calves. This will help increase circulation as it softens and rejuvenates your skin. You can use the pumice stone with the scrub for extra effect on rough spots. This scrub feels great on your feet. You can use any leftover scrub in the shower on rough knees and elbows, too. Rinse feet well and pat dry with the towel.

9. Clip nails neatly if needed, leaving some nail to file. File nails to follow the shape of the nail bed.

10. Place some olive or safflower oil on your hands and massage into feet tops and bottoms. Be generous with the oil without being drippy. Pay close attention to your cuticles, massaging oil into each toe. If needed, push cuticles back gently using an orange stick (a special wooden stick shaped for cuticles). Don't try to remove or cut cuticles.

11. Place soft cotton socks on your feet and leave on overnight. If you don't want to leave the oil on, you can wash your feet at this point using a mild soap. You will still retain the beneficial softening properties of the oil. Make sure to wash and dry your feet well, so your feet aren't slippery when you walk. When you're ready to apply polish, gently wipe your nail beds with an acetone- and methanol-free polish remover and then dry off. You can then apply polish.

There are no steadfast rules to this pedicure. You can add or subtract steps or use natural, chemical-free products of your choice. It's fun to do at home, it's inexpensive, and you'll get great results.

> Save money and your health by doing your natural pedicure at home.

A Word About Nail Polish

Nail polish is notorious for containing many hormone-disrupting chemicals. The main ones are phthalates, formaldehyde, and toluene. All three of these are known to be possible carcinogens and can lead to other illnesses, like diabetes. Your nails and nail beds are pathways to your bloodstream, so look for polishes that are free of these chemicals. There are plenty of companies that are offering water-based and solvent-based "natural" formulas that don't contain these nasty synthetics.

I love Scotch nail polish. "Scotch Naturals" was created by a mom who wanted a healthier polish for her daughter. She was determined to create a polish product that worked well, allowed her daughter to be a girly-girl, but didn't put her at risk for illness. What dedication! Her nail polish formulations are phthalate- and formaldehyde-free. The moms that bought Scotch polishes for their daughters ended up using it as well. Responding to requests from her new market group, Scotch now offers both kid and adult colors. The kids line is called Hopscotch Kids. You can find them both online at: www.ScotchNaturals.com.

Cancer Revealed to Me a Whole New Side of My Autistic Son

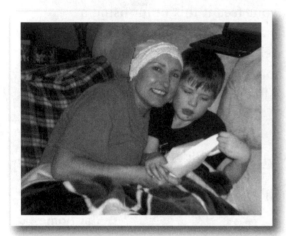

Ben enjoys a cuddle with Mom.

When I was first diagnosed with breast cancer, my biggest concern was how my two teenaged children, Kaitlyn and Donovan, would take the news, and how they would adapt to having a sick mom around the house. I was not so concerned about my six-year-old son, Ben, who has autism. While he is bright, his verbal skills are very limited. Generally, he talks only enough to express his basic needs. Given Ben's weak language skills, I reasoned that he would not really understand what was happening to me, and, even if he did, being "in a world of his own" he would not be affected by my plight. I could not have been more wrong!

While he says very little, Ben has learned to use the computer to express himself. Several times after my diagnosis, he surprised me by bringing me typewritten notes with messages like: "Dear Mom, you are nice," and "Dear Mom, I love you." Sometimes I would find his notes lying around the house, with other messages, such as "Mom is sick," or "Mom is hurt."

On a rare occasion, Ben will catch me off guard by speaking a full, meaningful sentence. Never was I more surprised than one night while putting him to bed, when he said to me, "Good night. Guardian angels watch over you and protect you."

Some might say he was just echoing something he had heard me say a hundred times before. True. But the miraculous part is that it is the one and only time I heard him speak those words, and it happened to be on the day that I was diagnosed with breast cancer.

Ben may look like he is "in a world of his own," but these gestures prove to me that he is a sensitive boy who is very much aware of what is happening in my world.

Not everyone is great with words. Just because someone cannot tell you how they feel when you are sick does not mean they don't care.

HEALTH TIP #5
Choose Your Words Carefully When Telling Your Kids About Your Cancer

Imagine this scenario: You bring your child to the doctor because you know something is wrong, but the doctor makes you wait outside during the exam. When she comes out of the room, she looks very concerned and whispers something to the nurse. She brings your sick-looking child to you and tells you everything's fine, but she wants to see your child every two weeks to treat him or her.

How would you feel? Angry? Confused? Worried? Ready to demand answers?

Your child has these same feelings when you've told them you are fine, but they see you going to doctor appointments, getting weaker from chemo, losing your hair, and squatting with your arms constantly wrapped around the commode.

Your desire to protect your kids from your cancer might cost you your relationship with them.

Experts in the field of child psychology agree that with kids and illness, age-appropriate honesty is the best policy. Letting them find out about your cancer from someone else, or trying to hide it, can lead to:

- fear of losing you

- worry that they caused the illness

- fear that they can catch the cancer

- worry that there is something a lot worse happening

- learning that cancer is something you don't discuss

- feeling that they aren't important enough to tell

- mistrusting anything you tell them

- a missed opportunity for your kids to support and help you through this time

Once you have come to terms with your diagnosis and feel you can tell your kids, find a time and a place where they feel comfortable, focused, and will be able to express themselves freely. If you feel you need others around you when you tell them, make sure your kids feel comfortable enough with them that they can be themselves and express emotion if needed.

> Maintain a healthy relationship with your kids. Remember, your children are going through this with you. Respect them enough to keep them in the loop.

Start with just the basics of what you know and the plan of action. For example: "The doctor found a lump in my body, and I need to have surgery to take it out. I might need medicine to make sure the lump, called a tumor, doesn't grow back."

Then let your kids take control of the conversation, asking questions if they want to, directing the conversation. Don't go into statistics, the unknown, or what *might* happen. And if you don't know something, be honest. Either no one knows, or you will find out the answer.

It is important that your children know that they can come to you at any time with questions or concerns to get truthful answers. You may want to arrange for others (family or close friends) who know about your illness to be available to them as well.

Some other things to remember:

- Side effects of treatment may make it seem like you are getting sicker. Be sure to explain this so it's not misunderstood.

- You might feel very comfortable at home with a bald head, but your "chrome dome" might embarrass your thirteen-year-old. Respect the feelings of your kids and have a hat handy for when your kids' friends come over.

- Showing your kids your scars, bandages, and drains might be *too* much honesty. You know your own children, but unless they ask to see this kind of stuff, it's best to keep it "under wraps."

- Kids can express worry in different ways: anger, being withdrawn, acting out, or a sudden drop in school grades. If you are seeing any red flags, use your pediatrician or the resources at your oncologist's office (social worker, support groups, and so forth) to look into the need for professional support.

- Consider the ages of your kids. If there is a big age difference between your kids, you may want to discuss this with them separately, but always make sure you do it on the same day so no one feels like they were "the last to know."

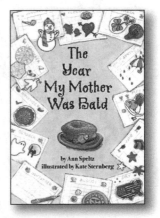

There are wonderful books out there to help kids deal with the issue of a parent having cancer. *When a Parent Has Cancer: A Guide to Caring for Your Children* by Dr. Wendy Harpham, who is a cancer survivor, a mom, and a doctor, is a great start. Another book I can personally recommend is *The Year My Mother Was Bald* by Ann Speltz. It is written as one girl's journal and follows her feelings as her mom goes through treatment, and it has a great list of resources in the back. I think this book would be great for boys or girls. My daughters were ten and twelve when I was diagnosed, and they read this book until the pages were ragged. Flash forward seven years, and I am cleaning out my younger daughter's room . . . and she still wants to hold on to that book.

Cancer Introduced My Teens to All Major Household Appliances

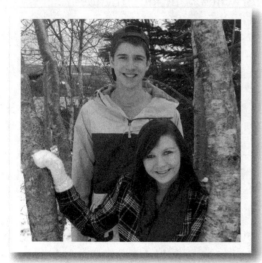

Kaitlyn and Donovan

My children are very fortunate in that they grew up with the luxury of a maid waiting on them hand and foot. For most of their lives, they didn't have to lift a finger to wash dishes, prepare themselves a meal, or even clean their rooms. The maid also doubled as a chauffeur, driving them to their friends' houses, parties, and other important social engagements. If you have not guessed it by now, the maid's name is Mom (I should add "slash" Ronnie, our babysitter).

You can just imagine my surprise when, shortly after my first chemo, I walked into the kitchen to find Kaitlyn emptying the dishwasher. I tried to hide my amazement and carry on a conversation as if this was a normal part of our day. After all, I did not want to scare her away! Just as I was making peace in my mind with the concept of giving up my maid's uniform to Kaitlyn, I spotted Donovan out of the corner of my eye taking a load of laundry upstairs. Up until that point, I could have sworn he did not even know that there was a laundry room in our house.

I suppose in a way that learning new skills such as cooking and cleaning was a perk for them. For example, Kaitlyn can now prepare an awesome Thai stir-fry, and Donovan has completely mastered the art of cooking chicken nuggets (flipping them at just the exact right moment!). It was definitely a perk for me to experience the proud feeling of having my teens step up to the challenge when I needed them, and to hear others tell me how lucky I am to have such thoughtful children. Cancer is a family disease, and sometimes I needed to be reminded that I was not the only one affected. Following my diagnosis many people commented on how well I coped with having cancer. I think it is my children who really deserve the accolades.

A difficult part of having cancer is relinquishing the role of caregiver to your children. Allowing them to help is like sowing the seeds of responsibility.

HEALTH TIP #6
Don't Just Sow Your Seeds, Eat Them, Too!

Seeds hold an amazing amount of potential. Just look at a tiny acorn and think how huge that potential is! The potential for nutrition is just as big, and with the variety of seeds available to you, you're sure to find some that you can easily use to enhance your healthy diet. Because seeds act like tiny little energy confetti, you only need to consume a small amount to get maximum benefits. Seeds all have their own unique flavor and work well with different kinds of foods. Sesame seeds, for example, work well with Asian dishes and are wonderful in salads, while sunflower seeds are great for snacking.

There are some extraordinary seeds that up until now were hard to find. Don't get me wrong; I love good ole sunflower seeds just as much as the next person, but I tend to look beyond the ordinary and toward the *extra*-ordinary to find the most powerful seeds with the most efficient form of cancer-fighting effects. Following are my top three "super seeds" with a brief rundown on what makes them so special:

Flaxseeds: Flaxseeds are light brown in color and look like a larger version of sesame seeds. When eaten whole, without being ground or crushed, flaxseeds provide a special kind of fiber in your diet that can help with constipation, which is great. But the real benefits are seen once they are ground, as they release cancer-fighting lignans and omega-3 fatty acids. Lignans can act as anti-estrogens, and it is believed that they can have some preventative effect on all cancers but especially breast and other hormone-related cancers. The best way to take advantage of all the health benefits of flaxseeds is to crush or grind them and use within twenty-four hours. After being ground they start losing their beneficial effects. Flaxseed oil can also be taken as a supplement as it contains the omega-3s but not the potent lignans. It's the lignans that are the potent cancer protectors, especially for hormonal cancers.

One ounce (about two tablespoons) of seeds has 150 calories, 12 grams of fat, 6,388 milligrams omega-3, 1,655 milligrams omega-6, 3 grams fiber, and 5 grams protein.

Big benefits of flaxseeds: omega-3s and healthy bowels.

Chia seeds: Cha-cha-cha-chia. Okay, you've got to remember Chia Pets! Yes, all those years of playing with those seeds (that got everywhere, and then Mom would yell) and we never realized what a nutritious, healthy toy we had. No one ever thought, back then, that we would be buying these to eat for our health! Chia seeds look a lot like poppy seeds. The chia gets its name from the Mayan word for "strength." When left in a liquid like juice or water for about fifteen minutes, they will absorb the fluid and thicken its consistency. That can make for better smoothies, but it also means that they expand in your stomach, making that "full feeling" last a bit longer, and that can be helpful if you're trying to lose weight.

One serving (one ounce) of tiny little chia seeds provides you with 42 percent of your recommended daily allowance (RDA) for fiber (11 grams) and 177 milligrams or 18 percent of your RDA for calcium. That's *three times* more calcium per ounce than milk. You don't have to consume one whole serving in one meal, as these tiny little things can be sprinkled just about anywhere and in any food throughout the day.

One ounce (about two tablespoons) of seeds has 137 calories, 9 grams fat, 4,915 milligrams omega-3 (that's equivalent to about ten omega-3 supplements!), 1,620 milligrams omega-6, 11 grams fiber, and 4 grams protein.

Big benefits of chia seeds: omega-3s, calcium, and fiber.

Hemp seeds: Yes, hemp—but don't think "pot" when you see these. The hemp plants grown for food and textiles like clothes and fibers are completely different from pot plants and don't contain THC (the drug component of the marijuana plant), so the high you get will be from knowing that you're eating healthy, not from anything in the seeds. Hemp seeds usually come shelled and are small and light. They have a bit of a nutty flavor and are great in cereals and oatmeal. Most people who are allergic to nuts and gluten can eat hemp seeds without a reaction. They are very high in protein so it's a good protein source if you're switching from eating animal-based proteins to a more plant-based diet.

One ounce (about two tablespoons) of hemp seeds has 162 calories, 13 grams fat, 2,436 milligrams omega-3, 7,728 milligrams omega-6, 1 gram fiber, and 10 grams of protein.

Big benefits of hemp seeds: high protein, no allergens.

> Just a little spoonful of any of these seeds here and there can add up to big health benefits for you.

Again, the easiest way to include these seeds in your diet is to add a sprinkle here and there as any amount is beneficial. If you want to include one serving of chia, for example, measure out one to three tablespoons in a small bowl and set it out so you'll be reminded to add a bit to your food during the day. When the bowl is empty, you're done.

These certainly are not the only seeds to provide a boost to your health. Take the time to explore other seeds like caraway, fennel, poppy, and pumpkin. (See more on pumpkin seeds in Health Tip #39.)

I Didn't Have to Go to Work

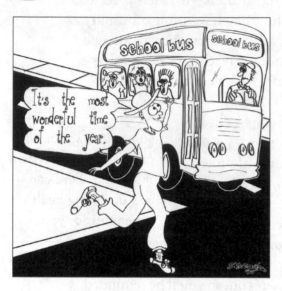

One of the most unusual perks of having cancer for me was being off work for more than a year. I work in the field of education, so every year since I was five years old, I had been heading back to school in September. It felt strange when September rolled around and I found myself putting the kids on the bus and going back home . . . strange, but GOOD! I couldn't resist the urge to skip down the driveway and sing, "It's the most wonderful time of the year." I got to enjoy the luxury of having the whole house to myself and really focus on getting well.

Recovering from cancer became my full-time job. It required secretarial skills, such as scheduling and rescheduling numerous appointments. I also kept detailed notes of my doctor visits and copies of my tests and scans. My research skills had never been better, as I combed the Internet in search of information to help me better understand my diagnosis and make informed decisions about my treatments. I educated myself on diet, nutrition, exercise, and the use of supplements. I also became a practitioner of alternative healing modalities, as I administered Reiki and angel therapy sessions to myself in my own personalized healing sessions. Not only did I make recovery my full-time job, but I also promoted myself to CEO of my own health!

If you are fortunate enough to have sick leave,
why not use it? Make getting well your full-time job.

HEALTH TIP #7
If You're Not Going to Work, You'll Have More Time to Work Out

For most of us, exercise is a four-letter word, right? We want so badly to believe that there is a path to fitness that involves sitting on the couch eating cookie dough.

Bad news: There is no substitute for exercise.

Good news: You don't necessarily have to grunt and sweat and be in pain (unless you're into that sort of thing) to get benefits.

Bad news: You can't pay someone to do it for you.

Good news: You can reduce your risk of cancer by as much as 40 percent if you exercise regularly!

There are many other benefits of exercise, including:

- more energy
- increased strength
- improved lung capacity
- improved mood by increasing endorphins, the body's "natural high" chemical
- better sex (because it improves your mood, gives you more energy, makes you stronger, and improves lung capacity)
- increased immunity power
- reduced risk of heart disease, stroke, diabetes, depression, obesity, arthritis, cancer, osteoporosis, high cholesterol, and high blood pressure
- promotes better sleep
- maintains proper weight
- helps control symptoms of menopause
- helps maintain strong bones

Bad news: You can't exercise while eating cookie dough.

Convinced? Okay, here are some tips to help you get started:

Find Your Niche

Humans are creatures of habit. The next time you take a shower, notice how you wash each body part in the same order every day. This is not a bad thing. Routines help us cope and help us to get things done, and we've learned from an early age that routines are comforting. Picking a certain time of day for exercise means fitting it into your schedule and making it a habit that you can live with and stick with, too.

You Don't Have to Sweat for an Hour

New studies show that you can break up the length of your workouts into sections. Twenty minutes on the treadmill in the morning, twenty minutes walking during your lunch hour, and twenty minutes walking the dog in the evening. Done! You will get more benefits from more strenuous exercise, but that's your choice. Just being more "active" has its benefits as well. Parking far from the door so you'll have to walk, taking the stairs instead of the elevator, and avoiding the moving sidewalk at the airport are ways to get exercise with minimal effort.

You Don't Need to Join a Gym

I don't know about you, but I HATE working out with others. All I end up doing is looking at all the fit people in their tight clothes with their bulging . . . um . . . muscles and getting depressed. One option to avoid this is to do at-home workouts, like walking in the neighborhood, doing an exercise DVD, or jumping rope. Check your local library to see if there are some DVDs for you to try so you can see what kind of routine appeals to you. Most shopping malls have walking groups that walk inside the mall before it opens. If you can resist the urge to stop and window shop, this might work for you. Your local hospital's cardiac rehabilitation program usually has information on mall-walking groups if you're interested.

Buddy Up

Studies show that if you exercise with someone else—a friend, a spouse, or family member—you are more likely to keep it up and it is more likely to be enjoyable. Gabbing always makes the time go faster. Whether it's with a friend or your family, exercising together makes it easier and you're more likely to participate, as you don't want to let the other person down by being a no-show.

Start Slowly

If you can't walk for ten minutes without getting tired, that's okay! Just do what you can, and, in time, you will build stamina and it will get easier. This is especially true after surgery or during chemo. Exercise will definitely help you during these times, but it's not the time to train for a marathon. Listen to your body . . . take it slowly . . . don't push it. You will get to a point in your treatment and recovery when you will be able to increase your intensity. Wait for it. If you're not sure what you should be doing, get some help either from a resource in your doctor's office or from a certified personal trainer that has had experience with cancer patients.

Make It Enjoyable

There are many activities to choose from when looking at starting an exercise program. You don't have to purchase fancy equipment or buy expensive clothes. Find something you like, and go with it. You can also mix it up for variety—biking one day, walking the next. Try ice-skating, rollerblading, or roller-skating at a roller rink for some serious fun. Yoga is also a great option, especially when recovering from surgery or illness.

Think of Your Exercise as Part of Your Treatment

Just like your medication or your follow-up doctor visits, exercise plays a big role in reducing your risk of declining health or future reoccurrence. Would you skip taking your medication because you just didn't have the time?

Keep a Chart

Charts help you see your progress. Just like kids who need to see gold stars on their behavior charts, adults need this, too, especially since you won't see the effects of your hard work right away. If you are starting an exercise program to lose weight, weigh yourself weekly, not daily. And remember that after you have about six weeks of exercise behind you, you will start trading fat for muscle. Muscle weighs more than fat. This means you can be getting fit and losing fat and inches, but you may not see it on the scale. When I first started working out, I lost 7 inches total on my body. I looked and felt better and my clothes fit better, but I didn't lose ONE POUND! If I had only looked at the scale, I would have thought I was failing!

> Exercise is the one common factor in people living longer, healthier, and happier and is a proven risk-reducer when it comes to cancer and other major illnesses like heart disease and diabetes.

There are many great resources for exercise. If you belong to a gym or fitness center, see if you can schedule several sessions with a certified personal trainer to get you started. Certified personal trainers have gone to school or have taken courses and have passed a test that make them experts in designing a safe exercise program specific to your needs. Some trainers will even come to your home if you don't have access to one at a gym. Just make sure they are certified and they have experience with whatever you happen to be going through, either chemo or surgery.

Visit these sites for more information on how to get started:

- Centers for Disease Control and Prevention: Physical Activity (www.cdc.gov/physicalactivity)

- President's Council on Fitness Sports & Nutrition (www.fitness.gov)

- Health Canada (www.hc-sc.gc.ca)

With any exercise program, you should always check with your doctor before starting one, especially if you are over forty years old or have a major illness, as you could have some underlying issue that might make certain types of exercise unhealthy for you.

When you get the green light to exercise, however you choose to do it, get started and don't ever stop!

I Didn't Have to Wax My Upper Lip

I was mortified when, just prior to starting chemo, my aesthetician suggested that I should get my upper lip waxed. Me? With facial hair? Well, she is the expert. I was haunted by thoughts of how it would grow back. Would it be all prickly and manly? Would I look like a fuzzy peach? My fears were unfounded, however, because once my chemo started, my upper lip remained as smooth as a baby's bottom, and my eyebrows looked perfectly groomed for months afterward (until they eventually just disappeared all together!).

For that "just out of the salon" look that lasts for months, have your waxings done before you start chemo.

HEALTH TIP #8
When That New Hair Finally Starts to Grow In, Here's How to Keep It Healthy

When I lost my hair to chemo, I wasn't as devastated as I probably should have been. Being presented with an experience not many younger women have (thankfully!), I was determined to "enjoy" it while it lasted and I did . . . by getting ready in 2.5 seconds, and getting out of speeding tickets. (Cops always have sympathy for the bald lady.)

Despite all the cool things about being bald, when my hair finally started to grow back I realized how much I had missed it, and I wanted to do everything I could to nurture and coax those wispy little strands back to being long, strong, and healthy. (Caution: The way the following information is presented might cause you to have flashbacks to a film you may have viewed in your eighth-grade science class, only there will be no quiz when it's over and you're free to pass notes if you wish.)

Hair, and its growth cycle, is really quite amazing. There are three phases of hair growth: anagen, catagen, and telogen.

The anagen phase is the growth phase, and the one involved with new hair production. In this phase, the hair follicle (the "root," where hair keeps its own personal blood supply) grows down deeper into the skin to get proper nourishment as the hair cells divide rapidly to push the hair shaft (hair as you know it) out of the pore and onto your head. The anagen phase is why we need to get a haircut. This phase lasts from two to seven years, is your "living, growing hair," and makes up most of what is on your head. Some chemotherapy agents love to target and destroy rapidly dividing cells and so the rapidly dividing hair cells make for a perfect target.

The catagen phase is a transitional phase where the hair stops growing, stops getting nutrients from the blood supply, and prepares to detach. It lasts two to four weeks.

In the last phase, the telogen phase, the hair rests for two to four months, completes the life cycle, and the follicle prepares once again to enter the anagen phase and grow a new piece of hair. As it does, the old hair is forced up and eventually falls out. We normally lose about 100 hairs every day from this process. Some forms of stress can force your hair into this phase prematurely.

The lengths of these phases are determined by heredity and genetics.

Okay, class, the film is over. Bobby, would you please turn on the lights?

When you finish chemo, and there is nothing to suppress hair growth, your hair will enter these phases once again. The first thing you might notice is that you begin to "get fuzzy." This happens because the growth of the cells that produce melanin, the substance that gives hair its color, lag behind the growth of the hair shaft. The initial fuzz you see will usually have no color and look white. (Although there are exceptions to the rule.) In this rebirth stage, all your hair is in the anagen phase, relying on the dermal papilla, or hair follicle "seed," to rapidly reproduce and push the hair shaft out. As the hair grows, it is coated with keratin, a protein coating, to strengthen it.

Notable, too, is the effect of Tamoxifen or other drugs on hair growth,

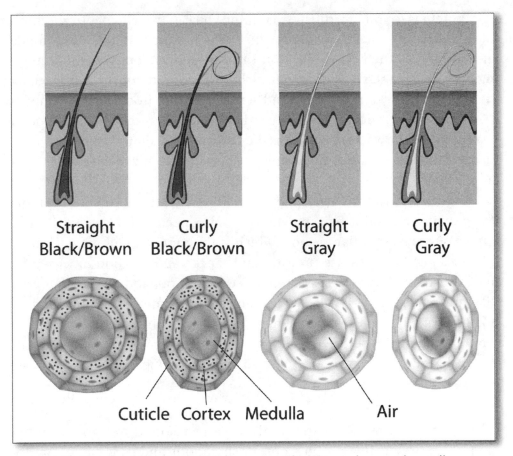

The "curly white/gray fuzz" that appears after chemo does not have all
the components it needs to grow hair with color or substance.

as some will find regrowth difficult or have bald spots or thinned hair while
taking certain medication.

Once construction is underway, your hair will continue to thicken and
fill in. During this time, you'll want to do everything in your power to insure
that you stay on the "mane train."

Diet

A healthy diet is crucial to healthy hair production. Protein and omega-3
fatty acids are key players in restoring hair growth.

Protein is found in virtually everything you eat, from apples to zucchini. Meat and dairy contain a lot of protein, but high protein animal-based foods are not always the best choice. You can easily meet your protein requirements by eating servings of protein-rich nuts, nut butters, seeds (especially hemp), lentils, quinoa, beans, and fermented soy products like tempeh. (Check with your doctor's recommendations on specific soy-based foods.) Avoid protein powders or shakes as they usually contain unhealthy soy fragments called isolates and are completely unnecessary if you are eating a balanced diet.

Omega-3 fatty acids are dietary fats that provide the body with the tools for growing beautiful hair, but they are also needed for general health. Omega-3s prevent inflammation, which is the root cause of many chronic illnesses like heart disease, arthritis, and cancer. You can find omega-3s in foods such as walnuts, flaxseeds, chia seeds, salmon, and dark leafy greens like spinach and kale. If you aren't getting enough omega-3s from your diet, look for quality omega-3 supplement capsules, as they are an easy, quick option for making sure you're getting the omega-3s you need, keeping in mind that dietary sources are preferred over supplementation.

Be Chemical Free

Your hair, like the rest of your body, doesn't respond well to chemicals and harsh preservatives. Watch out for shampoos and sprays that can dry and damage your brand-new hair with ingredients like alcohol and potentially cancer-causing substances like sodium laureth sulfate, DMDM hydantoin (formaldehyde), and preservatives like parabens (look for "paraben" in the name—for example methylparaben). Artificial colors and DEA (diethanolamine) can also be harmful. There's a lot to look for, but there are wonderful companies out there that are making hair-care products for health-conscious people like you. Avalon, Aubrey Organics, John Masters Organics, and Lavera are some good companies that value nature and what it has to offer your hair. Lavera's Orange Milk Volume Shampoo for fine hair might be just what your hair needs when it's in that starting-over phase. Visit www.lavera.com.

Magic Potions

If you want to help soften and reduce breakage on that new hair you've grown, you can make a wonderful mixture of oils that work specifically on your hair to strengthen and nourish it. You will need equal parts coconut oil, castor oil, and jojoba oil. Coconut and castor oils can be found in most grocery stores, and you can usually get jojoba from health food stores or online. (You can sub out the pricey jojoba oil for olive or almond oil if you can't find it.) Mix one ounce (two tablespoons) of each oil in a ceramic microwave-safe bowl or glass measuring cup. Gently warm the oils in the microwave for 30 seconds on high, stirring after 15 seconds until all the oils are combined and the coconut oil is melted. (Coconut oil is solid at room temperature.) The mixture should be warm, *not hot.* If you want to, add 10 drops of peppermint essential oil (not peppermint extract or flavoring) as peppermint can increase scalp circulation, smells really nice, and can lift your mood.

Essential oils can be found at health food stores or online. Make sure you're buying "essential oil," which is an oil taken directly from a plant and not a synthetic fragrance oil, which is a chemical substance made to smell like a plant. Try to get an oral-medication dosing syringe from your pharmacy for easy application to your hair or use a plastic "hair coloring" type bottle with a tapered tip and available at most beauty supply stores.

> You can help your hair back to life, just be kind and gentle and keep it natural.

Apply to your scalp in sections, and then work the oils through to the ends of your hair (or fuzz) saturating the whole strand. Apply a shower cap and let those nourishing oils soak into your scalp and hair for fifteen minutes to one hour. The longer you leave it on, the better your results will be. Then wash the oils out with a mild organic shampoo. You may need to wash twice to get the oils completely out of your hair.

Save any leftover mix in a sealed bottle at room temperature. You can use the oil treatment once or twice a week to keep your new hair soft and flexible, and continue to use it well into your "luxurious locks" phase. This mixture will help your hair strands and will also help to condition the scalp, allowing you to provide a healthy "growing field" for your precious little sprouts.

Washing

Don't wash your hair every day if possible. When that fuzz showed up I couldn't wait to go out and buy ten different shampoos and matching conditioners so I could actually wash my "hair" (to use the term loosely). But your shampoos can't compete with the natural oils that your scalp produces, as they are the number-one best oils to nourish your scalp and hair. If you wash your head every day, you will be stripping those beneficial oils away. Let's face it: how dirty can peach fuzz get anyway?

Brushing

Only brush your hair twice a day using a soft brush or wide-toothed comb. Frequent brushing and tugging might be pulling out hair that isn't ready to leave your scalp. And that's just plain mean!

Yes, having your hair back is very exciting, but take it slow and treat it right. Baby your baby hair, baby. Those tender first strands will grow up to be hair that would make even Rapunzel jealous. (Note: These healthy hair-growing tips are meant for HEAD hair only.)

I Got to Try Out
New Eyebrow Shapes

You don't realize how important eyebrows are to your look until you lose them. That became obvious to me shortly after I lost my eyebrows due to chemo. Kaitlyn was telling me about her weekend plans, and I looked at her with "raised eyebrows" in order to communicate to her: "Oh, so you really think I am going to let you go on a road trip with your friends?"

While this was the effect I was going for:

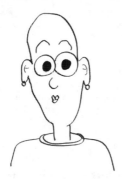

This is how I actually looked:

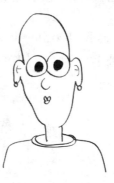

So, needless to say, without my eyebrows to communicate my displeasure, she ended up going on the road trip.

A similar incident happened about a week later. I went to Donovan's room to look for my phone charger and was horrified at the mess I saw there. I looked at him with "furrowed eyebrows" to show my displeasure and let him know it was time to clean up. However, rather than this:

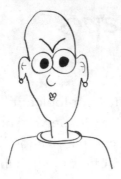

I looked more like this:

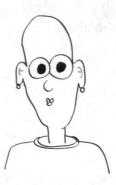

Without my eyebrows to back me up, it was pointless to tell him to clean his room.

So I figured it was high time I invested in eyebrow cosmetics and experimented with some new looks. I tried:

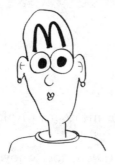

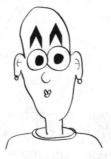

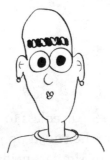

The McDonald's arches   The Jack-O-Lantern   The fuzzy caterpillar

But finally settled on this look:

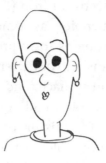

If you are in the market for new brows, try an eyebrow powder, which looks more natural than an eyebrow pencil.

HEALTH TIP #9
Would You Raise Your Eyebrows if I Offered You Some Weed?

What if I told you that one of the healthiest foods found anywhere can most likely be found on your front lawn? Can you guess what it is? Hint: It's the one plant that you curse at daily, spend hundreds of dollars to kill, and is the top reason for widespread outdoor chemical use.

Yes, dandelions!

Poor dandelions get a bad rap. No one likes seeing them in their yard, and, with nicknames like blowball, swine snout, and cankerwort, it's no wonder why you may have left this plant off your shopping list.

Dandelion leaves are loaded with vitamins and iron, and there's not a bad thing I can say about them. One cup of chopped dandelion leaves contains only 25 skinny little calories, no fat, and 535 percent of the recommended daily allowance (RDA) for vitamin K. Vitamin K is important for healthy blood and necessary for vitamin D absorption. That same pesky weed will provide 112 percent of your RDA for vitamin A, a powerful antioxidant and health promoter, and 10 percent of your RDA for calcium. (Moooove over milk!) And if that's not enough to change your mind, it is one of the best greens for iron (9% of the RDA).

The leaves are on the bitter side, as some dark greens are, but that's a good thing, as the bitterness helps to improve digestion by encouraging enzyme production and cleansing your liver. The bitterness blends nicely with assorted baby greens and spinach, and when used with other greens, actually improves the flavor of your salad. A lemon-based dressing complements the bitterness nicely. Try mixing one tablespoon of extra virgin organic olive oil, two teaspoons of fresh lemon juice, one teaspoon of honey, and one clove of crushed fresh garlic. Add a pinch of sea salt and dash of pepper, whisk for one minute, and pour over greens for a fresh and healthy option to your usual salad dressing.

Dandelion leaves also act as a natural mild diuretic and a mild anti-inflammatory, reducing generalized swelling and blocking inflammation, the root cause of many chronic illnesses.

The root of the dandelion is the subject of a growing number of studies for its role in fighting cancer. A 2012 research grant was awarded to the University of Windsor in Canada to test dandelion extract tea on leukemia patients. Initial research showed that treating a very aggressive form of leukemia (chronic monocytic myeloid leukemia) with dandelion root extract caused significant self-destruction of the blood's cancer cells. Using these results, the university applied for a more extensive grant where they created a very basic dandelion tea that could be tested on the different leukemia cells in the lab. To the researcher's surprise, the dandelion mixture caused the leukemia cells to commit suicide while keeping the healthy cells alive and well. There are anecdotal great success stories of patients using dandelion root tea to fight leukemia. There are currently research applications in the process that, if approved, would allow for human trials using dandelion root to treat leukemia and, in the future, hopefully other cancers as well. Are dandelions gaining your respect now?

There are many commercially sold dandelion root teas available in stores and online. Read the label carefully to make sure the ingredients are pure, and there is nothing harmful listed, and always check with your healthcare provider when adding anything herbal to your diet on a regular basis.

The dandelion community is growing, and dandelion lovers are constantly posting information online. One of my favorite recipes is from Clara Cannucciari. She is a delightful ninety-four-year-old great-grandmother who shares her childhood recipes from the Depression era on YouTube and in her cookbook. (Do an Internet search for "Clara's dandelion salad," and watch the YouTube video.) She explains the process of washing the leaves, also gives some insight into how she learned to make this recipe, and shares how freshly harvested food from your yard (before pesticides and weed killers) is not only healthy but also free! She is adorable, and, even if you don't make the recipe, you'll learn something from Clara. A viewer asked her how she stays so young-looking. She said, "Maybe it's because I eat a lot of olive oil and natural foods." Clara also said that growing up they "ate a lot of vegetables and ate meat kind of sparingly and I think it was better for us."

If you've never tried dandelions before, use commonsense precautions. Dandelion allergies exist (same goes for anything else in nature), but they are very rare. If you've picked dandelion flowers for your mom as a kid and didn't get a rash, it's pretty safe to say you won't react, but there is never a 100 percent guarantee. If you have known gallstones, or bile duct obstruction, you should avoid dandelion as it promotes the flow of the digestive enzymes, which is healthy for most but could worsen gallbladder disease symptoms if you're one of the lucky ones with gallstones. The high vitamin K content can alter bleeding time if you take blood-thinning medications.

While I suppose you could, it's probably best not to eat the dandelions in your yard because they have probably been the "going place" for neighborhood dogs, and if you've sprayed or treated your yard with any kind of fertilizer or weed killer, the toxic effects can stay in the soil for many years. Eating chemical weed killer kinda cancels out any beneficial health effects. (Ya think?)

> Open your mind and your kitchen to a fresh, healthy, cancer-fighting dandelion salad.

Specialty health food stores or farmers markets are the best places to buy organically grown dandelions. Since they're so easy to grow, they're usually pretty cheap, too, and, because they are grown on farms, the leaves are huge, beautiful, and flavorful.

Have a little respect, please, for the common pesky dandelion, for as you are blowing those fluffy seeds into the air while you're making a wish for better health, part of the answer might be sitting right in your hand.

Cancer Gave Me Something to Hope For

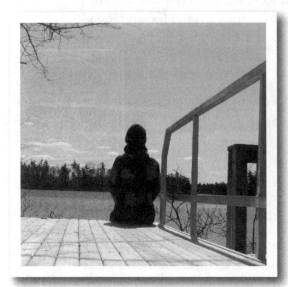

By modern-day definition, *hope* means to wish for something, without the certainty that it will be fulfilled. It is an unsure optimism. The Bible, however, gives a different meaning to the word *hope*. In biblical terms, hope is an indication of certainty; a strong and confident expectation. It is not just wishful thinking; it is a sure belief that what you hope for will come to pass.

I throw around the word *hope* on a daily basis, in the modern sense of the word: *I hope it doesn't rain; I hope the stain comes out of my new dress; I hope I get a refund on my taxes.* All of these are things that I desire to happen, but I have no confident expectation that they will happen (especially the tax refund!). If these wishes do not come true, it's really no big deal. Hoping for life on that other hand—well that's a different matter. It is here that I employ the biblical definition of the word *hope*.

> "Refusal to hope is nothing more than a decision to die."
> —Bernie Siegel, MD

Jesus said, "Therefore I tell you, whatever you ask in prayer, believe that you have received it, and it will be yours" (Matthew 11:24). In this quote, Jesus assures us that when we have faith, and truly believe that we will receive, our prayers are certain to be answered. The power of prayer, then, lies not in the asking but in the belief that what you ask for will be granted. That is hope. In that sense, cancer gave me something to really hope for. I did not "wish" for a full recovery, I "hoped," with certainty, that my prayers would be answered.

HEALTH TIP #10
I Hope You Know the Difference Between Omega-3 and Omega-6

If you don't know the difference between omega-3 and omega 6-fatty acids, you're not alone. But once you learn about your 3s and 6s, this is one secret you won't want to keep to yourself.

Omega-3 essential fatty acids are nutrients that your body relies on to function. They are involved in all new cell growth. They are also concentrated in the brain to improve and maintain brain health and are necessary for healthy skin and hair production.

The "essential" part means our bodies don't manufacture this fatty acid, and we need to get it from outside sources.

The real magic of omega-3 is that it reduces inflammation. The inflammatory process is responsible for most of the human body's chronic maladies such as heart disease, arthritis, inflammatory bowel disease, cancer, and others.

In April 2009, a Harvard School of Public Health study found omega-3 fatty acid deficiency ranked as the sixth highest killer of Americans, responsible for 72,000 to 96,000 preventable deaths yearly. Not many people are aware of this fact, and, while some people know that omega-3s are "good," they have no idea why or how to get them.

Omega-6 Versus Omega-3

Omega-6 is also an essential fatty acid found in things like corn, eggs, beef, milk, and milk products as well as polyunsaturated oils. Your daily healthy intake of omega-6 to omega-3 should be at a ratio of 2:1, or at the very least 4:1. Our dietary ratios are currently more like 20:1, as dietary consumption of omega-6 fatty acids has increased tenfold over the past thirty years. The same way omega-3s reduce inflammation, omega-6 fatty acids *increase* inflammation.

Polyunsaturated oils were pushed on the public because it was believed that they were healthier than saturated fats for your heart. But studies now indicate that this may or may not be true. Furthermore, the use of polyunsaturated oils has been directly linked to increasing tumor activity. A 2009 Purdue study funded by the National Institute of Health studied the action of cancer cells when exposed to certain fats. The findings indicate that cancer has a tendency to spread in the presence of a high-fat diet in general, but particularly diets high in polyunsaturated fats or omega-6s. Monounsaturated fats had no effect. (Olive is a monounsaturated fat.) An unhealthy increase in the intake of omega-6 and decrease in omega-3 in the diet has been shown to be a risk factor for many other illnesses as well, like arthritis and inflammatory bowel disease. These are the same conditions that a dietary increase in omega-3 fatty acids prevents. Can you dig it?

A shift in the omegas in the right direction (more 3 and less 6) can therefore have a huge impact on your overall health and the prevention of a long list of diseases, including cancer.

To decrease omega-6s:

- Limit corn products. Corn products (much of them genetically modified) make up a large portion of the American diet and that includes corn oil. When you can, ditch those corn chips, corn flakes, popcorn, corn bread, corn tortillas, and anything else made with corn. Read your labels, because you'll be surprised where corn is lurking.

- Limit dairy. There are great alternatives for cow's milk such as almond milk, coconut milk, and rice milk. Plant-based milks can also have more calcium than cow's milk and less fat. Choose the unsweetened versions when you can. There are wonderful plant-based mayonnaises, butters, and yogurts out there as well, and they taste exactly the same or better than their dairy-containing counterparts.

- Limit or eliminate eggs and egg products.

- Limit or eliminate beef and chicken, particularly industrial-produced (factory farm) corn-fed versus organic grass-fed meat products.

- Limit or eliminate soybean oil, safflower oil, and other polyunsaturated vegetable oils and switch to *olive oil*, a monounsaturated oil that is neutral (monos do not affect inflammation). You get even more benefits if the olive oil is extra-virgin organic. Technically, EVOO stands for extra virgin olive oil, but I like to use EVOOO, which is extra-virgin, *organic* olive oil. *Extra virgin* means it's minimally processed.

To increase omega-3s:

- If you eat fish, increase fish intake—mackerel, sardines, or salmon (wild fish if possible)—to two to three times a week.

- Increase deep-green, leafy vegetables—spinach, kale, and other dark greens.

- Include algae supplements, which are loaded with omega-3s, and can be grown organically. (Please check with your health provider to see if these are right for you.) There are many different kinds to choose from. If you're not sure, consult your naturopath or healthcare provider for the proper kind.

- Include walnuts and freshly ground flaxseeds as they are rich in alpha-linolenic acid (ALA), which converts to omega-3 fatty acid in your body.

- Include chia seeds in your diet as one tablespoon of chia seeds can have as much omega-3s as five fish oil capsules. Simply toss them in salads, shakes, or cereals.

- As a last resort, include fish oil capsules in your daily regimen. While flax seed oil capsules are also an option, fish oils provide a better form of omega-3 that is more easily metabolized by the body, Flax seed oil also lacks the beneficial cancer-fighting part of the flax: lignans.

So how do you know that your new "omega diet" is working? There are blood tests available that will measure the ratio of omega-6 to omega-3 fatty acids in your body so you can see how close your levels are to desirable. You can obtain the tests kits from a mail-order company, supply a small blood sample at home, and mail it in for results. It's not enough just to measure the omega-3s, as some tests do. You must measure the ratio of omega-6 to omega-3, as it is the ratio that determines your risk of inflammatory illness.

Counting every single milligram of fatty acid that you consume so you can look at the ratios for the rest of your life would be a bit ridiculous, but if you're moving toward a cancer-fighting diet, it would be a good idea to count your omega-3s and omega-6s for a few days so you can see where your levels are to identify where to make changes. Once you know where omega's lurk, it's easier to make good dietary choices. A great place to find the omega-3 to omega-6 content of your favorite foods is at www.nutrition data.com.

A Bit About Omega-3 Fish Oil Capsules

Eating the whole food is the best way to get omega-3s, but you may choose to use supplements in your daily dietary routine. Omega-3 fish oil capsules are one way to get the omega-3 fatty acids that your body needs to be healthy. New research indicates that two grams of omega-3 supplements daily (usually four capsules) can actually change the length of your telomeres, which are the structures that tell your healthy cells to live longer. Fish oil is sold in 1,000 milligram capsules, but not all 1,000 of those milligrams are omega-3 fatty acids. Fish oil also contains docosahexaenoic acid (DHA) and eicosapentaenoic (EPA), which are great for your heart. That means that only about 500 milligrams of that capsule are actually omega-3s.

Please note that not all fish oils are created equal.

- Some companies make their fish oil from all kinds of fish—sardines, mackerel, salmon, tuna, and anything else they can catch in the wild, or in a fish farm. Farmed fish have a lot more contaminants, pesticides, and PCBs (pollution byproducts) than wild-caught fish.

- To remove the contaminants, some companies put their fish oil through a process called molecular distillation. This process uses high heat and chemicals to break apart the omega-3 chain and essentially gives you the important parts of the fatty acid in pieces. (I generally avoid "processed" anything.) Not the most efficient way for your body to use it, but better than nothing.

- Some companies add vitamin E to the capsule to keep the oil from going rancid. Most unstable fish oil capsules will say on the bottle, "Refrigerate after opening." With quality capsules, this is not necessary. (My personal recommendation is Wholemega by New Chapter, but there are many others.)

If you take anything away from reading this health tip, it should be the following:

1. Increase your dietary sources of omega-3 fatty acids by eating more veggies and high omega-3 plant-based foods like chia seeds, or if you must by eating fish or taking omega-3 capsules. If you decide to take a fish oil capsule, research it so you know what you are taking, how pure the fish oil is, how the oil is processed, and the philosophy of the company that is supplying your supplements.

2. Try to reduce your intake of omega-6 (corn products and vegetable oils) to avoid encouraging the inflammatory process that may put you at risk for dozens of chronic illnesses by throwing off your omega-6 to omega-3 ratio. This does not mean you need to completely cut out foods that are high in omega-6, like healthy protein-rich hemp seeds for example, but be mindful of your intake so you can still hit that 4:1 (or even better 2:1) omega-6 to omega-3 ratio. Switching out food during your day like olive oil for sunflower oil or flax crackers for corn chips are simple small ways to tip the scales in your favor and have a significant healthy effect.

> Increasing omega-3 fatty acid intake and decreasing omega-6 intake can have dramatic health benefits that can reduce your risk of a long list of illnesses, including cancer.

3. Please talk to your health provider if you decide to start taking any supplement, as fish oils can interfere with some medications, particularly blood-thinning agents.

Cancer Made Me Realize My Own Strength

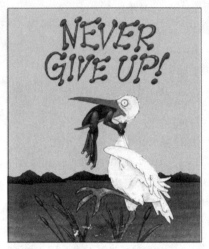

There is nothing like a battle with cancer to prove to yourself just how strong you really are. Ten years ago, if I could have looked into the future and saw forty-four-year-old Florence: divorced, single parenting three children, dealing with the many challenges of having a child with autism, and then facing cancer on top of that, well, I probably would have said, "Hand me a rope, would ya?" But I would have been underestimating the strength of forty-four-year-old Florence. Not only did I handle it, but I experienced some of the most joyful moments of my life in the process! It is true: God never gives us more than we can handle. But God, if you are listening, "I GET IT! I'M STRONG! Now go pick on someone your own size."

Celebrate your own strength!

HEALTH TIP #11
Celebrate Healthy Fats

Cooking was a lot different when you were a kid. Back then your mom's choices were:

- pot roast or steak?
- crisco or lard?

- baked or fried?

Now that we know a thing or two about healthy eating, the choices are:

- sweet potato or carrots?
- wild or brown rice?
- olive oil or canola oil?

That last one can be confusing. There are so many different oils on that supermarket shelf. Heck, you can see twenty different kinds of olive oils alone! Let's try to sort out the main points:

Oils are made of fats. Oil that comes from a plant is the fat that is extracted from that plant. Oils contain 100 percent fat. There are no proteins, carbs, vitamins, or minerals in oil.

Fats are necessary for human life. They keep our nervous system in check and provide us with "essential fatty acids," which provide fuel for heart and skeletal muscle and are necessary for many of your body's metabolic processes. We need fats in our diets to help with vitamin metabolism, hormone balance, and to aid with digestion. You could not survive on a diet of 0 percent fat.

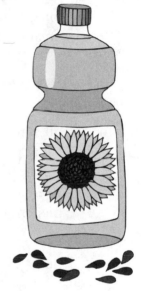

There are different kinds of fats that make up all oils. The differences have to do with the slightly varied chemical compositions. The three basic fat categories are saturated, monounsaturated, and polyunsaturated. These three types of fats are present in differing percentages in all oils. For example, olive oil contains 14 percent saturated fat, 12 percent polyunsaturated fat, and 74 percent monounsaturated fat. These fats can be further broken down into specific fatty acids. Omega-3 and omega-6 are two types of fatty acids present in oils, but there are many more.

It is widely accepted by numerous worldwide health organizations that diets high in saturated fats lead to heart disease and cancer. (And the jury is still out on whether plant-based saturated fats like coconut oil do the same damage, as the studies were conducted only with saturated *animal* fats.) Polyunsaturated fats, once thought to be "healthy," may not be, as they tend to be high in omega-6 fatty acids that promote inflammation and disease. If there were a "best" category for fats, monounsaturated fats would be the healthiest as they have been linked with lower risk of stroke, heart disease, and cancer even when eaten in less than moderate quantities.

That said, oils in general should be the smallest part of your diet. Even though olive oil is one of the healthiest, you don't want to slather it all over everything you eat or use it as the main ingredient in your morning smoothie. The lowest incidence of cancer is shown to come from a diet where 10 percent or less of its calories come from any kind of fat. In an average diet, that's about 200 calories or 22 grams/day which is far less than most people consume.

The oils lowest in saturated and polyunsaturated fats and highest in monounsaturated fats are olive, canola, and peanut. (Avocado oil is also high in monos but is not as easily accessible.) Civilization has been extracting oil from olives for more than six thousand years. Olive oil is my favorite for general everyday use. I try to buy cold-pressed EVOOO (extra-virgin organic olive oil) as it has the best flavor, quality, and health benefits.

Terms to Know When Buying Oils

Cold-pressed or expeller-pressed: This has to do with how they get the oil out of the plant. Cold-pressed means the plant or seed is squished using pressure and the oil is extracted leaving whatever is not oil behind. Cold-pressing does not use chemicals and high heat to force the oil out. Therefore, this maintains the oil's composition, so it's healthier and of higher quality.

First pressed: This means pressing just once to obtain the oil. It is not run though again.

Refined vs. unrefined: Refining means processing. This can be in the form of heating, filtering, or with chemicals. The more refined the oil, usually the higher you can heat it (as with frying), but it lacks the health benefits, as refining can alter the structure of the oil and change the final fat composition.

Virgin vs. extra virgin: Okay, all you Madonna fans, sing it with me: *Like an extra-virgin . . . pressed for the very first time.* Extra-virgin oil is produced from the first press of the fruit or seed. It is the purest and best-tasting oil. Virgin oil is still minimally processed, but it has a higher acidity, which gives it a different flavor. (So I'm told. If I had a master chef's taste buds, I might be able to tell the difference.) Virgin and extra virgin, as it applies to olive oil, are higher in monounsaturated fats and other beneficial fatty acids making them the healthiest choice.

Pure olive oil (or olive oil): When it says "pure olive oil" or just plain "olive oil," the oil contains a combination of virgin olive oil and processed pomace. Pomace is produced from processing the leftovers from the virgin olive oil extraction. It has a weaker flavor, but can stand up to frying and high-heat cooking or baking. If the bottle is labeled "100% pure olive oil" it is the lowest quality, but it can often be a lot less expensive. "Light olive oil" has nothing to do with calories. It is made from refined or processed olive oil that causes the color to be light.

> When choosing your cooking oil, take the time to pick the best one for your health!

"High oleic": This is an oil that contains more than 80 percent monounsaturated fat. The higher mono content has been bred into the seed itself by altering the way it grows. Unlike genetically modified organisms (GMOs) or genetically modified foods, these plants are hybrids of the original. As long as the oil is not chemically modified, or processed, it's a very healthy choice because of the high monounsaturated content. Since the patent has expired on growing high oleic plants, you will probably see more on the market. Any type of plant can be made into a high oleic hybrid, including corn and soybean oil, but a large percentage of those crops are GMOs, which you may want to avoid. Always buy organic high oleic oils if possible as single, one-ingredient foods labeled "organic" can never be GMOs.

Some Other Oil Facts

- When using oils for dressings, choose cold-pressed, unrefined oils to get the best flavor.

- Avoid heating oils to their "smoke point" (the point where the oils begin to burn and produce smoke). This means the oil is changing chemically and can be harmful if done often. It also affects the taste. Certain oils are better than others for frying. Canola has the highest smoke point out of the top three healthiest.

- Store oils in airtight containers in a dark place to prolong life and preserve the antioxidant health benefits. When oil is packaged, a thin layer of nitrogen is added to the top of the bottle to replace the oxygen. When the oil is opened and exposed to air, the aging process begins. Sometimes vitamin E is added to prolong the oil's life and will be listed on the label as "vitamin E" or "tocopherols." Refined oils high in monounsaturated fats last up to a year after opening. Oils high in polyunsaturated fats keep about six months. Saturated fat oils like coconut and palm have years and years of shelf life. That's why the food industry loves them so much!

- Try to buy organic oils whenever possible. Pesticides are "fat soluble" and usually collect in the oil part of the plant.

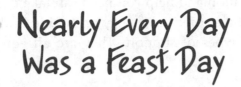

Nearly Every Day Was a Feast Day

Iam very blessed to have a great support network of family and friends around me. This comes in particularly handy when you consider that I am a single working parent, mother of three, and my youngest has autism. Needless to say, I NEED the support!

During the week following my chemo treatments (and longer if needed), my support team would kick in full force, taking turns making dinners for me and cleaning up afterward. And I'm not talking mac-'n'-cheese here, my friends—these were delicious three-course meals. So even on the days when I didn't have much of an appetite, I always managed to eat some of these feasts that had been lovingly prepared for me.

Call upon your support team to cook for you. Don't have a support team? Then find one! There are many organizations, church groups, and other volunteer groups out there who are dedicated to helping people like you.

HEALTH TIP #12
Need a Hand?

No matter how self-sufficient you may be, everyone needs support when going through a difficult time. Many can find what they need from family and friends, while others find great benefits from support groups and online chat rooms.

Finding and developing a great support system not only benefits your mental health, but it can also actually improve the outcome of your illness.

Getting the information and help you need can take the stress off you and allow you to spend that precious energy on getting healthy.

There are four types of support. They are all equally important for regaining health.

1. **Emotional support:** having someone understand what you are going through, listen, and maybe give a hug or two

2. **Instrumental support:** things that you may need, like a ride to your treatment or a prepared dinner

3. **Informational support:** knowledge that will help you to make optimum healthcare decisions; these can come from a doctor or from someone who has walked in your shoes

4. **Appraisal support:** opinions of others on how you're doing with the choices you've made—pats on the back, if you will

Studies show that patients with nonfunctioning or nonexistent support systems have less positive outcomes with their illness than those with strong support systems.

Examine your support systems. Are you taking advantage of what they are offering? Or are you more likely to think, *I don't need any help.* Think about the four types of support mentioned above. Are you lacking in one or more of these key types of support?

Here are some links to check out. If you're looking for local resources, you can use these links to find those as well.

Worldwide

- National Cancer Institute (www.cancer.gov) gives information on global cancer issues, topics, and research.

- Cancer Support Community (cancersupportcommunity.org)—formally the Wellness Community and Gilda's Club Worldwide—is an enormous organization that provides support, education, and hope to those affected by cancer.

- Cancer Index (www.cancerindex.org) provides links with close to 100 different support groups worldwide as well as links to treatments, preventions, and medical centers for all types of cancers.

- Oncochat (www.oncochat.org) is an online support system for those with cancer. Here you can share information with other cancer patients and survivors from around the world.

- Association of Cancer Online Resources (www.acor.org) provides lists of information and support that will allow you to access what you need.

In the United States

- Cancer Hope Network (www.cancerhopenetwork.org) matches you one-on-one with a cancer survivor who has gone through a similar experience.

- Imerman Angels (www.ImermanAngels.org) matches you one-on-one with a cancer survivor. Connect through phone calls and e-mails.

- American Cancer Society (www.cancer.org) provides information about doctors, treatments, and services.

> Make sure you are using every support system available to you to improve your outcome.

In Canada

- The Canadian Cancer Society (www.cancer.ca) provides information about cancer and cancer-related services; connects you to a peer support system; and allows you to be part of an online community.

- The Canadian Cancer Advocacy Network (www.ccanacc.ca/) provides information and support for caregivers, patients, and their families.

- Cancer Advocacy Coalition of Canada (www.canceradvocacy.ca/) advocates for prevention and treatment issues, as well as the emotional, physical, and financial needs of patients and survivors.

There's plenty of help and support out there for you. It's up to you to take the first step in getting it.

The Use of Medicinal Marijuana

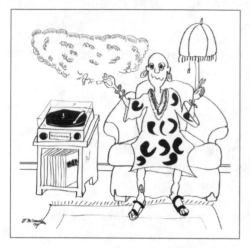

Let me make one thing clear: I am not the type to scrimp on drugs. When it comes to natural childbirth, for example, I am completely against it. If there is a drug out there to ease pain and suffering of any kind, you can give it to me (I'm talking legit, prescribed meds of course). After all, that is why God created pharmaceuticals.

When I was diagnosed with cancer, one of my biggest concerns was about the side effects of chemo. I was fine with losing my hair, but just the thought of being sick made me sick. I was so relieved when my oncologist explained to me the variety of drugs available to cancer patients: steroids, diuretics, and anti-nausea pills, to name a few. If all else failed, she could even prescribe medicinal marijuana!

Suddenly, I had visions of myself in a long, flowing skirt, my arms weighed down with bangles, puffing contentedly on a joint as I listened to Bob Marley tunes. I even briefly considered getting the peace symbol tattooed on my ankle. However, my daughter Kaitlyn put an abrupt end to my fantasies when she said, "Mom, don't even think about trying to be one of those COOL cancer patients. You can't pull it off." And so, my friends, I am sad to say that while the use of medicinal marijuana is a perk of having cancer, for me it was a missed perk. Although I do think I AM cool enough to pull it off!

Cancer treatments can have some nasty side effects, but there is no need to suffer in silence. Explore with your doctor the many options available to ease unpleasant symptoms and side effects.

HEALTH TIP #13
No Rolling Papers? Try Ginger for Nausea Relief

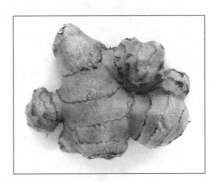

Marijuana is not the only botanical that can help ease chemo side effects. My "nondrug" of choice was ginger!

The Chinese names for ginger, gan jiang (dried ginger) and sheng jiang (fresh ginger), mean "to defend," suggesting that ginger helps to defend or protect the body from ailments. In modern China, ginger is used in almost half of all Chinese herbal prescriptions. Herbalists believe that even modest amounts of ginger in the diet can strengthen the lungs and kidneys, and it is a proven anti-inflammatory. The body's own response to inflammation is the root cause of many chronic illnesses like heart disease, diabetes, and cancer. So "anti" inflammatory agents, such as ginger, are good for the body. (And with the way ginger tastes, your mouth won't mind either.)

Ginger ale consumption on airplanes is always high. One theory among flight attendants is that people have found that it relieves motion sickness and settles the stomach. (During my chemo-run, never was I seen without my ginger ale in hand!) Researchers agree. *The Lancet*, a well-known medical journal, reported that consuming ginger before a long flight was equally as effective as taking the most popular pharmaceutical treatment, dimenhydrinate (Dramamine), at preventing motion sickness. Luckily, ginger is one root that is easily found in markets, either as a whole root or in powder form. Given the choice of taking a natural, delicious-tasting root or a drug, I would hope that choice would be a no-brainer.

There are many ways to "get your ginger on." You can sip ginger tea, suck on ginger candy, eat ginger cookies, or drink ginger ale.

My favorite way to eat this delicious root is in soup. This quick and easy carrot ginger soup really relieves any kind of stomach upset, provides healing antioxidant vitamins A and C, and was a staple during my chemotherapy treatment:

> Ginger is a useful, natural, and yummy way to help with nausea. But don't wait until you feel sick to try this delicious cancer-fighting food.

CARROT GINGER SOUP

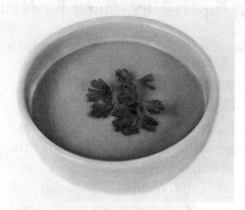

YIELD: 8 CUPS

2 tablespoons extra-virgin organic olive oil (EVOOO)

1 medium onion, peeled and chopped

6 cups vegetable broth (organic if possible)

2 pounds of carrots, peeled and roughly sliced (organic if possible)

2 to 3 tablespoons grated fresh ginger*

1 cup almond or coconut milk (coconut is creamier)

Sea salt and white pepper, to taste

Parsley sprigs, for garnish (if you're a garnisher)

*Fresh is always better, but powdered or in a tube will work too.
If using powdered, use $1^1/_2$ tablespoons.

Directions:

In a 6-quart pot, heat oil and onions over medium heat, cooking and stirring until onions are limp and transparent (about 10 minutes). Add broth, carrots, and ginger. Cover and bring to a boil. Reduce heat and simmer until carrots are tender when pierced with a fork (about 13 to 15 minutes).

Remove from heat, let sit for 10 minutes, and then transfer to a blender. Be careful! Don't fill the blender more than halfway. It may take several batches to do it this way, but when you are blending hot foods, there is a real danger of heat explosion (and with that comes a huge mess). Leave the hole in the lid to the blender open, and loosely hold a dishtowel over the opening to allow the steam to escape. Pulse the blender a few times before letting it run on "puree." Puree all contents until very smooth, and return to the pot. (You can use an immersion or hand blender, if you wish; just blend very well until smooth. There should be no visible pieces.)

Add your choice of plant-based milk and stir over high heat until almost boiling. Add sea salt and pepper, to taste. Ladle into bowls and garnish with parsley (if so desired).

This soup also freezes well. I find this soup tastes even better to me when it's not very hot, just warm. Medicine never tasted so good!

NUTRITION PER 1 CUP SERVING:

Using whole coconut milk: Calories: 150; Protein: 1 gram; Carbs: 6 grams; Fat: 9.5 grams; Sodium: 705 milligrams

Using almond or low-fat coconut milk: Calories: approx. 120; Protein: 1 gram; Carbs: 6 grams; Fat: 4 grams; Sodium: 705 milligrams

1 serving, either way, also has more than 300% of your RDA for vitamin A, a powerful antioxidant and cancer fighter.

Note: Reduce your sodium to almost zero by making your own vegetable broth without salt, or cut the sodium in half by using half broth and half water in the recipe.

I Didn't Have to Worry About My Guests Finding a Hair in the Food I Prepared

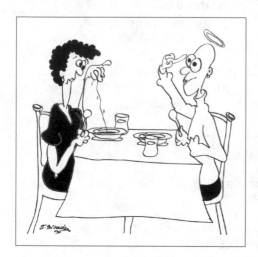

When I first learned that I would be "on chemo," I wasn't exactly sure what "on chemo" meant. I knew that I would be sick, and I would lose my hair, but as to how this chemo would be administered was a mystery to me. Would I have to get it every day? Would I be sick for the entire four months?

Although it was not pleasant by any stretch of the imagination, it was not quite as bad as I had envisioned. While treatments differ depending on the type of cancer, I received a total of six rounds of chemo. Each IV (intravenous) treatment lasted about four hours, and treatments were spaced three weeks apart. Basically, for a week to ten days following a treatment, I was knocked on my arse—well, more accurately, my back. Then I'd feel myself start to come around and, thankfully, for the last week, I usually felt well enough to live a normal-ish lifestyle. I took advantage of my "good week" to do things with my kids, spend time with my boyfriend Shawn, and try to repay my support team in some small way for all the fabulous stuff they did for me!

During one of my good days, as I was preparing a meal for a few of my friends, I instinctively reached for my apron and hair net. Then I laughed. Getting a hair in the food I was preparing was one less thing I had to worry about. And if someone happened to find one, I could innocently say, "Hey, it's not mine!"

This may be a small perk, but it was enough to make me laugh. It is good to appreciate the humor in situations such as this.

HEALTH TIP #14   Appreciate Your Liver

As I write this, I am "detoxing" right now. (Are you getting a visual?) So are you. Part of the process of your body's metabolism is the excretion of toxins. (Just look in the toilet, and you'll see some.) But there are also toxins outside your body like pollution, radioactive particles, UV rays, pesticides in food, contaminates in water, and chemical exposure from personal-care products that bombard your system every day. All toxins are harmful to you, and your efficient body is constantly trying to expel these toxins to maintain health and prevent illness. And it all goes on, completely unnoticed, while you go about your daily routines like going to work or picking up the kids from school.

If you are overexposed to toxins and your body can't keep up with clearance, or if you have unhealthy intestines or a tired liver, your body will be unable to clear these poisons from your system. That can open you up to a breakdown of proper functioning called "illness" or "disease."

"Detoxing" is a hot topic right now, and there are many people on the Internet and on TV who would love you to believe that, to rid your body of toxins, you need to buy their product so you can detox quickly and have instant health. They promise you that you will feel great, lose 20 pounds, and have more energy than a five-year-old at Disneyworld. And you'll have it in three days! News flash: You can't change your entire health in three days. But you *can* make the decision to change and start taking the first steps toward that change in three days.

Proper detox can only happen if you have two body parts in perfect working order: your intestines and your liver. Without healthy pipes (bowels) and a healthy filter (liver), your body is unable to process contaminates that attack us around the clock. The health of these organs is even more important when going through chemo as it is up to your liver to metabolize those huge doses of chemotherapy drugs. Having an unhealthy liver and colon can lead to toxins collecting in your brain and fat cells, and circulating through your entire body causing chronic illness and disease.

An **unhealthy person** allows toxins to enter his or her body through:

- smoking

- processed, high-sugar, high-chemical foods

- chemicals in their environment, like BPA from plastics or chlorine in their water
- pesticides in their foods
- pharmaceuticals
- chemicals in their personal-care products

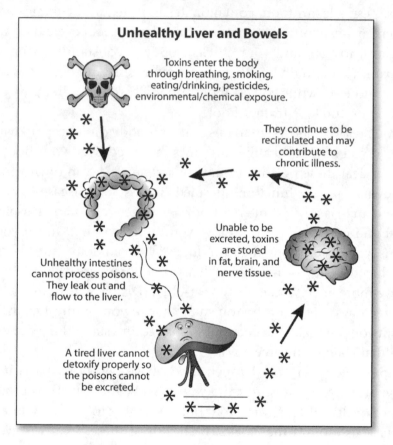

Unhealthy Liver and Bowels

Toxins enter the body through breathing, smoking, eating/drinking, pesticides, environmental/chemical exposure.

They continue to be recirculated and may contribute to chronic illness.

Unable to be excreted, toxins are stored in fat, brain, and nerve tissue.

Unhealthy intestines cannot process poisons. They leak out and flow to the liver.

A tired liver cannot detoxify properly so the poisons cannot be excreted.

A **healthy person** is someone who:

- eats clean, whole, nonprocessed foods, with no chemicals
- limits pesticide exposure in foods
- exercises regularly
- limits unnecessary pharmaceutical use

- drinks plenty of dechlorinated pure water
- is conscious of toxins in the home

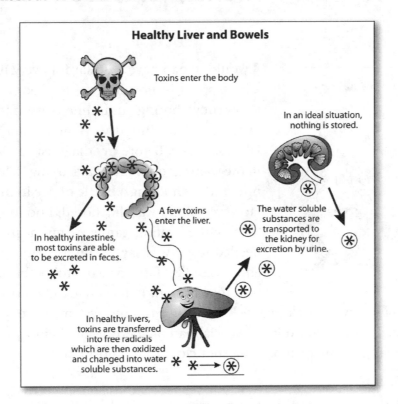

Healthy Liver and Bowels

Toxins enter the body

In an ideal situation, nothing is stored.

A few toxins enter the liver.

The water soluble substances are transported to the kidney for excretion by urine.

In healthy intestines, most toxins are able to be excreted in feces.

In healthy livers, toxins are transferred into free radicals which are then oxidized and changed into water soluble substances.

You can fix your intestines by fixing your diet and your lifestyle. For example, eating a whole food plant-based diet and meditating every day promotes healthy intestines, which results in healthy pooping, which, in turn, results in a healthier you!

It's a bit overwhelming when you realize you need to change the habits you've grown accustomed to for many years, so you may be tempted to look for quick and easy solutions in this category. But the real "health" will come from a lifestyle committed to clean, whole foods, adequate water intake, exercise, a relaxed mind, and avoiding chemicals . . . not from an enema bag or a three-day "cleanse."

> Don't look to a detox kit for your answer to health. Instead, change your lifestyle and make long-term investments you can bank on. Remember, according to the Tao proverb, the longest journey begins with a single step.

I Got Fast-Tracked for Blood Work

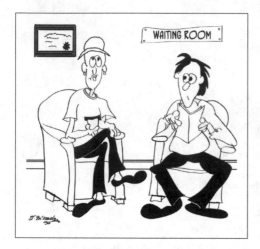

I would like to have a dollar for every minute I have spent in hospital waiting rooms. We all know how boring and time-consuming it is waiting to have blood work and other routine lab tests done. Before my diagnosis, I would sit in the waiting room for hours, trying to look dignified while holding a bottle of pee in my hand. However, after I was diagnosed, I no longer had to play the waiting game. At my hospital all I needed to do was say, "I am a chemo patient," and I would get fast-tracked. I think the rationale was that they didn't want us chemo patients hanging out with "sick people" since our immune systems were low. Hey, it worked for me! I also had a special parking permit for chemo patients so that I was guaranteed a parking spot close to the hospital.

Use your chemo status to your advantage. Find out if your hospital will fast-track your routine lab tests, or give preferred parking. If you are forced to wait, use your time wisely. Bring an inspirational book to read, listen to your favorite tunes, or do a meditation.

HEALTH TIP #15
Even Ironman Needs Iron

As you're watching the blood pour into that glass tube from your arm, think about this: Your blood is pretty cool. Blood plasma is the river that everything floats in; white blood cells attack germs; platelets help you to form clots when you cut yourself; and red blood cells carry oxygen to every cell of your body to support life. All of that is going on every day inside you.

The components of blood all work together to keep you going, but it's the red blood cells, in my humble opinion, that are the true "super cells." When red blood cells don't work, it affects every system in your body. *Anemia* is the term for "tired red blood cells." What would make these super-cells slump? Two reasons are chemotherapy and radiation, as chemo attacks healthy red blood cells and radiation attacks the factory (bone marrow) where the red blood cells are made. (Damn those treatments.) Luckily, once the treatments are over, your anemia should continue to improve.

Another cause of anemia is low iron.

Iron is necessary for the production of the oxygen-carrying part of red cells. Low iron equals low oxygen equals one tired and depressed person. It is especially important for those undergoing treatment for cancer to eat a balanced diet high in iron-rich foods to top off iron stores during and after treatment.

And, um, no, I won't tell you to eat liver.

The general population equates "meat" with "high-iron" foods. But iron is present in countless numbers of fruits, vegetables, beans, nuts, and legumes as well. In fact, one cup of oatmeal has more iron (10 milligrams per cup) than three ounces of beef liver (7.5 milligrams).

Animal-based foods and plant-based foods have different kinds of iron. Iron from animal sources is called heme iron while plant-based sources have non-heme iron. They're both iron, but heme iron is absorbed at a higher percentage than non-heme, so you don't need as much of it to meet the daily requirements. That can be good *and* bad. Iron is recycled from old red blood cells stored in your body, and it's not excreted. Too much iron causes oxidation leading to heart disease and cancer. One study showed that lung cancer rates were 300 percent higher in red-meat eaters than abstainers, and another study showed that 88 percent of metastasized breast cancer patients had elevated iron levels. In today's society we are seeing more iron *overload* issues than iron deficiencies among meat eaters. Symptoms of high iron can include heart palpitations, joint pain, and fatigue.

Plant-based foods, on the other hand, contain non-heme iron. Less of the iron you eat is absorbed, but if you are eating a well-balanced five fruit/veggie serving a day, you will get all of your iron without the iron overload. You can also increase your absorption of nonheme iron by cooking in cast-iron pots and pans and including foods high in vitamin C like citrus, berries, and peppers with the meal. Yes, throw some mandarin oranges and red peppers (high vitamin C) into your spinach salad (high iron) to kick-start the iron absorption! Just for fun, here's a comparison of iron contents from animal- and plant-based sources:

Animal sources:
3 ounces of beef tenderloin = 3 milligrams of iron
3 ounces of chicken breast = 1.1 milligrams of iron

Plant-based sources:
1 cup boiled black beans = 3.6 milligrams of iron
1 cup lentils = 6.6 milligrams of iron
1 cup cooked spinach = 5 milligrams of iron
2 ounces pumpkin seeds = 8.4 milligrams of iron

I could go on for days. . . .

The daily requirement of iron for women not pregnant or lactating is 18 milligrams per day. Over age fifty-one? Cut that in half as older folks (I said *old-er* . . . not *old*) don't excrete iron as fast as youngsters do.

Some other foods that will help you keep your stores at the proper level are dandelions, almonds, whole-grain bread, peas, all beans, kale, apricots, dates, and many more.

Note: Don't ever take iron pills or vitamins containing iron unless you have had your blood levels checked for deficiency. Extra iron in pill form is not extra healthy.

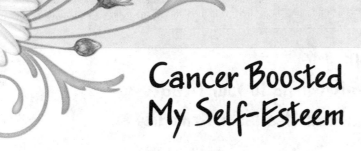

Cancer Boosted My Self-Esteem

As a child, I was the poster child for low self-esteem. I was painfully shy, anxious, and could not shake the feeling that I was just not quite good enough. This feeling continued into my early adulthood. Even in my first job as a teacher, I was desperately lacking confidence despite having graduated from university with honors degrees. Over the years, my self-confidence and self-esteem slowly improved; however, never have they been better than since my diagnosis of cancer.

You must be wondering, how can cancer possibly *boost* my self-esteem? Well, since facing this challenge, I have gotten so many words of encouragement and praise from people I know (and even some I don't know), such as:

- "You are such an inspiration."

- "You are the strongest woman I've ever met."

- "You are the most positive person I know."

- "If anyone can beat this thing, it is YOU."

It kind of took me by surprise to learn that other people perceive me in this way. I really did not see myself as being strong, inspirational, or more positive than the next person. Hearing these words of encouragement made me see myself in a whole new light. (Good thing I have two teenagers to keep my ego in check.)

When people tell you positive things about yourself, BELIEVE them. They are not just making it up because you have cancer; they are just more comfortable saying it to you at that time.

HEALTH TIP #16
All That Praise Going to Your Head?
Try Some Natural Headache Remedies

Headaches are one of the most common pains that make people reach for the pill bottle. Being a cancer survivor, I can't help but have just a little smidge of worry when I get a headache. But then I remind myself that headaches are very common and having one headache does not mean I am headed for the MRI machine.

The most common headaches are muscle tension–related from necks being asked to stay in one position (like when you're on the computer too long). But headaches can also be due to lack of sleep, high blood pressure, sinus pressure, dehydration, hormonal shift, or needing a new eyeglasses prescription.

Only a small number of headaches are serious. If any of the following apply to you, head to your nearest emergency room or call your healthcare provider:

- You develop a new persistent headache (especially if you have a history of cancer).

- You experience an abrupt, severe headache, which may be like a thunder-clap.

- Your headache is accompanied by a fever, stiff neck, confusion, seizures, double vision, weakness, numbness, nausea, or speaking difficulties.

- The headache occurs after a head injury, especially if the headache gets worse.

- You have a chronic, progressive headache that is precipitated by coughing, exertion, straining, or a sudden movement.

- You have a headache that becomes more frequent and is not easily relieved by pain medication.

Most headaches will respond to pain relievers like acetaminophen or ibuprofen. (However, use them wisely as overuse can actually *cause* headaches.) But before you reach for the pill bottle, why not try some of these natural cures first?

- Turn up the heat! Heat relaxes muscles and can take the edge off a tension headache. Try a heated neck wrap or towel or hop in a warm bath or shower.

- Cool it down! Some headaches respond to ice packs, especially on the forehead or the back of the neck. Remember to wrap your ice source in a cloth or towel before applying.

- Water me down! Dehydration is a common but often overlooked cause of headaches. Make sure you're drinking enough water: at least 50 to 64 ounces (1.5 to 2 liters) per day. Try getting in four 8-ounce glasses before lunch, but don't forget to continue water consumption throughout the day to stay hydrated.

- Stick it to me! Acupuncture can be effective for recurring chronic headaches (after your doctor has made sure there is not a serious cause). Always find a certified acupuncture therapist.

- Rub me the right way! Massage, whether it is by your partner or done professionally, is a great way to relieve muscle tension. (Especially if it leads to a happy ending, which can actually relieve headaches as well.)

- Get minty fresh! The scent of peppermint has been shown to relieve pain. Keep some peppermint tea on hand or spritz some peppermint water (hydrosol) on your face when a headache hits, or place 2 to 3 drops of peppermint essential oil on a cloth (like a washcloth) and place the cloth on your forehead while lying down to breathe in the scent.

> Try some natural, healthy remedies to help your next headache.

- Use pressure to relieve pressure! Acupressure is the method of stimulating certain points on your body to bring pain relief to certain other parts. To relieve tension headaches, massage your temples and between your eyes.

Another pressure point is the fleshy part between your thumb and first finger or between your first and second toes. A skilled acupressure therapist can show you the right way to get results.

- Breathe! Practice some deep breathing to help you relax. Sitting comfortably, take a slow, deep breath in, hold it for two seconds, and slowly release. Try visualizing the breath in as going straight to your headache and the breath out as blowing your pain away. (That's called *visualization*.)

Your headaches don't have to be a pain in the neck . . . or anywhere else if you know what to do to relieve them.

Cancer Helped Me Discover New Beauty Tips

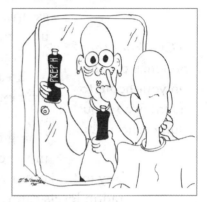

One of the many unpleasant side effects of chemo is puffiness around the eyes. When you have several liters of chemicals pumped into your body, it has to go somewhere. Imagine my dismay when I awoke one morning to find bags the size of shopping bags hanging beneath my eyes. And to make matters worse, my boyfriend Shawn was on his way to visit me!

I searched through my bag of creams and serums to find a solution, but none looked promising. Then I spotted the Preparation H, and I remembered a tip I had read in a beauty magazine. Hey, it works to shrink hemorrhoids, so I decided to give it a try. The puffiness disappeared right in the nick of time, just as Shawn was arriving at the door. I noticed his nostrils flare a little as he leaned in to kiss me. Hey, I may have smelled like an ass, but I looked darn good! (Disclaimer: Do not, and I repeat, do NOT try this at home—but if you choose to ignore my warning, then be careful not to get it in your eyes.)

Just because you have cancer does not mean you can't look good—
especially when you are greeting a welcome houseguest!

HEALTH TIP #17
Get Rid of an Unwelcome Houseguest

We all know that the leading cause of lung cancer deaths is smoking. But the second leading cause of lung cancer might surprise you. It's radon.

Radon is a radioactive gas that is in the environment all the time. You are probably breathing it in right now, but it is in such small doses that your body can handle it.

Sometimes, small cracks in your home in the floors, walls, and foundation can allow high levels of radon from the soil under your house to leak into your home and accumulate there. Homes that are tightly sealed with lots of insulation are at higher risk because the gas stagnates and can't escape. You and your family then end up living with this unwanted guest, being exposed to radon for months and months.

Breathing in radon damages the lining of the lungs. Long-term exposure increases cancer risk. The lung cancer risk is much higher in those who are exposed to radon *and* who smoke. Going outside at night to see if your house is the one glowing in the dark is not the way to detect radioactive radon. The only way to find out if your home is radioactive is to get a radon test kit. Because radon levels can vary with things like the weather, testing needs to be over a period of time. Some tests measure the radon for up to ninety days and store the information so it can then be sent to a lab to be analyzed. You can also have a professional test your home. It is estimated that in the United States, one out of fifteen homes has unhealthy radon levels.

> Check for the presence of radon in your home to identify a serious lung cancer risk.

To fix the problem, the cracks or openings allowing the radon to enter your home are sealed. There are companies that specialize in this type of work.

Unlike your obnoxious Aunt Gladys, radon is one houseguest you don't have to tolerate. For more information go to www.epa.gov/radon or www.hc-sc.gc.ca and search "radon."

People Were Nicer to Me

When people found out I had cancer, EVERYONE suddenly became nicer to me! Friends and family came out of the woodwork to cook, clean, and help out with the kids. This was especially the case after I lost my hair and began to "look" the part of a cancer patient. As an added bonus, when I wore a hat or other headdress that gave away my baldness, even strangers were super nice to me, giving up their parking spots, letting me go ahead of them in lines, and dishing out the compliments like crazy. For a while there, I thought every guy in the supermarket was hitting on me. But alas, it wasn't me; it was my bandana that was attracting the attention.

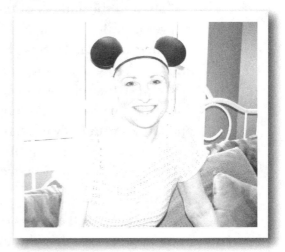

Goofing around with my baldness.

I will admit, though, at first I did not appreciate all of that attention. I felt as though people were looking at me with pity, and the last thing I wanted was to be pitied! One day while lined up at the supermarket check-out, I had a conversation that changed my perspective. An older gentleman very nicely asked about my condition and then proceeded to tell me about his wife who had been diagnosed with breast cancer twenty years earlier and was still doing well. He wished me all the best and said that he would pray for my recovery.

> Nearly everyone has their own story of how cancer affected their lives, which allows them to empathize with yours.

What I recognized in this man was not pity, but rather empathy. Because of his own experience with cancer, he could sympathize with mine. Following that conversation, when I noticed people looking at me differently, I no longer felt as if I was being pitied. Instead, I considered that those people might have had their own story of how cancer affected their lives, which allowed them to relate to mine. They really were just being nice.

HEALTH TIP #18
It's Nice to Be Nice . . . to the Nice

Can being nice to someone actually be healthy? According to several studies, and the authors of the book, *The Healing Power of Doing Good*, the answer is yes!

There are actually researchers who study the effects of kind acts on health and well-being. They find, time after time, that being good is good for you. When you are helping someone else, you are unable to focus on yourself and your own stress-provoking thought patterns. This breaks the stress cycle and allows your body to relax and focus on just that one thing. Helping, in some cases, is like a form of meditation.

Some of the positive effects of lending a hand are:

- Getting a "helper's high," which is a rush of euphoria followed by calmness similar to the effects of meditation. This produces the same kind of endorphins (our body's natural painkiller and feel-good chemicals) that you get with exercise. (A runner's high without the run!)

- reducing feelings of despair and isolation by providing hope, not just to the one helped, but to you as well

- improving depression and symptoms of depression, such as lethargy, insomnia, and chronic pain

- increasing your immune response

You can also choose to be a volunteer in an organization to help a group of others. Volunteering in a group setting has the extra benefits of:

- increasing social and relationship skills by connecting with others in a positive setting (Who knows, you might even meet your special someone!)

- helping you to be more outgoing

- increasing self-confidence

- showing your kids that you can make a positive change with your actions when volunteering as a family

- learning job skills and improving your career (Habitat for Humanity taught me how to use a nail gun without shooting myself in the foot.)

- providing fun and fulfillment (When volunteering at a community garden, you literally get to "reap" the benefits of your work.)

It's hard to allow people to do things for you. When I was in the midst of my chemo treatment, accepting help meant admitting I *needed* help. I was raised to be self-sufficient and self-reliant and taking help meant I was "weak" and "needy." But I realized (very quickly) how nice it was to have that hot meal ready or get my groceries delivered to my front door. It was not only nice—it was needed. And that didn't make me weak or needy. It just made me human.

> You don't need an excuse to be nice, but getting healthier is a nice one!

By allowing people to be nice to you, you are actually doing THEM a favor. Now consider the many ways you can be nice to others by allowing them to be nice to you. The next time someone says, "Let me know if there is anything I can do to help," have your list ready:

❑ Cook a meal.

❑ Help with housework.

❑ Watch your kids for a while.

❑ Pick up prescriptions.

❑ Mow your lawn.

❑ Walk your dog.

❑ Drive you to and from appointments.

❑ Sit with you through a chemo.

❑ Pick up groceries.

❑ Pick up your mail.

❑ Run errands.

Allowing others to help is helpful in more ways than you realize. For more information on the specifics of feeling good while doing good, check out *The Healing Power of Doing Good: The Health and Spiritual Benefits of Helping Others,* by Allan Luks and Peggy Payne [iUniverse.com, Inc., 2001].

An Excuse to Escape Dish Duty

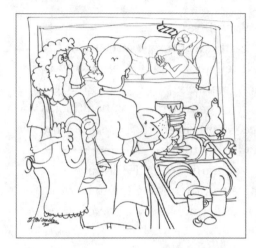

While I love big family dinners, I hate the cleanup afterward. I hate it so much, in fact, that I have earned myself the nickname "Eat and Run." I don't pride myself on being afflicted with the eat-and-run syndrome, but when that turkey coma kicks in, I fall victim. As I shamefacedly slept off those extra calories, I am sure that snide remarks were being made behind my back about my dirty-dish avoidance. But that was before cancer. Even when I half-heartedly offered to help with the dishes after my diagnosis, I just got shooed away to a welcoming couch. I almost felt sorry for my sister, Sherry, one Sunday when she hinted about her hysterectomy in an attempt to escape dish duty. But, hey, by that time, it had been seven weeks since her surgery; she'd milked that baby for all it was worth! Now me, on the other hand, I figured I could probably get another year out of my situation if I played my cards right. Christmas dinner at Mom's that year was never so relaxing.

Cancer gives you a ready-made excuse to avoid dish duty.

HEALTH TIP #19
Need Another Excuse? Think About the Toxins

Are you sick of loading and unloading the dishwasher? Well the truth is, it might be the dish soap that's making you sick. The chemicals in your dish soap may get your dishes squeaky clean, but do you really need toxic chemicals to do the job? Whether you are washing the dishes by hand or loading them into a dishwasher, the dishwashing product you use may contain substances that are harmful to your health. Here are three of the most common and the most dangerous toxins found in dish detergent:

Triclosan

Triclosan is a chemical antibacterial agent that is widely used in dish detergent and hand soap as well as children's toys, clothing, deodorants, and even toothpaste. This "germ fighter" may be killing more than just unwanted bacteria. Triclosan is absorbed through the skin and remains in your body for up to twelve hours. There is evidence that triclosan can find its way to your fat cells where it can accumulate and interfere with the body's thyroid metabolism. (Your thyroid regulates a multitude of body functions.) Even the American Medical Association issued a statement at their annual meeting that "the use of common antimicrobials (triclosan) . . . as ingredients in consumer products should be discontinued." It is noted to be a highly potent allergen, causing dermatitis and worsening asthma. Triclosan is also among over 200 chemicals found in umbilical cord blood of newborns in the United States.

In 2012, the U.S. Environmental Protection Agency (EPA) began studying the harmful effects of triclosan due to excessive reports of toxic side effects and growing research that cite hormone related effects especially to the thyroid gland. They plan to review the registration process for this chemical (to possibly reclassify it as harmful) in 2013, but it may not be until 2015 until this is completed.

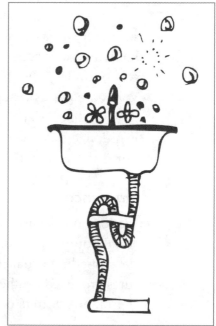

Triclosan is also devastating to the environment. As it washes out from the drains into the water systems, it destroys the bacteria that maintains the delicate biological balance of rivers, lakes, and streams, and kills fish and other vital water plants. It also reacts with the chlorine as it goes through the water treatment facilities and forms new cancer-causing compounds as it comes into your home and out of your faucets. Because of this, many governmental water-management agencies are calling for widespread reductions in public triclosan use. In March 2013, Minnesota announced that their state agencies will no longer purchase any products containing triclosan.

Yes, you don't want germs on your dishes, but using plain ol' soap without the fancy chemical germinators kills them just as effectively.

Bleach

Chlorine bleach is found in most automatic dishwashing detergents, but it is highly unnecessary. Bleach (real name: sodium hypochlorite) is a disinfectant found in cleaners for use throughout the house. It's cheap, and the "bleach-y" smell makes us think that things are really so very germ-free. But do we really need something that kills 99 percent of viruses for your dishes?

Chlorine bleach is a potent irritant to your skin. If you've ever gotten bleach on your skin you notice that your skin feels slippery. That's the chemical reaction you're feeling as the bleach pulls the oils from inside your skin up to the surface.

There is also evidence that the use of chlorine in the household forms several toxic gasses such as chloroform and carbon tetrachloride, which are known carcinogens. These gasses fall into the category of volatile organic compounds (VOCs). Created by the mixing or breakdown of chemicals, VOCs are gasses that we breathe every day in our homes.

Hey, battery acid is a dangerous chemical classified as a corrosive. Bleach is a dangerous chemical classified as a corrosive. What is bleach doing in our dish detergent?

Fragrance

We love our soaps to smell like anything but soap, don't we? Gentle rain, floral bouquet, citrus squeeze. The manufacturers know their stuff and have developed a virtual cornucopia of scents to delight us. The chemical mixtures are listed on the label as "fragrance," but because of lax labeling laws, the manufacturers don't have to tell us which chemicals are contained in said "fragrance." Most "fragrance" contains synthetics like formaldehyde, benzene, and toluene—all carcinogens. Until current labeling laws are changed, there is just no way of knowing how many carcinogens you are being exposed to during dish duty.

Don't you just love chemistry? So what do we do now that we've thrown away all our dish detergent? Luckily, companies like Seventh Generation and the Honest Company have found ways to produce dish detergents and cleaners that are safe and effective. Just look for ingredient labels to be plainly printed on the bottle and avoid the three bad ones just mentioned. Beware when you don't see ingredients clearly disclosed or see labels that say "made with natural ingredients," as this could mean 1 percent of the product is natural and 99 percent isn't.

If you hand wash your dishes, just use plain castile soap. (Find liquid castile soap in the natural or "organic soap" section of your market.) Liquid castile soap is made with plant oils, usually coconut, castor oils, and others, and can come in many scents. I love Dr. Bronner's liquid castile soaps (www.drbronners.com), as they come naturally scented with essential oils. (Essential oils come from plants and are not made from chemicals in a lab.) With scents like peppermint and eucalyptus, who needs chemistry?

Note: Even when you are using "natural" soaps you should always wear gloves when washing dishes to avoid any potential irritation or skin reaction.

If you use an automatic dishwasher, use safe detergent without chlorine bleach and synthetic fragrance. You can boost the cleaning power of any detergent by sprinkling several tablespoons of simple baking soda (sodium bicarbonate) over the dishes before you hit the start button. (You really can't "overdo" using baking soda as it dissolves in the water to make the water "soft" so the detergents and soaps work better.)

For a homemade automatic dishwashing detergent, you can use this recipe from www.diynatural.com:

- 1 cup Borax (natural mineral; buy in most grocery stores in laundry section)

- 1 cup washing soda (sodium carbonate; found in laundry section)

- $1/2$ cup powdered citric acid (from citrus foods; buy online or in health food stores)

- $1/2$ cup kosher salt (table salt can also be used, but kosher salt has no chemicals)

Mix everything in an airtight container and use about 2 tablespoons per load in the main washing cup. (I sometimes add just a dash to the prewash cup as well.) I've used this recipe, and I love it. Keep it in a tightly sealed container and away from moisture. Every area that you can eliminate toxins from in your environment is a victory for your health.

Clean up your act by switching to a
natural detergent soap for your dishes
to avoid needless chemical exposure.

Cancer Helped Me to Stop and Smell the Roses

One of the more pleasant perks of having cancer was having quality time to spend with my dog, Patches. I recall walking Patches one beautiful fall day, the sky was cloudless, and there was just enough chill in the air to put a spring in my step. On my walk, I noticed some late-season wild roses in bloom, and I took the time to literally stop and smell the roses. Their heavenly scent seemed to fill my body with a healing vibration.

Before cancer, I probably would not have taken the opportunity to go outside and enjoy such a perfect day. Even if I was not at work, I would be looking around the house at the mounds of laundry, mutant dust bunnies, and stacks of unopened mail all vying for my attention. But that day I said, "The housework will always be here, but this beautiful day won't. I'm taking Patches for a walk!" And I am glad I did. The following day was a chemo day, and I knew that over the following week or so, I would draw upon that pleasant memory many times to help me through the rough days, and I did.

Even if you do not feel well enough to take a walk, get outside and enjoy the fresh air. There is something about being outdoors that revs the spirit and makes you happy just to be alive.

HEALTH TIP #20
When on a Nature Walk, Don't Forget the Blackberry

Leave your phones at home, because I'm talking about the superfruits. Blackberries may just be my favorite weapon against cancer. Most varieties of berries contain the same healthy benefits. Mainly, they are all very high in antioxidants and specific plant-based, cancer-fighting chemicals. The antioxidants in berries make it easier for our body to process the toxins we come in contact with every day and protect our immunity. Also contained in that succulent little fruit are substances like quercetin and ellagic acid, which may have direct tumor-killing actions. Animal studies conducted at the Ohio State University Comprehensive Cancer Center show that a diet consisting of 10 percent black raspberries slowed tumor growth. The results of the animal study were so dramatic that funding was secured to study the effect of the berries on people with esophageal cancer.

Eating blackberries . . . that's my kind of research trial!

Researchers say the key lies in the combination of cancer-fighting substances in the berries. Berries contain more than ten different substances that can fight or protect from cancer. The belief 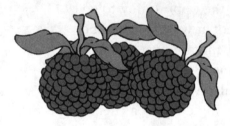 is that it's not one particular part of the blackberry that fights the cancer, but it's the action of the different substances working together that have the cancer-killing effect when eaten as a whole food, which is a good argument for focusing your cancer-fighting efforts by eating healthy foods rather than relying on too many supplements.

In the news recently, there has been the suggestion that taking aspirin may have some protective qualities from certain types of cancer. Interestingly, berries contain salicylic acid, the same anti-inflammatory component in aspirin that is believed to protect from cancer. It won't be long before doctors are saying, "Take two pints of berries and call me in the morning."

Any berry has benefits, but to get your money's worth, look for the darkest colors, like the blackberry, blueberry, and cranberry. Organic is always better because the pesticides can settle into the nooks and crannies of the berry and be hard to wash off, but don't let that stop you from enjoying them. The benefits of those gorgeous juicy morsels far outweigh the negative pesticide effects.

Freeze-dried berries are great to have around to throw into shakes or cereals, and you don't have to worry about them going bad or being mushy.

Berries are also great in recipes. Try this blueberry salad dressing for a healthy change from fatty, boring ranch:

BLUEBERRY DRESSING

YIELD: 1 CUP OF DRESSING

$1/2$ cup frozen or fresh blueberries

$1/4$ cup agave nectar

1 tablespoon balsamic vinegar

Black pepper, to taste

1 tablespoon soy sauce

$1/4$ cup extra-virgin olive oil

Serving size: 2 tablespoons

Each serving has 72 calories
and 6.7 grams of fat

Wash blueberries (if fresh) or let defrost in fridge according to package directions if frozen. Blend blueberries, agave, vinegar, pepper, and soy sauce in a blender till smooth. After ingredients are blended into a smooth liquid, set blender on slow speed and slowly drizzle in the oil to emulsify. Serve on a healthy salad of dark greens, nuts, seeds, veggies, and fruit. (Courtesy of Healthful Habits, Inc.)

Hippocrates said, "Let food be your medicine, and medicine be your food." So be sure to include cancer-fighting berries in your diet whenever you can!

I Didn't Have to Buy a Halloween Costume

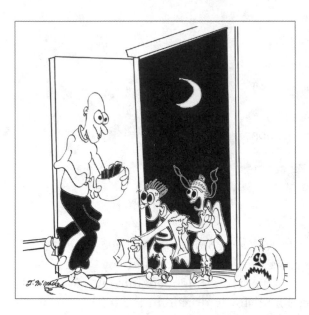

I love Halloween, but I often agonize about finding the perfect costume. I love to see the look on the children's faces when I open the door wearing my costume to hand out treats. Some years I would go the scary route and dress up as a wicked witch or a bloodthirsty vampire. Other years I would pretty myself up as a garden fairy or a blue butterfly. My all-time best costume, however, was when I had cancer and I didn't dress up at all! I ask you solemnly, is there anything scarier looking than a bald, middle-aged woman?

Work with what you've got! Go bald and attach some pointy ears for a very realistic space alien look; wear a diaper and carry a baby bottle; or paint your head to look like a Jack-O-Lantern. The possibilities are endless.

HEALTH TIP #21
Blood Is Fun on Halloween, but Not in Your Morning Routine

I wasn't trying to rhyme, but if it helps you to remember this health tip when you're brushing your teeth, then all the better! Blood in the sink after you brush is the telltale sign of unhealthy gums. Other signs of gum disease or *gingivitis* are gum redness, swelling, and tenderness. It's estimated that about 78 percent of people have some signs of gum disease. It's probably no big news flash that daily flossing will reduce your risk of gum disease, but what you may not know is that flossing can prevent heart disease, stroke, and possibly even cancer as well. Skeptics, please read on.

Dental floss, when used correctly, disturbs the colonies of bacteria that live in between your teeth and gums. (Disgusting, isn't it?) Bacteria can enter your bloodstream through your gums at any time, but it's more likely to happen if your gums are inflamed, as in gum disease. Once bacteria finds its way into your blood, it can settle on the inner walls of your arteries anywhere in your body. If it decides to settle in the very tiny arteries, like the ones that feed your heart muscle with blood, it can have serious consequences. Over time, and through a series of events, this could cause the arteries to narrow, cutting off the blood supply to your heart muscle and eventually causing a heart attack.

A heart attack from ignoring your dental hygienist sounds like a stretch, but studies show that those with heart disease had high levels of bacteria in their mouths. Many factors affect your risk for heart disease, from your genetics to what you eat. But the thought is, if a high level of bacteria in your mouth is associated with heart disease, then reducing the bacteria might reduce your risk of heart disease.

Another part of the story involves a blood chemical called C-reactive protein (CRP). The liver produces CRP in response to any inflammatory process going on in the body. The presence of CRP leads to the production of chemicals and enzymes that might act on the lining of the artery wall, which can lead to the narrowing of that artery. Depending on where the artery is, it can eventually cause a stroke or heart attack.

It is unclear whether the high CRP is a result of the gum disease or the heart disease is caused by other factors, so it's a classic case of "who dunnit." But there are several studies that do show, without a doubt, that those who have gum disease also show thickening of the walls of the arteries. This has been shown across the board in those who do not have any other risk factors for heart disease such as smoking or high cholesterol.

So what does this have to do with cancer, you ask?

In a study that followed 2,000 breast cancer patients for more than seven years, they found that women with high CRPs have lower survival rates. Remember, CRPs rise as a reaction to inflammation. Less inflammation, lower CRPs. Inflammation—that is, the body's physiological response to inflammation—is related to an increased risk of many illnesses including cancer. Inflamed gums cause your body to "respond" by releasing certain chemicals into your blood. Eliminating any source of inflammation, like the inflammation you get with chronic gum disease, in theory, would help reduce the risk of those illnesses.

Another study followed 48,000 men for fifteen years to look for disease progression based on lifestyle. Those with gum disease were twice as likely to get pancreatic cancer as those with healthy mouths. The men with cancer were also found to have high CRP levels.

While there are no definitive studies proving that flossing reduces your risk of cancer per se, the dots are there waiting to be connected. Connect them—and then go floss.

Do It Right:

- Flossing should be done at least once a day—twice is better. Flossing after meals is great, too. Any more than that may border on obsessive.

- Choose your preferred floss type—waxed, unwaxed, dental tape, green, red, striped, whatever. For those with a keen palate and a keen sense of humor, there are even floss flavors like bacon, cupcake, coffee, and waffle. Or if you really feel funky, you can floss with absinthe-flavored floss to start or end your day!

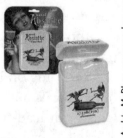

© Archie McPhee www.mcphee.com

- Make sure you get in between each tooth AND the far back (where there is no "in between").

- Move the floss along as you go by using a new section of floss for each tooth.

- Bury the floss by getting below the gum line.

- Don't worry if your gums bleed at first; they will get stronger and you will see less blood with repeated flossing, until eventually the bleeding will stop.

> Floss for dental health, but also for overall health!

- Rinse well with cool water after flossing.

- It doesn't matter if you floss before or after you brush.

- You can use conventional string floss or disposable dental floss picks (although my dentist tells me the string kind is better). There is even a water jet flossing attachment for your showerhead! What a great multi-tasking tool!

Cancer Introduced Me to Some New Saints

Being raised Catholic, I kinda have a thing for the saints. From the time I said my first novena at the age of ten, St. Theresa and I have been BFFs. I refer to her as my multipurpose saint, as I can call on her for any reason. Sometimes, however, it is necessary to pull out all the stops and throw in a prayer or two to the patron saint of your cause. When my sister, Lynette, was having trouble selling her house for example, we called upon St. Joseph, the patron saint of selling houses. Shortly thereafter, the house sold! (I'm not so sure if her Jewish husband is privy to this information.) Any time I am traveling and the road conditions are risky, I call upon St. Christopher, patron saint of travelers, to accompany me on my journey. Even if I find myself in a situation that seems beyond hope, I can always call upon St. Jude, patron saint of hopeless causes.

It did not surprise me in the least when, following my diagnosis, fellow Catholics started lunging at me with prayer cards. It turns out that there is not just one, but actually two patron saints of cancer: St. Peregrine and St. Michael of the Saints (to distinguish him from just plain old St. Michael). Not wanting to pick favorites and offend anybody up there, I prayed to both of them.

A prayer is a powerful thing, sometimes so powerful that you can actually feel the energy of the words as you say it. I found that to be the case for this prayer in particular. Please pause for a moment, and if you are so inclined, offer a prayer to St. Michael of the Saints:

We praise you, Most Holy Trinity, for having sent us St. Michael of the Saints to be our friend and intercessor in the fight against cancer.

Grant us, we pray, a humble faith that we may follow in his holy footsteps and believe without a doubt in your generous gift of healing.

With humble and childlike trust, we ask your Divine help through St. Michael of the Saints in this urgent necessity.

May this gift of bodily health bring us peace and joy, which are but a foretaste of heaven, and may we be counted one day among your saints in glory.

Father, your world is ill with cancer and frightened. We pray you ease the suffering of those afflicted, give loving hands to those who care for them, and light the way for those who seek its cure.

Merciful Father, extend your healing hand so that we may cry out: A cure, at last!

In Jesus's name we pray, Amen.

Whether or not you affiliate yourself with a particular religion does not matter. A prayer can be as formal as the Christian one written above or as simple as the "God bless you" we utter when someone sneezes. It is not the words, but the intent behind those words that carries the power. So no matter what your beliefs, turning to "God" (whatever that term means to you) can be very comforting in your time of need.

The most powerful prayer is a prayer of gratitude. No matter what is happening in your life, there is always something to be grateful for. Give thanks for all that you have.

HEALTH TIP #22
I Am Thankful for . . . Fungus

Yes, fungus. But I'm talking about fungus in the form of beautiful mushrooms! Experts estimate there are more than 14,000 varieties of mushrooms. Many are used in cooking, 1 percent of them are deadly, and some are used for . . . *ahem* . . . "recreational purposes."

Nearly 4,500 years ago, the Egyptians believed that mushrooms were the plants of immortality. As it turns out, they may be right. The use of edible mushrooms is currently being studied as a way to fight many illnesses and conditions including breast, gastric, colorectal, and prostate cancer, HIV/AIDS, high cholesterol, high blood pressure, and diabetes.

The varieties that seem to possess the most power for fighting illness are *Lentinula edodes* or shiitake (pronounced shi-TOK-ee), *Grifola frondosa* or maitake (pronounced mi-TOK-ee), and *Ganoderma lucidum* or reishi (pronounced RAY-she), although it seems that all mushrooms possess a little bit of "magical health" fairy dust.

> If you choose to take mushroom capsules, please check with your doctor, as they can alter your blood sugar (in a positive way!) and can also affect blood-thinning medications.

The most exciting thing to come out of the mushroom newsroom is the potent anticancer effects of the "turkey tail" mushroom. The turkey tail (*Trametes versicolor*) is a flat-looking, multicolored mushroom that is proving to have extremely potent anticancer properties. One component of turkey tail is the polysaccharide krestin (PSK). Currently, Japan, China, and Australia use PSK with other cancer therapies as legitimate treatments for cancer to reduce recurrence and lengthen survival time. Because of a glitch in how the U.S. Food and Drug Administration (FDA) regulates drug approval, the concentrated PSK can never be used in the United States as a cancer treatment. But you *can* buy quality turkey tail supplements that contain PSK.

Here's a word about mushroom supplements (okay, several words): Why take a supplement? While I love mushrooms, I don't eat them every single day, so I take a capsule. There are dozens of mushroom supplements (pills) out there, with various combinations and different varieties of mushrooms. You can find "wellness" mushroom compounds that combine ten to twenty different mushroom varieties into one capsule, or you can find them in groups or separately. You can buy a combo of shiitake, reishi, and maitake, which comes together in one pill, for example. It's important with mushrooms to always know what you are buying and who grew what you are buying. It's always best to buy organic foods in general, but it's even more important with mushrooms. Make sure you see a certifying agency seal on the package, and that the package doesn't just say "organic." You want your mushrooms to be pure.

A great company for certified organic mushroom supplements is Host Defense (www.hostdefense.com). Host Defense was the company that supplied turkey tail supplements for the study subjects in an eight-year research study funded by the National Institutes of Health (NIH) that showed an improvement in the immunity and a reduction in recurrence of breast cancer patients who underwent chemo and radiation therapy. There were no adverse effects of the supplements. These results have been well documented all over the world. If you want some "sugar to help the medicine go down," you can take your organic turkey tail extract in a bit of pure Vermont maple syrup (www.maplemedicinals.com). C'mon, folks, it doesn't get any easier than this!

Dozens of studies have been conducted worldwide using mushrooms. These are just some of the things mushrooms can do:

- They allow our blood to hold more antioxidants, which increases immune response and helps healthy cells to live longer.

- They improve the function of insulin and help to maintain proper blood sugar levels.

- They give healthy cells a little invisible suit of armor so they can resist invasion.

- They help men's hormones, namely testosterone, remain at healthy levels, keeping the prostate happy.

- They directly lower total and LDL (the "bad") cholesterol in the blood.

- They possess antiviral properties.

- They possess antifungal properties (yes, a fungus that fights fungus!).

- They enhance immunity in HIV/AIDS patients.

- They alleviate inflammation associated with inflammatory bowel disease.

- **Mushrooms actually shrink cancerous tumors and prevent them from recurring!**

You can go to Memorial Sloan-Kettering Cancer Center's website to read about all the benefits of mushrooms and other botanicals (www.mskcc.org/cancer-care/intergrative-medicine).

Mushrooms are just like any other plant-based food, basically composed of water, fiber, vitamins, minerals, protein, and sugar. The water and high fiber help with digestion and staying "regular." Mushrooms also contain:

B Vitamins: In the form of pantothenic acid, which helps in the production of hormones and plays a part in the health of the nervous system, and riboflavin, which helps maintain healthy blood cells. There's also niacin, which helps the digestion, skin, and nervous system.

Minerals: Mushrooms contain copper, necessary for making healthy red blood cells, and selenium, which is an antioxidant that helps protect the body's cells from damage and destruction, helps rid the body of heavy metals like mercury, and helps the immune system. Also, mushrooms are among the richest nonanimal sources of selenium, which is great for those wanting to eat a more plant-based diet.

Amino Acids: Ergothioneine (ET) is an amino acid necessary for living and growing. It functions as a antioxidant and an anti-inflammatory, which helps to prevent a variety of chronic illnesses like heart disease and cancer, and has been shown to help manage chronic pain.

Electrolytes: Just like the potassium you get from eating bananas, mushrooms have potassium, which helps blood pressure and heart cell function as well as general muscle health.

Sugar: The sugar contained in mushrooms is very different from the sugar in an apple. Beta-glucans are the glucose-containing structures in mushrooms that have incredible immune-stimulating effects. Beta-glucans are the components of mushrooms that are responsible for resistance against cancers, allergies, and infection. While beta-glucans are also found in yeast, oats, and barley, it is the beta-glucans found in mushrooms alone that have the special antitumor and anti-infective properties. Beta-glucans have also been shown to protect against radiation sickness and have been studied to combat the side effects of certain chemotherapy drugs.

> Adding mushrooms to your diet is a funky way to fight cancer.

Protein: Protein builds muscle and promotes cell health. It is important to include protein-rich foods in your diet especially if you are cutting down on animal products. Most varieties of mushrooms generally contain 3 grams of protein per cup.

Mushrooms are fungi, just like the fungus that was responsible for the number-one medical discovery in the history of medicine and the most widely used antibiotic in the world, saving millions of lives—penicillin!

The great thing about eating mushrooms is that you can throw them into just about anything you eat: sauces, salads, stir-fry dishes, and more. There are many varieties available in your local market, and you can even buy kits to grow them yourself, which would eliminate worry about where they were grown. (They're easy to grow, as they grow in the dark!) You can find lots of kits and great information at www.fungi.com.

Other varieties of mushrooms have benefits also, like the portabella and button variety, so try to include any kind of mushrooms in your diet when you can. Your cancer will hate you for it.

Please note that none of the mushrooms mentioned
for the promotion of health are hallucinogenic!

I Got First Pick of "the Fodge"

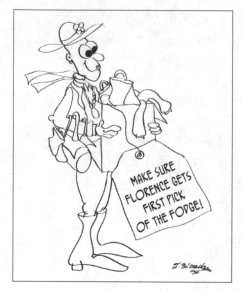

First of all, let me begin with a definition of the word "fodge" as I believe it to be a term unique to my hometown of Lawn, Newfoundland: *Fodge (noun). Hand-me-downs. Goods handed down to a person after being used and discarded by another.*

I am the oldest of five sisters. My youngest sister, Lynette, who lives in Miami . . . well, let's just say that she married well. A couple of times each year, Lynette will send home a fodge of designer clothing, makeup, shoes, and purses, which is descended upon by the females in my family like a pack of wolves. Prior to getting cancer, I was lucky to walk away with half a tube of Dior mascara. Trust me, you would not want to come between my nieces Krissy and Cassie when there is a Chanel purse on the line! Things can turn ugly pretty quickly. You can only imagine how moved I was then, when Mom and Dad came to visit with a big box from Florida and a handwritten note from Lynette saying, "Make sure Florence gets first pick of the fodge!" I had Coach purses coming out the yin yang!

It is okay to use your cancer to get free stuff.

HEALTH TIP #23
Find a Healthy Place for Those Get-Well Gifts

We know they mean well and they love us, but it's hard to find a place for all those candles, figurines, and crystal pink "hope angels" that friends and loved ones give us during our illness. Generally speaking, we all acquire lots of "stuff" from many different places in the course of our lives. Some of it is treasure and some of it is trash.

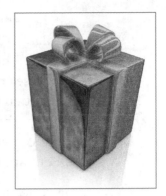

According to the rules of feng shui (pronounced "fung-shway"), the ancient Chinese art of object arranging, how we choose to display our "stuff" can have a profound positive impact on all the areas of our lives.

Feng shui is not a superstition or a new age religion. (And besides, I don't think any religion anywhere forbids home decorating.) It is the traditional Chinese practice, started around 1,100 BC, which states that in order to enhance your positive life force, or chi (pronounced "chee"), you must exist in harmony with nature, clear your surroundings, and in turn, clear your life of negativity. Negativity could present itself as a simple picture in your home that reminds you of something unpleasant, or as an annoying, uncomfortable chair. By clearing and rearranging your surroundings, you allow the chi, or life energy, to flow freely and harmonize with your environment, thereby allowing good things—health, positive relationships, good fortune, and more—to come into your life.

The interesting thing about this ancient art is that of all the aspects of your life, such as wealth, family, and creativity, it is the *health* aspect that remains the center of all the other areas. Health touches all other areas of your life and has a direct and profound effect on each one.

This makes perfect logical sense. If you don't have your health, including physical, mental, and spiritual health, then all the other things, like career, love, and family, will suffer. Your health must come first and be the primary focus of your life. In feng shui, the health sector is the "building block of all general well-being."

This grid is called a Bagua template. You can use this "map" to find the sections in your house or the sections in a particular room that relate to each aspect of your life. A good compass will help you find the true north and south and will guide you to each of the sections. By arranging things according to the template in each section of your home, it can positively affect those areas of your life.

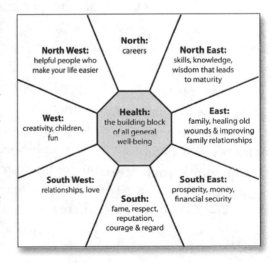

The center of your home represents the "health" section of the Bagua template. It is the area that holds and sustains your physical and emotional energies. There are certain items, properly placed, that will enhance your "health sector." Luckily, these items are just the kinds of things you probably have gotten from well-wishers! Making an arrangement with the following things in the center of the room, like on a coffee table or on a small table in the center of your home (like in the hallway or against a center wall), will enhance this sector. You can pick and choose from the list:

- a collection of potted plants (the greener the better)

- crystals or rocks (a great place for the pink crystal angel!)

- shades of yellow (it can be those dandelions your child picked for you)

- pictures of mountains or the world (you must have at least twenty get-well cards with mountain scenes on them, don't you?)

- bowls of fruit (Great! You just got that fruit basket from your neighbor! Extra points if it contains peaches, as these are the Chinese fruit associated with longevity and health.)

- religious objects (angel, saint, Buddha, or cross figures would work well here)

- humorous touch (any fun photo or item, but I'll leave it up to you whether that whoopee cushion your brother gave to you makes the cut)

Feng shui gives you an unconventional way to use gifts from well-wishers to improve your health.

You don't have to include all these items in the center area, but with a list like this, you can certainly come up with a nice arrangement using lots of your "stuff." And this way, the gift givers are really helping your health!

There is so much more to feng shui than just placing objects on a table. People spend years learning the intricacies of mastering it. If you are interested, there are many books and online resources you can find to learn more about this interesting and life-enhancing art. There is even a *Feng Shui For Dummies* (no offense).

Happiness is a "free chi."

I Could Watch My Favorite Movie Anytime I Felt Like It

What was a grown woman doing watching *Mama Mia* in the middle of the day . . . for the third time in a week? Hey, I had cancer. *Mama Mia* made me feel good.

Shortly after my diagnosis, my daughter and I headed out to Walmart to stock up on DVDs. I figured that I would have plenty of downtime (both literally and figuratively) in the coming months, so I would need something to keep me busy. I am also a firm believer that laughter is the best medicine. Studies have shown that laughter boosts the immune system, relaxes muscles, reduces pain, elevates mood, and relieves anxiety and stress. (Not to mention, watching movies provides a great distraction from thinking about the Big C.) Some cancer centers actually use a form of therapy called laughter therapy as a tool to promote healing with their patients. Given the health benefits of laughter, you might want to consider getting yourself a "prescription" for Netflix.

Need a pick-me-upper? Watch your favorite feel-good movie.

HEALTH TIP #24
Watch the Movie, but Ditch the Microwave Popcorn

I don't think there is anything that smells better than buttery microwave popcorn; do you? But the smell of popcorn popping on the stove or in an air popper can be just as enjoyable—and a little less toxic. Aside from the unhealthy hydrogenated oils and palm oils that are used in the popcorn mixture inside the bag, the popcorn bag itself can pose the biggest risk of all.

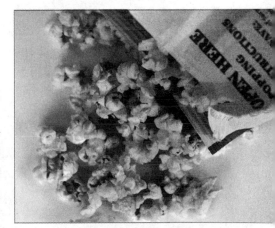

Plastics that line the inside of the microwave popcorn bag contain per-fluorinated compounds (PFCs). This group of chemicals and its cousins, perfluorooctanoic acids (PFOAs), act as the water and oil repellent on the inside surface of the bag. Exposure to PFOAs is known to cause cancer as well as liver and hormone disruption and has recently been associated with lowering the effectiveness of childhood immunizations by affecting the immune system to the point where it inhibits the production of anti-bodies. (The purpose of the immunization is to increase antibody produc-tion.) Anything that weakens the immune system opens the door for illnesses of all kinds.

Exposure to PFCs is not limited to popcorn bags as it is present in many food containers (such as fast food french-fry boxes) and is even present on stain-resistant carpets and clothing; recent testing shows that PFCs exist in high levels in the air supply of many office buildings. We all are exposed to it, as a random blood sampling of the general population showed that 90 percent of us have an ample amount of PFCs pulsing through our veins.

Because PFCs accumulate in our body and can take decades to excrete, and because of the rising concern over recent research, the U.S. Environmental Protection Agency (EPA) has been devising a "PFC action plan" to deal with the increasing evidence that PFC exposure is dangerous and harmful. However, some of the U.S. EPA's action plans can take over ten years to complete, so it's up to you to be aware and eliminate it where you can.

Cut down on chemical exposure by switching to stove-top or air-popped corn to get your popcorn fix.

Okay, I can tell that a little toxic plastic probably won't be enough to keep you from those light fluffy pieces of buttery heaven. So, let's talk about what makes those pieces so buttery.

The main chemical used to make artificial butter flavor is diacetyl. The EPA initially approved diacetyl for flavoring because it appeared that it was safe when used in foods. But when it is high-heated, like in manufacturing, or when making microwave popcorn, it emits a toxic gas that causes bron-chiolitis obliterans, a potentially fatal, nonreversible lung disease that caused the death of a handful of "popcorn addicts" and has sickened hun-dreds of factory workers. Bronchiolitis obliterans has become known as "popcorn lung."

After an investigation in 2007, most manufacturers removed diacetyl from their popcorn products. But don't push the "start" button on that microwave yet. The chemicals used to replace diacetyl are just as bad, and it is believed that the lung problems will continue to exist, especially for the one who first opens the bag and inhales that heavenly but toxic vapor.

Sorry to be such a Debbie Downer, but there is hope! You can pop your own corn using organic ingredients (of course!). Here's how it's done:

1. Place a 3-quart or larger pot with a lid on the stove.

2. Pour 2 tablespoons of oil (cold-pressed and/or organic oil if possible) in the pot with 4 kernels of organic non-GMO popcorn and cover.

3. Turn heat to medium-high and watch the pot. When the first kernels pop, pour in $1/2$ cup of kernels and cover pot.

4. Shake pan over the heat, keeping it moving and venting the steam ever so slightly. When popping slows down to 2 to 3 seconds apart, turn heat off and leave pot covered until popping stops. Pour into a bowl and season with toppings. While butter certainly is an option, a healthier choice would be seasonings like sea salt, cinnamon, or garlic powder. You can always use Earth Balance plant-based butter or something similar to keep your snack plant-based, healthy, *and* delicious.

While the intake of corn products in general should be limited because of many health factors (most corn is genetically modified and it is high in omega-6 fatty acid), there is a huge happiness factor with this delicious comfort food.

Speaking My Mind

As far as indicators go, I was not considered to be at high risk for breast cancer. There is no family history, I am healthy, I exercise, I don't smoke, and I generally take good care of my body. The biggest risk factor for me was stress, largely brought on by years of holding back my thoughts and feelings, and swallowing anxiety. While science has not confirmed a direct link between stress and the onset of cancer, there is ample evidence to show how stress can impair the functioning of your immune system. Whether or not stress caused my cancer (I do believe it played a role), there is no doubt that I needed a strong immune system to recover from it. Therefore, an important part of my survival plan involved stress management.

I am sure that you have heard the analogy of the oxygen mask in an airplane. If the mask drops, you are to secure your own before you try to help other people; otherwise, you may lose consciousness. When I got cancer, I realized that I needed to take care of myself first and foremost; otherwise, there was a chance I wouldn't be around to help the others in my life who need me.

A critical component of taking care of myself involved (and still does) reducing the stress in my life. Rather than keeping things bottled up, I learned to honor my feelings by speaking my truth. I abandoned my old pattern of avoiding conflict at all costs, in favor of standing up for myself in a respectful way. I also added a new word to my vocabulary—"No"— sometimes followed by, "That doesn't work for me." The funny thing is, while I feared that people would not like me if I put my own needs before theirs, the opposite is true: I am shown more respect than ever before.

Be kind to your body, mind, and spirit by standing up
for yourself and speaking your truth in a respectful way.

HEALTH TIP #25
Speaking My Spirit

How important is spirituality to your health? If recent research is correct, the answer is *very* important.

We are all spiritual beings, whether you want to admit it or not. Spirituality can have different meanings, but basically it is your core belief system developed by your connection with others and is the essence of what brings meaning to your life.

The evidence for the connection between health and spirituality has grown over the years. It doesn't really matter what form of spirituality you practice—be it one of the organized main religions, personal meditation, or just an appreciation for nature. But one thing is clear: your physical health can improve by getting in touch with your spiritual side.

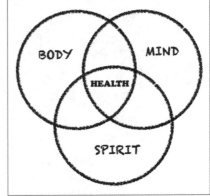

How does spirituality make you healthier? In part, it seems to have to do with a reduction in stress. Reducing stress improves immunity and reduces the incidence of illness. Spirituality usually includes some form of meditation, which has been shown to directly improve the immune system. It can also offer a sense of hope or faith, which is a positive feeling that can have healing physical effects. Spirituality can provide you with a connection to others and gives a sense of purpose to your life.

If spirituality is already a big part of your life, I suggest you make it bigger. If you've never explored your spiritual side, there are scads of books and resources to help get you started. The best way is to find someone who has a spiritual side that you admire and ask them what they do. Spirituality just may be the missing piece of your health that you were looking for.

> Explore your spirituality as another avenue to better health.

Cancer Made Even My Most Embarrassing Moment Seem Trivial

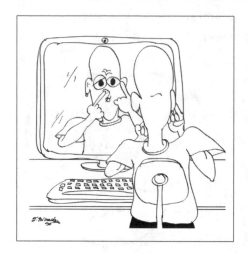

After having my saggy boobs examined, poked, prodded, and squashed, few things in life can embarrass me anymore, as I learned soon after meeting Shawn. Hey, I may have been forty-four, but no matter what the age, new love is a magical time, and a time when we want our new partner to see only the very best of us. This came as a bit of a dilemma for me when, just six months into our relationship, all of my hair fell out. Let's just say, the honeymoon was far from over. How could I possibly keep that magic alive while looking like Uncle Fester? Why, of course, a wig. And might I add, a "red hot" wig! That would keep the spark going for sure.

My relationship with Shawn was a long-distance one, but thanks to the Internet we were able to connect every day through video on Skype. We usually planned our Skype dates in advance, which allowed me time to put on my hair and makeup, and make myself presentable.

One day Shawn surprised me by ringing in when I was in full chemo attack mode. Not a pretty sight. However, I did manage to rush into the bathroom and hastily pull on my wig and apply a swipe of lipstick before answering his video call.

Much to my relief, while I could hear Shawn on my computer, I couldn't see him. Turns out he was calling from his office computer, which does not have a camera. I thought, *Great he can't see me*, since my wig was lopsided, and I was wearing orangey lipstick.

"That's okay, Honey," I said to him, while tearing off my wig and throwing it across the bed. "We can still talk, even if we can't see each other."

I then proceeded to use my computer screen as a mirror, tugging and pulling at my face to see how I would look with an eye lift, a nose job, or maybe a chin tuck. (Come on now, we've all done it!) You can only imagine my horror when Shawn said, "Florence, do you realize that *your* camera is still on and I can see you? I thought it best to tell you that before you start to pick your nose or something."

With a forced smile I replied, "Of course I knew it was on. I was just checking to see if you were paying attention."

**Life is serious enough, with or without cancer.
Learn to laugh at yourself.**

HEALTH TIP #26
Force a Smile and It Will Stick

Consider this: A four-year-old smiles 400 times a day, while an average adult smiles only 14 times. Kids just find reasons to giggle. Let's face it; it doesn't take much to get them going. Coincidently, most kids also seem better able than adults to cope with the stresses of life. *Hmmm.* Maybe they're on to something.

There is some truth to the old adage "laughter is the best medicine." Laughter and smiling are simple and easy ways to reduce stress in your life and may lead to an increased immune response that can help combat illnesses like heart disease, ulcers, and cancer, just to name a few.

Smiling does more than just show your teeth. The simple action of forming your mouth into a smile:

- uses fourteen facial muscles

- sends a message to your brain that says, "Everything is okay."

- sends a message to those around you that you are approachable, improving your inter-personal interactions

- reduces your stress response

Now, if you are looking for some really heavy-duty physiological responses, just L-O-L. Laughing does the following:

- exercises your lungs, chest, and the tiny artery muscles that regulate blood pressure

- releases chemicals in your brain that improve your mood

- improves your immune system (when done regularly)

- reduces your stress response

No one knows the healing benefits of laughter more than Dr. Patch Adams. An actual medical doctor, Dr. Adams learned during his medical training that laughter was the key to speedy recoveries, especially with chil-

> Take notice of how many times you smile today. Increasing your "smile time" just may decrease your "sick time."

dren. It was not unusual to see him in the hospital adjusting his honking red clown nose and carrying a rubber chicken instead of a stethoscope. He currently teaches medical school students and other professionals about the use of "high-dose laughter" when practicing medicine. Check out some hilarious and heart-wrenching videos by searching "Dr. Patch Adams" on YouTube and rent *Patch Adams*, a wonderful movie with Robin Williams that tells his story.

One oncology nurse I spoke to said she tells her chemo patients to smile if they are feeling nauseated. More times than not, she's seen it help relieve nausea when nothing else did.

The interesting thing is that it really doesn't matter if you have something to smile about or not. Your body cannot tell the difference between a forced smile or a nervous laugh and the real thing. You still get the great physiological and mental benefits from both.

I used the smiling technique to help me cope with several painful medical procedures during my cancer treatments, and it definitely helped. It also threw the doctor off completely. "Okay, Susan, this is going to hurt a bit." "Great doc!" I would say with a smile.

The simple act of smiling or laughing can be done anywhere at any time and is one of the easiest health tips there is.

Cancer "Shaved" Ten Minutes Off My Shower Time

*B*eing a mother, I have had to hone the ability to shower, wash, and condition my hair, plus shave various body parts, all in under twenty minutes. However, while I was on chemo, I no longer had to bother myself with hair care or removal of unwanted body hair, and my shower time was cut in half. Having shorter showers was a definite perk of having cancer, and I made use of the extra grooming time by stepping up my skin care. Even though cancer treatments can wreak havoc on your skin, my skin had never looked better!

If your shower routine is shortened, don't give extra bathroom time to your kids. Rather, use those precious grooming minutes on skin care.

HEALTH TIP #27   Skin Care 101

*I*f beauty is only skin deep, then all the more reason to work on getting great skin! It's not just chemotherapy and radiation that can damage your skin, but cold, sun, and exposure to everyday chemicals like chlorine can dry you out as well.

Your skin is the largest organ in your body (okay, technically, it's *on* your body) and protects you from viruses and bacteria that would kill you if they ever crossed the skin barrier and invaded your other organs. It also provides you with your fifth sense, touch, and your sixth sense. Yes, your sixth sense . . . your skin's "*arrector pili* muscles" cause those goose bumps you feel when you sense imminent danger.

Skin, also known as epidermis, is made up of a series of layers that contain your skin cells as well as your sweat glands and hair follicles. But it's the oil glands that do the hard work of keeping your skin soft and healthy. When oil production can't keep up with demand because of environmental factors, or when your skin is damaged as in radiation or sunburns, your skin becomes dry, flaky, and may even crack. Getting your gorgeous silky-soft skin back will not only help you to look fab in that summer dress, but that skin barrier will be able to do a better job of keeping you healthy and illness-free.

Skin cells are always rapidly reproducing. We replace all the skin on our body every thirty days or so. Rapid replacement also means rapid death. In fact, much of the "dust" you see in your bedroom and on your sheets is dead skin cells. This is actually good news because you have a chance to improve the look of your skin relatively fast by including healthy skin-care habits in your daily routine.

There is an inner layer and an outer layer to your skin. So it would make sense that you must treat both. To heal your skin from the inside, be conscious of what you put in your mouth. An overall healthy diet consisting of whole plant-based foods is generally good for skin, but these nutrients are particularly important:

- **Omega-3 fatty acids:** Omega-3s are essential to overall health and are specific to healthy skin. Omega-3s are found in walnuts, wild salmon, dark greens, various seeds including flaxseeds and chia seeds, and edamame or whole soybeans. (Always check to see if it is okay to eat soy with the type of cancer you have.) You can also take a quality omega-3 supplement. (See Health Tip #10 for more information.)

- **Flavonoids:** Flavonoids are a group of substances that are high in antioxidants and help your body to produce healthy cells. In parts of your body that produce rapidly, like your skin, it is important to provide the "construction crew" with flavonoids so they are equipped with the proper tools. Look for them in dark red berries and red grapes (here's where you can justify that one glass of red wine, too!), kale, broccoli, apples with the skin on, and yes, dark chocolate! Yippee!

- **Vitamin C:** Just ask Dr. Linus Pauling, a well-known scientist who devoted his life to chemistry and uncovering the benefits of vitamin C, and he would tell you that healthy skin regeneration depends on it. In fact, my surgeon prescribed 1,000 mg of vitamin C daily after my double mastectomy to help with general healing. You can find your "C for citrus" in the logical places, such as oranges, lemons, and limes, but vitamin C is also abundant in bell peppers (yellow have the highest), kiwi, and strawberries.

- **Folate:** Folate is one of the B vitamins found naturally in foods like beans, green leafy vegetables such as kale and spinach, sunflower seeds, and beets. You may see "folic acid" in the ingredients list of fortified baked goods and cereals. Folic acid is the synthetic or artificial form of folate. Folate strengthens and protects skin and has been shown to enhance the reduced risk of skin cancer when other precautions for skin cancer are taken, such as wearing sunscreen.

While you're eating healthy to heal your skin from the inside, you'll need to treat the outer layers of your skin by replacing the oils that it so desperately needs. However, if you try to replace your natural oils by slathering it with "baby-type" oils, you'll get nowhere. "Baby-type" oils are made of mineral oil. Mineral oil is derived from petrochemicals and fossil fuels just like motor oil and gasoline. Structurally, mineral oil is very different from the oils produced by your skin, and, since your body does not recognize it, most of it does nothing for your skin besides smother it. If absorbed, your body rejects it, and it does not benefit your skin in any way. (That's why mineral oil is given as a laxative—it goes right through you!) When you apply mineral oil or lotions that contain mineral oil to your skin, it mostly sits on top of your skin. It looks nice and shiny, and your skin *looks* moisturized, but that oil does not provide any nutrition for your hungry skin. (By the way, petroleum jelly is the same thing as mineral oil; it's just in a jellied form instead of liquid.)

Plant-based oils are best for moisturizing your skin. In particular, coconut oil, macadamia nut oil, grapeseed oil, and olive oil. These oils and others like them contain very similar fats to your own skin's oils, which allows your body to absorb them and use them as nourishment for repair.

For wonderfully moisturizing body oil try this recipe. Use organic oils when possible. You should be able to find all these oils in your local supermarket:

- 2 tablespoons coconut oil

- 4 tablespoons grapeseed oil (or macadamia nut oil)

- 2 tablespoons olive oil

Place all oils in a glass measuring cup and microwave on medium heat 30 seconds at a time, stirring after each 30 seconds until the coconut oil is melted (about 1 to 2 minutes). Pour into a clean 4-ounce plastic bottle with a flip top. (You can usually buy empty plastic "travel" lotion bottles at pharmacies.) After you step out of the shower, **while you're still wet**, apply *thin* lines of oil to arms, legs, and shoulders, paying extra attention to rough knees and elbows, and massage in well. (This recipe is probably too heavy for use on your face.) Avoid applying to your feet as there is a danger of slipping if you apply it to your feet after showering.

Take your time massaging the mixture in for a minute or two, as your skin needs time to absorb the oils. Then, gently towel dry. You won't ever need to apply any lotion after this. Continued use will keep your skin smooth, supple, sexy, and, more important, healthy. And you don't have to worry about *these* ingredients being absorbed into your body. Food for your body, food for your skin!

Your skin is a vital organ. To keep it healthy, make sure you're feeding it right.

If you want to look for a good commercial lotion to use, please check the ingredients list. If "mineral oil" is on the list, keep looking. A good lotion will contain plant-based oils, botanicals, and no synthetic fragrance, coloring, or chemical preservative like parabens. If you wouldn't put it in your mouth, it doesn't belong on your skin.

Your poor skin gets attacked from every angle. One of skin's environmental hazards is chlorine. Chlorine is present in all tap water as a byproduct of disinfection and purification. Chlorine exposure from bathing dries your skin out terribly. Installing a chlorine filter on your showerhead will filter out this harsh chemical and prevent damage to your skin, hair, and nails. Chlorine-filter showerheads are easy to install and maintain, and there are many on the market. Just search the Internet for "chlorine filter showerheads" or visit a home improvement store and choose the one that best fits your style and pocketbook.

Chlorine exposure from swimming pools can also affect your skin. If you just swim once in a while in a chlorinated pool, not much damage is done. But if you swim daily or several times a week for exercise, it can be very drying, and you may be absorbing that harmful chlorine through your skin. You might want to consider applying the oil recipe mentioned above to your skin before you swim. This will provide a layer of protection to your skin while you're exposed to the chlorinated water. If you have a chlorinated pool at home, you may want to check into one of the chlorine-free options for keeping it clean, like salt or ozone purifiers.

Cancer Allowed Me Time to Do the Things I Love to Do

I will be the first to admit that not every day with cancer is a good day. But there were days between chemo treatments that I felt "almost normal." During those days I took advantage of my time off work to do the things that I *love* to do: gardening, reading, writing, or sometimes just grabbing a snack and watching Netflix. Before getting cancer, I was reluctant to allow myself such guilty pleasures, but I came to view these activities as a necessary part of my survival plan. I continue to make "me" time an important part of every day.

Make doing the things you LOVE to do
an important part of your survival plan.

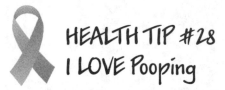

HEALTH TIP #28
I LOVE Pooping

Yeah, I'll admit it. I love pooping. I'm proud to say I'm #1 at #2. I like to think of myself as the "Kung-poo Master." I'm proud because bowel habits tell the story of overall health. If your diet and lifestyle are healthy, chances are you won't experience any bowel issues like constipation, diarrhea, bloating, or gas. But since it's not exactly a common topic of conversation, you may think your bathroom habits are normal and healthy, when they're anything but (or should I say, "butt"?).

To get to the "end" we have to start at the beginning. Your BM starts its journey as food. Digestion begins in the mouth, as food is chewed and mashed and mixed with enzymes that start the process. The mixture then is pushed down into the stomach where it's mixed with more enzymes, and there is more mashing and churning. That mixture then goes into the small intestine, where nutrients are absorbed by the intestine walls, and into the blood and is distributed to all the cells of your body for proper functioning and growth.

Anything that can't be digested by the body goes on to the large intestine. Your large intestine is about as long as you are tall. As the waste moves through your colon, water is absorbed back into the body and reabsorbed back into the colon if needed. Eventually, everything collects in the sigmoid colon, and then the rectum. Truly healthy rectums are filled and emptied daily.

If everything is working properly, a nicely formed, light brown, somewhat soft, bowel movement is pushed out of the anus (mostly by the internal contractions of the rectum) and voila! A turd is born! (Honestly, I don't know why this isn't the topic of more dinner conversations.)

Stool consists of 75 percent water, 8.3 percent dead bacteria, 8.3 percent live bacteria, and 8.4 percent indigestible fiber.

This is the way the story is supposed to go, but many factors affect "The Duke" and his journey, and the process may take various twists and turns and get stalled along the way for many reasons.

How Do You Poop?

Think about your usual bathroom experience. Which one most often applies to you?

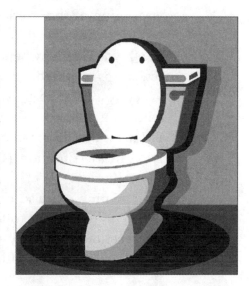

What happens: You feel like you want to go, but it only happens twice a week or less. When it does happen there are grunting sounds followed by tearing eyes and a huge sigh of relief when it's over. Sometimes you feel a bit dizzy when you're done. Your poop, even though you've worked very hard at it, is only a tiny hard marble (or many marbles), and it makes a splash when it hits the water. You might see a little bit of bright red blood in the toilet or on the tissue.

What this says: Your diet probably consists of fries and donuts washed down with coffee. In fact, caffeine is your drug of choice. (Large amounts of coffee, more than two cups a day, on a regular basis, dehydrate your body.) You can't remember the last time you ate a raw food, and ketchup is your daily vegetable. Water isn't water unless it's cola. Your exercise is walking to the couch so you can flip on the TV. You probably have a lot of bloating and cramping and are always complaining that you are tired. Your medicine cabinet is filled with laxatives and antacids.

To get a "zen BM" start with your water intake. This is a simple way to improve your bowels. Since your poop contains mostly water and fiber, you can't poop if you don't get enough of either one. Since water is shifted from your bowels to your cells to help your body function, a dehydrated body means dehydrated stool, and there won't be enough water to help move things along. This is one of the main causes for constipation.

The smaller and more "marblelike" your poop is, the more stressed you are. The more relaxed the colon is, the longer (not bigger) the stool is. Chronic stress will slow down the nonvital organs in your body and redirect the action from your digestion to your heart, lungs, and brain. There's reason number two for not going #2.

When you see a very small amount of bright red blood in the toilet or on the toilet tissue, it could mean you have hemorrhoids (bulging and weakening of the arteries near your rectum) or tiny tears in your rectum (like paper cuts on your butthole) that you can get from too much straining. If you have any persistent bleeding, or when you see more than just a few drops of blood, you should get checked by a professional right away. When you strain to go, you are performing a "valsalva maneuver" (pushing with your airway closed). This strained action puts pressure on the heart. For most healthy people, this is not a problem, but if you have an underlying heart condition (that you may not be aware of), it could be very unhealthy.

Straining can also cause little tears in your retina, causing you to see "floaters" (not in the toilet—in your vision). This usually corrects itself and is not serious. But really, if you're pushing so hard that you are making your eyes bleed, don't you think it's time for a change?

What happens: Your poop is formed, but you see "stuff" in it. Sometimes your poop sinks and sometimes they float.

What this says: You've eaten something that your body can't digest. The outer shells of corn kernels, for example, are made of cellulose, which is totally indigestible by your body. If you pulled those kernels out (I don't recommend this), you would find the inside of the shell is gone because the inside is digestible. Sometimes you'll see fibers from vegetables, or shells from seeds in your stool as well. If you swallowed a coin, or a pebble, that would be in there too. (Any frantic mom whose child swallowed any of these can attest to that.)

Floaters—turds that float in the bowl—are poops with gas in them. If you drink a lot of carbonated drinks, you will most likely have floaters. Sinkers don't have as much gas. Either is fine. It just depends on your diet.

What happens: You poop fine, but sometimes it's a strange color, like green or black.

What this says: You eat colorful stuff. Dark green veggies like spinach will turn your poop greenish. Artificial blue dye, like in Gatorade and blue ice pops, will turn your poop a bright green (almost like "glow in the dark" green). Beets will turn your stools much darker (and will turn your pee a beautiful sunset color!).

> Your healthcare provider should always evaluate persistent black or light-colored stools.

Not all colors are normal. Light- or clay-colored stools could mean there is a problem with your liver, and you should be evaluated by your healthcare professional. Yellow stools can sometimes mean there is a blood disorder, as it is the broken-down "dead" red blood cells that are digested that give poop its brown color.

Black, sticky stools mean that you are breaking down and digesting living red blood cells—that is, you are bleeding somewhere in your digestive tract. (Those vampires must have some black stools, eh?) Dark stools can also be the result of certain medications or iron supplements.

What happens: You know poop stinks, but this is unbearable!

What this says: You are probably a meat eater. Digested meat is stinkier than digested veggies. Certain other foods like spicy beans produce gasses in your bowel that produce noxious smells as well. Doody also is loaded with bacteria; *E. coli* is the main one. The presence of bacteria is normal and is actually necessary for normal poop production. These bacteria produce gasses when they grow and reproduce. It is these gasses that smell.

If the smell is bad but strange, and you see fatty snot in your poop, you may have fat collecting in your stool. This is not normal as fat is normally digested and processed in your stomach and small intestines. If there's fat in your BM, something in that process is not working, and it should be checked out by a healthcare professional.

What happens: You go three times a day, and it's very soft or liquid. You feel bloated and get cramps a lot.

What this says: This probably happens when you have a deadline at work coming up or have to give a speech. Acute stress, or high-level stress for a short period of time, can cause your body to become hyperactive and this also translates to your bowels. If the stool is pushed through your intestines too quickly, there is no time for the water to be reabsorbed into the body, so the extra water comes out along with the other waste.

A virus can also cause inflammation of the bowel and spasms, causing the stool to be moved along too fast. Intestinal viruses usually move through your system in a few days.

Prolonged loose stools can cause severe dehydration. Any prolonged diarrhea that lasts for more than a week or that is accompanied by fever or blood should always be evaluated by a professional. *Diarrhea in children is particularly dangerous as they can become dehydrated very quickly.*

Many occasional loose stool problems are diet related. Dairy is the usual culprit. Sweeteners like sorbitol or xylitol are also to blame.

What happens: You usually poop daily and usually at the same time. Your poo is soft but formed, and it is described as a snake rather than a short sausage. It is light brown to medium brown in color. There is no pain or effort in production. There is no "plopping" sound.

What this says: You have mastered the art of truly Zen bowel movements. You are healthy and get plenty of water (as a general rule, 64 ounces or 2 liters daily, consumed throughout the day). Raw fruits and veggies are a main staple of your diet. You don't eat a lot of dairy, white starch (white rice, white pasta, bread), or processed food. You exercise regularly and are able to control your stress.

Bravo! You are the Kung-poo Master!

Healthy bowels will also reduce your risk of colorectal cancer. Guidelines for colorectal cancer screening start at age fifty. See Health Tip #38 for suggested screening tests.

Here are some fun poop facts:

- You can have from 5 to 25 pounds of stool in your body depending on your size and type of diet.

- Close the lid on the toilet before you flush! The flushing agitates the water (and feces) so that tiny droplets of water can be hurled up to 20 feet. (I'm betting it's less than that to your toothbrush, isn't it?)

> Your health depends on your ability to eliminate waste. Make sure your bathroom experience is a beautiful thing.

- Using witch hazel, an inexpensive, natural, soothing agent can ease the pain and inflammation of hemorrhoids. Soothing witch hazel soaked pads can be found in pharmacies or online.

- Bird poop is white and pasty because birds can't urinate, so their digestive tract mixes everything together and it all comes out at once—right on your freshly washed car!

- Some say processed, "chemically enhanced" foods never really leave your digestive tract. That means, depending on what you were fed, you probably have some food from when you were a baby in your gut right now.

Important note: *If you think there is something wrong with your bowels, please see your doctor. None of this information should be used to diagnose or treat you.*

Riding Shotgun

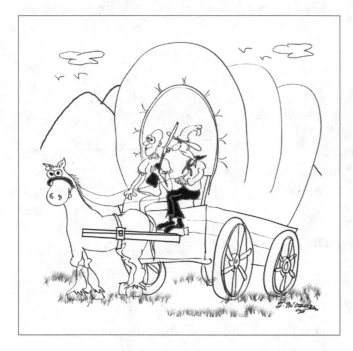

Before I go driving anywhere with my teens, I am sure to hear one of them yell, "Shotgun!" This statement gives the person saying it the privilege of sitting in the front seat of the vehicle. I assume the expression originated in the days of the covered wagon, when the person sitting next to the driver carried a gun for protection and, therefore, was known to be riding shotgun.

After getting cancer, I didn't have to call "shotgun." No matter how many people were packed into a vehicle, I automatically got the coveted spot. Even Mom, with her bad knee, would climb into the back of a two-door vehicle so that I could ride shotgun. It may have been a small perk of having cancer, but it was a perk all the same.

Perks such as riding shotgun may be a small bonus when you have cancer, but each of these conveniences makes life a little easier.

HEALTH TIP #29
Make Breakfast More Convenient with Simply Scrumptious Granola

You've heard it countless times: "Breakfast is the most important meal of the day." After your nightly hibernation, it fuels your body and brain, improves memory, and improves your mood. Some have, what seem to be, valid reasons for skipping it:

- no time
- not hungry

- trying to lose weight
- breakfast is boring

Sorry, but I can shoot every one of those excuses down with one word: granola.

You may have seen granola recipes that put you in the kitchen all day toasting your oats and slowly baking over and over. Forget those. The recipe on the following page is quick and easy, and you can tailor it to your tastes by adding what you like. Instead of almonds or walnuts, try pecans. Instead of sunflower seeds, try crushed cashews and sesame seeds. Explore different ingredients and make a granola with your signature.

Now about those excuses . . .

No time for breakfast? Make some ahead, bag it, so you can just grab it on your way out.

Trying to lose weight? Skipping breakfast has actually been shown to cause weight *gain* because you're hungrier before lunch and tend to snack more. This granola has more than 7 grams of protein per serving and will stay in your stomach longer to keep your hunger away.

> Don't skip your chance for a quick nutritious breakfast. Try this easy, healthy granola!

Not hungry? Just one whiff of this heavenly mix and you will be.

Think breakfast is boring? You can dress up this granola with a different blend of dried or fresh fruits every day. You can even eat it hot! How exciting!

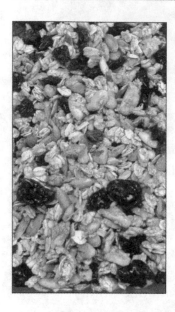

SIMPLY SCRUMPTIOUS GRANOLA

YIELD: 5 CUPS

3 cups old-fashioned rolled oats (not instant)

$3/4$ cup sliced or slivered almonds or chopped walnuts

$1/2$ cup unsalted sunflower seeds, raw or roasted

$1/2$ cup raw, shelled pumpkin seeds (also known as pepitas)

$1/2$ tablespoon wheat germ or almond meal (optional)

$1/2$ tablespoon ground cinnamon

$1/4$ teaspoon salt

2 tablespoons canola or similar oil

$1/2$ cup pure maple syrup (Grade A amber if possible)

1 cup dried fruit such as cherries, cranberries, apricots, dates, figs, etc.

Preheat oven to 325°F. Mix all the dry ingredients, except for the fruit, in a large bowl. Mix oil and maple syrup in a smaller bowl and blend well. Add the wet to the dry ingredients and mix to coat thoroughly. Spread on cookie sheet that has been sprayed with a light coating of oil. Bake 30 to 40 minutes, mixing the granola two or three times to brown evenly. The browner it gets, the crunchier it will be.

Remove from oven and let cool. The granola will be soft and sticky when it first comes out, but will crisp as it cools. Once it has cooled, add your dried fruit of choice and mix well. Choose dried unsweetened dark berries like cranberries or blueberries for extra cancer-fighting benefits.

Store in an airtight container, and it will keep for two weeks. You can double this recipe to make more if you like. You may find you need to bake mixture an additional 5 to 10 minutes and stir more often to brown the doubled amount.

NUTRITION PER $1/2$ CUP SERVING:

Calories: 330; Fat: 16 grams; Fiber: 4.3 grams; Carbs: 40 grams; Protein: 7.3 grams; Cholesterol: 0 grams

---

You can take this on your hike or eat it as a healthy snack. Besides providing protein, it has fiber, which helps you be the king or queen of your bathroom "throne."

Cancer Made Me Feel Grateful for My Chores

WAIT! Hear me out. One day during my treatments, I cooked supper for my children and cleaned up afterward—all by myself. And it felt wonderful! I appreciated my support team and was quite happy to allow them to cook and clean for me when I needed it. But when I felt well enough to do it myself, I actually felt grateful for my chores (well, except for washing the dishes).

Maybe I should look at washing dishes like Buddhist teacher Thich Nhat Hanh: "Washing the dishes is at the same time a means and an end—that is, not only do we do the dishes in order to have clean dishes, we also do the dishes just to do the dishes, to live fully in each moment while washing them."

I will be sure to share those words of wisdom with my sisters at the next big family dinner. After all, who am I to deprive them of the opportunity to live fully in the moment?

Don't get too comfortable in the sick role. When you can do for yourself, DO for yourself, and be thankful that you can.

HEALTH TIP #30
Please Say, "Thank You"

Those two little words are more powerful than you think as they can have a big impact on your health.

The definition of gratitude is expressing thanks to someone who has done something nice or helpful, or just being thankful for a situation.

Taking note of things or people that you are grateful for (some might call this "counting your blessings") can actually improve your health and well-being.

Gratitude research is a growing body of science with some interesting findings. In one study, for example, participants were split into three groups. One group was told to keep a journal of all the things they were grateful for over a ten-week period. The other group was told to write down all the things that caused them aggravation, and a third group just wrote down events as they occurred with no emphasis on being positive or negative.

Those who wrote down things they were grateful for experienced more overall optimism and actually had fewer doctor visits than the group that wrote down things that aggravated them, suggesting that when you notice the good, you feel good.

In another study, the psychological impact of different positive activities was measured in individuals by questionnaire. The one activity that had the biggest impact on happiness was writing a letter of gratitude to someone in their lives that the individual felt was never properly thanked. The beneficial effects of this one act lasted for months!

This is also one of those "double whammy" actions as you *and* the person being thanked get benefits. Who doesn't like being told they're appreciated?

> Expressing gratitude is not just for Thanksgiving Day; it's for every day.

Interestingly, gratitude is the one emotion that cannot be directed toward yourself. Therefore, it forces you to look outside yourself and redirects focus on someone else, allowing your brain to take a rest from thinking about troubles and issues you have.

The easiest way to say thank you is just to say it. It doesn't matter if it's in person or over the phone; expressing appreciation works as long as you're sincere. Small gifts are nice, but a hand-written thank-you note is often more valued. (Brownie points if the card is handmade.)

Being generally thankful for your life, nature, and the people in it can be expressed by keeping a journal. Think of several things every day that you are thankful for and write them down, or just stop and take a few minutes to focus and meditate on the things that elicit gratitude.

Cancer Connected Me to a Powerful Prayer Network

Norman Vincent Peale, in his bestseller *The Power of Positive Thinking* said, "When you send out a prayer for another person, you employ the force inherent in a spiritual universe."

When I first discovered I had cancer, I stepped my own prayers up a notch and asked everyone I know to pray for me. While I have always been a deeply spiritual person, I am also very scientifically minded. Even though research is mixed on this topic, there are studies that show that even in double-blind studies, patients who are prayed for fare significantly better than those who are in the not-prayed-for group. There are other studies that show that prayer does not make a difference. I have a problem with these studies. If you are praying for someone you don't know and will never meet as part of an experiment, are you going to pray with the same fervor as you would for your daughter who has cancer? Probably not. I think there is something to be said for the quality of the prayer, a factor that cannot be controlled for by science.

My parents are big believers in the power of prayer. One afternoon they came to visit and found me lying on the couch crying my eyes out. A colleague of mine who had been diagnosed at about the same time as me had just died from breast cancer. I felt so sorry for her family and worried about what the outcome would be for me. I could see the pain in my mother's eyes as she held me and rocked me in her arms. But dad would have none of it! "What are you crying about?" he said very matter-of-factly. "Your mother and I have all that cancer prayed out of you by now."

After each chemotherapy treatment, I would post my "chemo status" on Facebook, and I was so pleased with the response. Whether it was a formal prayer, a "thinking of you," or just "wishing you well," all were good intentions and therefore forms of prayer.

Even if you are not a spiritual or religious person,
what do you have to lose? If you are sick,
pray and ask others to pray for your recovery.

HEALTH TIP #31
Prayer Is Good Medicine

The research is solid that prayer as a form of meditation can help the one who prays (pray-ers), but does being the subject of the prayer, or being the one who is being prayed for (pray-ees), have its benefits as well?

Research is limited and conflicting at best. How does one measure or prove the power of prayer for someone else? The subject of "intercessory prayer" (praying for the well-being of someone else) has been studied by only a handful of researchers. Some studies would work this way: Researchers would take a group of "pray-ers" and tell them to pray for a specific person and their physical outcome to a specific surgery or illness. Success was measured by the level of improvement in their condition. Sometimes, the patients knew someone was praying for them, and, in other cases, it was kept a secret. In some instances, there were significant health improvements in the prayer recipient group, showing shorter recovery times and less need for invasive therapies. In most cases, the physical outcomes of the pray-ees showed no measurable improvement.

But this is a tricky subject to study. There are many variables and things you really can't measure. Like how "well" the pray-ers prayed. I mean—were they multitasking? Like praying while driving or when a commercial came on the TV? And then there's Flo's point about not knowing the person who is the subject of your prayers. Emotional connections might make a difference when praying for someone in your family versus a stranger.

While intercessory prayer has mixed results, the power of prayer for the pray-ee has been well documented. Harold G. Koenig, MD, director of Duke University's Center for Spirituality, Theology, and Health, is an expert in researching the influence that religion and faith have on health and well-being. His book—*The Link Between Religion and Health: Psychoneuroimmunology and the Faith Factor*—is the product of a meeting with twelve of the world's leading psychoneuroimmunologists, theologians, and physicians that took place at Duke University in 1999. His book contains almost three hundred pages of research results and statements from these specialists that reinforce the relationship between "mind and body," using religion as the main component of the "mind." Time and time again, a direct correlation was proven between faith, prayer, and better physical health.

An interesting point in the literature is the differentiation between *intrinsic religiosity* and *extrinsic religiosity*. Dr. Koenig explains the difference between the two in this way: "*Intrinsic* religiosity reflects a deep commitment to one's faith, which is reflected in an integration of religious beliefs and practices into one's life. In contrast, *extrinsic* religiosity is essentially utilitarian and involves the use of religion to reinforce one's social status or to justify one's way of life."

The religious beliefs and practices he is referring to include faith and prayer. In other words, you can't just "phone it in." You can't just "talk the talk," you also have to "walk the walk." Merely walking into a place of worship won't give you instant faith. The same way walking into a gym won't give you a smokin' hot bod. Prayer or spiritual meditation is something that must be practiced and nurtured. But once mastered, it can have a profound positive influence on your health.

> Prayer, in general, is an easy way to improve your health and sense of well-being. And you can always send your prayers to those who need it. Nothing negative can ever come from it.

Getting started might be the hardest part. If you already belong to a place of worship, you could consult a spiritual leader for some help. If you're a "self-study," there is a wonderful book by Helene Ciaravino titled *How to Pray: Tapping into the Power of Divine Communication*. This nonthreatening, nondenominational guide is simple to read and even easier to understand and follow. This book is great if you're someone who wants to connect to the divine using prayer, but doesn't know where to begin.

Consider prayer just one more tool for your "anti-cancer, living-better tool box."

Cancer Made Me Appreciate My Pooch

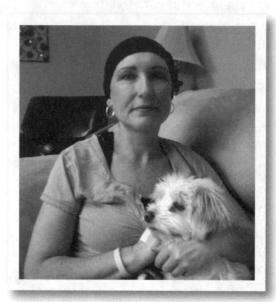

Flo and Patches

My dog-loving friends would be mortified to hear that during cancer treatment I actually fantasized about killing my dog, Patches. One night, for example, she woke me from a sound sleep with a shrill whine and the clickity-clack of her sharp nails tap dancing across my laminate floor. I faked I was asleep for as long as possible, but soon realized I was not going to get any rest until I let her out to pee. At this point in my story I would like to send a sincere apology to my neighbors, in case they looked out at 2 AM that night and saw a bald woman, clad only in her underwear (thanks to my hot flashes), yelling, "Hurry up and pee, would ya!"

But I digress. Patches proved herself to be a faithful and loving companion throughout my cancer treatments. She never left my side. As I was fading in and out of consciousness postchemo, I could always count on seeing her furry face, black lips, and big brown eyes looking at me when I opened my eyes. She had been with me for nearly ten years, but that was the first time that I truly enjoyed her company. Too bad it took getting cancer to make me really appreciate having her around.

If you are battling cancer, this might not be the best time to get a new pet. But if you already have one, cherish the relationship with your furry friend.

HEALTH TIP #32
Pooch, Pussycat, or Python, They All Have Health Benefits

Okay, the python is a bit of a stretch, but I'm sure there are those who love their pet python as much as Flo loved Patches. And why shouldn't they? Pets offer us a never-ending supply of unconditional love, and that love has a positive effect on stress, which in turn has a positive effect on your health.

Among dozens of studies on pets and health are those that find:

- Pet owners have a lower risk of dying of heart disease than non–pet owners.

- Fifteen minutes with a pet (dog, cat, or watching fish—not sure if snake handling was included in the study) actually caused chemical changes in the body that improved moods and reduced stress.

- People who own dogs are more physically fit than non–dog owners because of the regular walks dogs require, and this can be of particular benefit to those recovering from surgery or a severe illness.

- Pet owners were found to have lower blood pressures than non–pet owners.

- Those who grow up with pets have stronger immune responses and are actually less likely to develop allergies as they grow older.

- People who have undergone major surgeries recovered faster if they had a pet at home.

So if you have a pet, whether furry, feathered, or scaly, taking a dose of companionship and love along with your antinausea meds might just be just what you need to get through those tough days. There are some precautions, however, for pet owners undergoing treatment for cancer or who have a compromised immune system.

> Embrace your pet to let go of stress.

- Litter boxes and cages should be kept out of the kitchen.

- Wash your hands thoroughly with plain soap and water after handling your pet.

- Get someone else to clean cages and litter boxes and pick up poop. (Hey Flo, I think I just found another perk!)

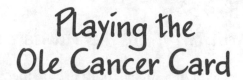

Playing the
Ole Cancer Card

I dunno, there is just something about having cancer that makes you think that you no longer have to play by the rules. For example, if my sixteen-year-old daughter, Kaitlyn, were to say, "Mom, you can't park here, it's a no parking zone!" I'd say, "But of course I can, honey, I have cancer." It is as if cancer had given me a newfound sense of entitlement. Besides, who was going to make me move my car if I happened to slip and say that I have cancer? Although my teen chastised me for this attitude, I found her on occasion playing the ole cancer card as well: "Sorry my essay is late, Mrs. Smith. Yesterday was Mom's chemo day."

Hopefully there will only be a short time in your life when you get to play the cancer card, so go ahead and take advantage of this perk! (Example: "Sorry I was speeding officer, I was just on my way to chemotherapy.")

HEALTH TIP #33
Go Ahead, Take Advantage, and Be Assertive

Consider, if you will, this scenario unfolding in the chemo room:

You are sitting in the chair, ready for chemo, but as the nurse hangs the bag, you notice it's a different-colored fluid than all the other treatments you've gotten in the past.

Which response best matches yours?

a. You say nothing because they're the professionals and should know what they're doing. It's not your job to know those things.

b. You pull your arm away and yell, "Hey! That's not my chemo! You're making a mistake!"

c. You ask, "Excuse me, but that doesn't look like Taxol. I just want to make sure that's what I'm supposed to get."

If you answered (a), you may be a passive patient. Passiveness is allowing anything to be thrown your way. You don't have any say in your treatment, because you don't want any and you would rather suffer in pain than "bother" anyone to get relief. You may not even know the names of the drugs you're getting, but you take them because you're told to do so. You see yourself as the "good patient," but in reality you are a victim. Passive patients have been shown to have less favorable outcomes than those who speak up and are involved in their treatment. (Please note: Being passive is not the same thing as having faith. You can have faith and be very *accepting* about decisions about your treatment plan.) The passive patient is not involved in planning their treatment journey. They are just passengers . . . in the backseat . . . with a blindfold on.

If you answered (b), you may be an aggressive patient. While you will definitely get attention, it probably is not the kind of attention you want. Insulting the people taking care of you is not the best idea in the world. Especially since they have to stick you with needles occasionally. Aggressive patients are often avoided and may miss getting valuable information they need for their care. Everyone gets angry now and then, but if you can't control the anger, and you find yourself pointing fingers at your doctors and their staff, you may want to examine your feelings. Anger can stem from a sense of losing control and may lead to the need to control your caregivers. Aggressive patients are the drivers with road rage, and often everyone just gets out of their way.

If you answered (c), you are the assertive patient. Assertive patients are outspoken without being rude. They are very involved in their care, know all their medications, and are active participants in their treatment plan. They have taken control of their health and have meaningful conversations with their healthcare providers about their treatment course. They ask questions and therefore get better and more pertinent information. Assertive patients actually have better treatment outcomes with fewer negative side effects. They are in the driver's seat, and they are responsible for setting the navigation system to take them where they want to go.

> Take charge of your health and your health care to make a positive impact on your health and your life.

Dr. Bernie Siegel, a celebrated author who was named one of the "Top 20 Spiritually Influential Living People on the Planet" in 2011, has been teaching survival behavior for decades. Dr. Siegel not only is an advocate for patient assertiveness, but he has written books on the miraculous results that being assertive has had on patients. Dr. Siegel states:

> The word "patient" derives its meaning from submissive sufferer. That is not a good thing to be when hospitalized or receiving medical treatment of any kind. You need to be a respant, or responsible participant, if you want to heal and survive.

> So . . . are you a patient? Or a respant? The choice is yours.

Sleeping In

Being an early riser by nature, I prided myself on the ability to get by with very little sleep. There always seemed to be so many things to do, and so little time to do them! Who had time for sleep? But after cancer, I rested as much as I felt my body needed it. According to Susan, getting the right amount of sleep is absolutely necessary for good health, so I had nothing to feel guilty about. In fact, even now, getting plenty of sleep is an important part of my survival plan. Ah, it feels great to roll over, look at the clock, and slip back into a deep and guilt-free sleep!

Listen to your body. If it tells you to sleep, just do it.

HEALTH TIP #34
The Art of Napping

Sleep is essential for good health. But does that include the thirty-minute snooze that you steal under your work desk at three o'clock in the afternoon? According to Harvard Medical School, the answer is yes.

If you are like the majority of working 9-to-5 people, your body's natural rhythm reaches a lull between 2:00 and 4:00 PM. This is the period of time when you feel you are dragging to get through the rest of the day, which leads some of us down the hall to get some coffee, do an "energy shot," or worse, grab a candy bar. But it turns out that napping may be the healthy answer.

A recent British study compared different ways of making it through the afternoon snoozies: either

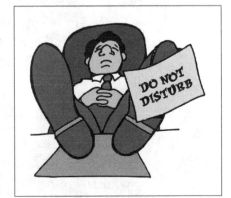

by getting more nighttime sleep, by drinking caffeine, or by taking a nap. The most effective way to make it through the day was the nap.

Harvard researchers have found that naps can improve memory, enhance learning, and spark creativity. Studies performed at NASA on pilots and astronauts showed an improved performance of 34 percent after napping, and 100 percent enhanced alertness. The science is so strong on this issue, that sleep researchers even advocate having policies that encourage napping at work. For example, at the Google headquarters, nap pods are placed strategically among their workspaces. The pods look like huge ice cream scoops. Putting your head in the "scoop" blocks out sound and light so you can catch some serious Z's. Some other employers that let their employees sleep on the job are Ben & Jerry's, Nike, Pizza Hut, and British Airways. Instead of the employees abusing their "rest rooms," it has actually increased productivity and employee satisfaction.

The longer you are awake, the less likely it will be for your brain to retain information. Napping resets the clock, so to speak, and your alertness is restored for a little while longer.

Getting some extra sleep seems to be especially important to those who work nights. In one study, air traffic controllers on the night shift were far more alert after taking a forty-minute nap, and it has been recommended to firefighters working the night shift that they take an extra nap in the late afternoon right before they start work to help with concentration and fatigue.

I would probably check with your employer first before settling in for your daily siesta. But if it's something that you are able to do, here are some tips:

- Try to get twenty to thirty minutes of sleep. Any more than that might have a negative effect of feeling groggy. Even a few minutes of sleep has been shown to help.

- Take your naptime in a quiet, cool, dark place if possible, to reduce the amount of time you spend falling asleep.

- If you plan to take a nap at 2 PM, don't have coffee at lunch. Caffeine takes some time to have an effect on your energy level and might sabotage your sleep.

- Don't nap after 4 PM or it might interfere with your usual night's sleep.

- If you plan to nap in the afternoon, include lunchtime foods that contain tryptophan, a food chemical that promotes relaxation. Some of these foods include pumpkin seeds, greens like spinach, turnip greens, and watercress, white and crimini mushrooms, and asparagus.

- Shake the stigma that people who nap are lazy. You're not lazy; you're smart!

Contrary to what you may have been told, taking a nap before 4 PM will not affect your ability to get a good night's sleep that night. For example, if you have trouble falling asleep usually, it will be no different whether you nap or not and the same goes for good sleepers. And while getting eight to ten hours of continuous sleep is the best routine for your health, napping has been shown to improve general health and reduce risk of heart problems in all types of sleepers.

> To combat fatigue during the day, consider taking an afternoon snooze.

The next time afternoon fatigue starts to set in, instead of reaching for the caffeine, reach for the pillow and eyeshades. You'll wake up refreshed and ready to tackle the rest of the day!

For more information on sleep, visit the National Sleep Foundation at www.sleepfoundation.org.

Early Menopause

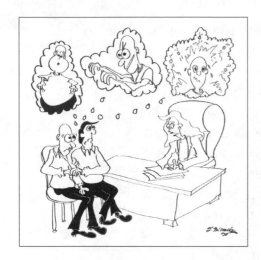

Hey, I know what you are thinking, ladies: *What is so perky about early menopause?* Those were my thoughts exactly when my oncologist told me about "chemopause": a side effect of chemo that causes the womanly cycle to come to an abrupt halt. Sitting in the pretty young doctor's office with Shawn by my side (very early into our relationship), I couldn't help but blush as she told us the likely side effects: mood swings, hot flashes, loss of libido, weight gain, and no more monthly periods (well, that part I was looking forward to). I would not have been the least bit surprised if my new love had suddenly bolted out the door, but I'm glad he decided to stick around. Sure enough, chemopause kicked in soon after treatments began, but fortunately my only unpleasant symptom was hot flashes—a small price to pay to get rid of the dreaded monthly visitor.

Many moons ago, while I was still married, I whined to my best friend that my hubby turned into a complete villain once a month, purposely doing things like slurping his soup in an attempt to drive me bonkers. In fact, when I thought about it, it seemed that everyone around me got kind of crazy at that time. "Does this happen at the same time every month?" my wise friend asked. "Yeah, usually just before my period," I confided. Ah, it suddenly dawned on me; they weren't trying to make me crazy. I had PMS. But those days are behind me now. As an added perk of chemopause, I no longer turn into a demon once a month.

Chemopause is not all bad. Just think of the perks:
no more periods and no more PMS.

HEALTH TIP #35
No More Living in a "Healthy Cage"

You must not eat any meat. You must eat broccoli every day. You must never raise your voice. You must be crazy if you think you'll find any of these statements in this book!

If you think of french fries when I say "vegetable," and the thought of exercise makes you want to cry, you're not alone. Changing everything you do, eat, and think every day is a tall order. And since we humans don't fare well with change of any kind, trying to stick to your "healthy living plan" can be like living in a dungeon for some.

Here's something to remember: when making a healthy living plan, you must consider your happiness.

Eating seaweed and drinking turmeric tea may not be the thing that gets you to your happy place; however, you should be willing to try some new things to see if you can work them into your plan. Your healthy lifestyle should never be stagnant but should be an ever changing, evolving process; evolving to the healthiest lifestyle possible for you.

Eating a plant-based diet, exercising four to five times a week, and meditating daily will help you feel better and fight illness, but if abstaining from that burger while all your friends are devouring theirs makes you feel trapped and causes anxiety, then go ahead and eat the burger. It's better to be happy eating the burger than to be miserable by not eating it. But maybe the next time you want that burger, allow yourself the idea of exploring other options, like a black bean burger. And when trying said black bean burger, try not to put any negative labels on it, like "I have to eat this dumb thing instead of the burger I love." Instead try to think, "I can still have the burger occasionally if I want it, but I'm going to try this to see if I feel better when I eat this one."

Of course, you don't have to say these things out loud.

Here's an anecdotal story, so take it for what it's worth. About four months into taking the medication for post–breast cancer treatment (the aromatase inhibiter, Femara) I started to get terrible joint pain and swelling. When I woke up in the morning, I literally could not walk. It would take me about twenty minutes or so to loosen up and walk normally. I was a forty-one-year-old with ninety-year-old joints. When I went to see the acupuncturist for a tune up, he suggested I cut down on dairy as that can seriously affect joint inflammation.

Now I loved my cow's milk. I mean LOVED it. I loved it on cereal, I loved it in shakes, I loved it in my tea—and what the heck was I going to dunk my chocolate chip cookies in? I probably was drinking a quart of cow's milk every day. But it was *skimmed milk,* so in cardiac nurse terms, I thought I was eating healthy.

So I heard his "no milk" advice and tucked it in the back of my head. (*Way* back there, along with learning how to play the harp someday.) But the pain kept getting worse. Finally, when I had to hold on to things to walk after getting out of bed in the morning, I made the decision to give up milk for two weeks to see what would happen. I switched to unsweetened almond milk, after tasting the various options, and I tried not to look at that beautiful white jug sitting there beckoning to me in the fridge. The first day was frustrating, but after one week, I was accepting it, and, after two weeks, my joints started to feel a lot better, but I wasn't even noticing that because the gastric bloating and stomach pains I had been living with had disappeared! That's when I was hooked. And that's when I was able to work on getting all dairy, such as cheese, yogurt, and ice cream out of my diet and out of my life. It was a process, but because I kept feeling better, it reinforced my choices. And with dairy, because of the proteins and other substances that make you crave it, it took about four weeks until I just plain didn't want it anymore. I never realized how good I could feel, and I didn't realize how dairy was affecting my body until I stopped it. After doing more research and discovering that casein (the protein in dairy) could contribute to developing more cancer, my mind was made up and I never looked back.

My point is, I tried this change for my health and I am happy with my choice. I'm not regretting it every time I pour almond milk on my cereal, and, in the end, I'm not following the advice of anyone but myself—my well-informed self.

Recently, I was reading about seaweed and all its benefits. Costco was actually sampling seaweed salad the other day. Someday I will be ready for that seaweed salad, but not today. And I'm happy with that choice . . . for now.

> Seek out new, healthy lifestyle changes without losing your "happy place," but realize what makes you happy now may change in the future.

Cancer Streamlined My Christmas Shopping

I had my sixth and final chemo in December 2011, shortly before Christmas, and it was by far the toughest one. For days I was mostly confined to my bed, with my dear little Patches never leaving my side. I found myself drifting in and out of stages of sleep and wakefulness, never knowing whether it was daytime or nighttime. My energy was at an all-time low. I recall wanting to go to sleep one evening, but my bedside lamp was on, keeping me awake. All I could do was look at the lamp and wish that I had enough energy to reach over and turn it off. Calling out to someone to help was out of the question. Even talking was too much work for me! I dreaded for anyone to ask me a question because that meant I had to search my dazed mind for an answer, and then speak the words, which left me feeling exhausted. I would always muster up enough energy in the evenings, however, to sit and eat with my family, ensuring that I was giving my body good nutrition to keep up my strength.

Needless to say, as Christmas approached, I had no shopping done. There wasn't a present to be found in the house (except stuff for my kiddies, which I had ordered online). And the strange thing was, I was as cool as a cucumber about it. After all, who was going to say anything if they didn't get a present from me that year? I mean really, how would it look if someone complained that their sister/friend/girlfriend/daughter with CANCER did not buy them a gift? So, they could call me a Scrooge if they wanted but they would only be making themselves look bad.

Christmas shopping can add unnecessary stress to your life when you are dealing with cancer. People will understand if you take a year off. (And if they don't, they are only making themselves look bad.)

HEALTH TIP #36
How to Eat Healthy Around the Holidays
and Not Seem Like a Health Freak

Stick sugar and fat in my face enough times, and it's likely to be gobbled up eventually. That's the danger when you're attending parties, holiday or otherwise. Going to a party with all that food sitting out is like being locked in a food fun house . . . distorted evil sights, sounds, and smells . . . colorful bubbling poison drinks . . . little spiked weenies being shoved in your face . . . smiling, evil, clownlike people who are tempting you to ruin your healthy eating streak!

You don't have to be a victim. And you don't have to seem like you're on some kind of starvation diet to those around you by carrying a little Ziploc baggie full of carrot sticks in your purse. There are some good strategies you can use when going to these types of functions that will help you stay on the healthy eating track. Choose the ones that work for you and will still allow you to have a good time at the shindig.

- **Eat before you get there.** You'll be less likely to eat the wrong things if you're not hungry. Your before-party snack should be something with a bit of fiber and protein like a small salad with added walnuts and seeds, or whole-grain bread with almond butter. Fiber and protein will keep you fuller longer and help you resist the urge to overdo it.

- **Don't have your one alcoholic drink right away.** If you're going to stick to the one drink max that is recommended by the National Cancer Institute guidelines, don't have it as soon as you get there. Chances are, during the night you'll have another, and maybe even another if you hang around long enough. Have your drink, but start off with sparkling water with a splash of fruit juice. Heck, stick one of those little umbrellas in there, too. It will still satisfy your taste buds, put you in a festive mood, and help you bide some time until you're ready for your drink.

- **Look at everything first.** Take a moment to take stock of what's on that hors d'oeuvre table. Make a mental note of what you'll have before you start making up your plate. Choose fresh whole foods like veggie sticks and fruit and limit creamy or cheesy dips. If you do choose dips, put a small amount on your plate and walk away as opposed to standing near it and "robot dipping" over and over.

- **Only put two things on your plate at a time.** If you fill your plate with a heaping mound of food, you'll eat it and be back for more. But if you only put two things on the plate at a time, you'll space out your consumption. Grazing, over time, allows you to digest what you're eating, and it forces you to fill multiple plates and make multiple trips.

> Make a plan for party eating, but don't stress about it if you don't follow it.

- **Hold a drink in your dominant hand.** Occupying your "grabbing" hand will make it tough to "grab" another cheese puff.

- **Above all, have fun.** Enjoy yourself. Keep these rules in the back of your mind, but don't let them ruin your evening. If you eat more than you planned, don't beat yourself up. There's always tomorrow to put you back on track.

Cancer Allowed Me to Keep Better Tabs on My Teens

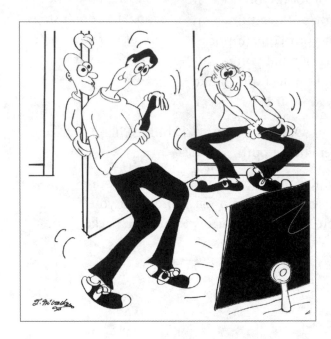

Life before cancer was a whirlwind. I would work all day, come home to prepare three different meals to satisfy my finicky eaters (Okay, I am not going to win Mother of the Year after that comment!), then try to spend some fun, yet educational time with my youngest child, Ben. That didn't leave much time for my teens, Kaitlyn and Donovan. However, cancer slowed the pace of my life and allowed me to become more involved in theirs.

I am not sure if that was exactly working to *their* advantage, however, as nothing could slip by me. Let's take, for example, the mysterious case of the flu that hit Donovan on the same day that the Xbox game Modern Warfare 3 was released. I think it was a bit of an epidemic among the guys in his school. I will give the devil his due; he might have even gotten away with it had he not posted to Facebook, "My life is now complete," with a picture of the game. Yes, I was creeping my son on Facebook. When you have cancer, you can get away with doing that.

> Cancer gives you a lot of downtime. Put it to good use by snooping on your kids.

HEALTH TIP #37
Put That Downtime to Even Better Use by Picking Up a Hobby

I should add "a stress-relieving and healthy hobby" such as fishing or scrapbooking to this tip title. I don't think entering hot dog–eating contests would qualify in this category!

It all goes back to stress relief. Reducing stress has been shown to reduce your risk for many illnesses including cancer. Most examples of stress relief have to do with being able to shift the focus of your stress away from what is causing the stress (thoughts about your illness, work schedules, family issues) and onto something completely different, even if it is just for a short time. This shift not only provides some short-term stress relief but has been shown to have benefits on overall well-being too when done routinely.

Hobbies that include physical exertion, like gardening and walking the golf course, have the added benefit of keeping you physically fit as well. This in turn can help you lose weight, thereby reducing your risk of cancer even more. (Pretty neat, huh?)

In addition to the physical benefits, hobbies also provide psychological benefits. Creating a finished product like knitted goods or a model airplane gives you a sense of accomplishment and self-worth. A hobby like painting or pottery making will also give you an emotional and psychological outlet. Many hobbies allow you to connect with others in clubs, furthering the healing benefits by providing health-promoting socialization and friendship. See all the things you can accomplish in your free time?!

You can go with the usual hobbies like rock and coin collecting, but here are a few inexpensive and enjoyable hobbies that you might not have thought of:

Goldfish keeping. Don't laugh. Raising goldfish is easy, inexpensive, and there are hundreds of beautiful goldfish varieties that you can explore. Believe it or not, there are goldfish shows, just like dog shows, that judge your goldfish on color and size, and, yes, even personality. This hobby eliminates stress on many levels:

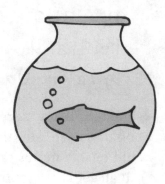

• Watching fish swim has been shown to reduce stress and even lower blood pressure.

• Pet keeping in general is shown to reduce stress. Feeding and taking care of the tank while you watch your goldfish grow will give you a sense of satisfaction. Don't be surprised if you find yourself getting emotionally attached to "Goldie"!

• Winning a blue ribbon in a goldfish show will increase self-worth and raise your endorphin levels. Endorphins are the brain's natural "feel-good" medicine.

• Joining a goldfish club will help you connect with others, which is a healthy form of socialization.

For more information on goldfish showing in the United States, go to www.goldfishsociety.org.

Disc golf. This is the "poor person's" form of golf because all you need is a few special discs (what you and I know as "Frisbees") and a disc golf course. Disc golf is played just like real golf, except the hole is a basket. The object of the game is to get the disc in the basket in the least amount of throws. The rules are pretty much like regular "club golf" and there are even pars for each "hole." The nice thing is, it doesn't matter how old you are or what your ability level is. Everyone can play. Playing disc golf will:

• Get you outside and moving, which is good for your health by communing with nature and increasing your activity level.

• Builds friendships by buddying up with a friend to play. If you don't have a disc golf partner, you can find one by joining a local club.

• Compete in disc golf tournaments to meet new people and have fun. All those things are good for general health and self-confidence.

For more information go to www.pdga.com (Professional Disc Golf Association).

Metal detecting. Here is a relaxing hobby that doesn't require any socialization and you can actually make money doing it! A metal detector is a handheld machine that is waved across the ground in order to find metal objects under the ground like coins, jewelry, and antique artifacts. Metal detectors range in price from $50 to $5,000, depending on how many bells and whistles you want it to have, or you can also get very good deals on used detectors on some of the Internet "garage sale" sites. Metal detecting has many advantages.

- It requires lots of focus—one might say "meditation"—on the sounds of the detector in order to find objects. Meditation in any form relieves stress.

> Hobbies are more than just ways to pass the time. They can improve your health too!

- You are exposed to a healthy outdoor environment either in a field, at the beach, or just in your own backyard.

- This hobby is usually done in solitude, allowing yourself time to "tune everyone and everything out," which can be very relaxing.

- There is a chance that you may find good stuff and it's fun when you do!

For more information about metal detecting and to get started visit www.gometaldetecting.com.

Bank Account Recovery

I was not the type of person who concerned myself with having lots of savings in the bank. Truth be told, my bank account was more often "in the red" than I would care to admit. After my chemo started, however, I experienced a phenomenon that I like to call "Bank Account Recovery." In other words, I stopped shopping so often. Each chemo treatment would knock me down for at least a week to ten days—days that I was rendered unable to shop. I was pleasantly surprised at the reduction in my banking transactions and the resulting bottom line. Folks, I'm not kidding you: by the time chemo ended, I had saved literally hundreds of dollars!

> Being on chemo is like an investment: on those days that you are not well enough to shop, consider it money in the bank.

HEALTH TIP #38
Invest in Cancer Screening

I know it's a "pain in the orifice," but routine screening for cancer is still the best way to catch it early. A routine mammogram caught my stage-3 breast cancer at age forty-one. Make it a point to check yourself and get checked by a health professional for the major cancers like colon, breast, prostate, skin, and cervical. The following are the guidelines to follow.

Skin Cancer Screening

Skin cancer is easy to screen because you do it in the privacy of your own bathroom. You should be checking your skin for anything new or unusual once or twice a year, but become familiar with your skin now, to notice areas that might pop up later. Remember your ABCDEs. If you see a mole that has any of the following characteristics have a health professional check it out to see if you need further assessment:

- Asymmetrical

- Borders are blurred or not defined

- Color is not uniform, but has dark or light patches

- Diameter is larger than a pencil eraser

- Evolving shape, color, or size of a mole

Those with any of the following risk factors should see a dermatologist for surveillance and further medical screening suggestions as you are considered a higher risk than the general population.

- a family history of melanoma

- the presence of atypical moles (moles that have ABCD or Es)

- previous melanoma

- skin that is fair, burns easily, and fails to tan

- numerous frecklings and common moles

- blue eyes or red hair

- a history of blistering sunburns

A partner or someone else (who is very close to you) should check the "hard to check" places like the back of your neck, your scalp, backs of your legs, and any other areas you can't see well in the mirror.

Colon Cancer Screening

The following tests should begin at age fifty.

- Fecal occult blood testing yearly. Samples of stool are placed on special cards and sent to the doctor's office to see if there is any blood hiding in the stool. You can also get these online and do the testing. If positive, you should see a health professional for further recommendations.

- Flexible sigmoidoscopy every five years. A flexible light with a camera is

~~shoved up your butt~~ gently inserted into the anus to allow the doctor to check for abnormalities in the rectum and lower part of the colon. This test is usually done in the doctor's office, and, as it's not particularly painful, you don't need to be put to sleep.

- Colonoscopy every ten years or at the doctor's recommendation. You are given a sedative while the doctor examines your whole colon and rectum with a lighted camera and takes pictures (8-x-10 glossies are available upon request). Polyps, which are small growths, can be removed and biopsies can be taken during the test. After age seventy, the risk of this test might outweigh the benefits and is decided on a case-by-case basis.

Prostate Cancer Screening

A blood test called a PSA (prostate specific antigen) can determine if further testing needs to be done. The right screening for you should be discussed with your healthcare provider.

- PSA should be done at age forty in men with more than one family member diagnosed with prostate cancer before the age of sixty-five.

- PSA should be done at age forty-five in men who are black and also those with one immediate family member diagnosed with prostate cancer before age sixty-five.

- PSA should be done at age fifty for most other men.

Breast Cancer Screening

In the future, I think screenings will involve more efficient methods that give more information, but for now these are the recommendations:

- At age twenty, start self-breast exams monthly. Go to www.breastcancer.org to see how. You may see some recent literature that says there is no benefit to self-exams. To that I say, "Tell that to all the women who found their breast cancer through self-exams." There is no downside to knowing your body and being able to find changes in it. There is no "risk" associated with self-breast exams no matter what nonsense you happen to read.

- A clinical breast exam, meaning a manual exam done by a healthcare professional, should be started in your twenties and be done every three years until age forty and yearly after that.

- At age forty, start yearly mammograms and continue for as long as you are in good health.

- Women at high risk either because of family history or genetic factors should be screened with MRI (magnetic resonance imaging) in addition to mammograms.

Cervical Cancer Screening

A routine pap test with an exam is recommended. A small swab of cells from the cervix is examined in a lab for abnormalities.

- From age twenty-one to age twenty-nine a Pap test should be done every three years.

- From age thirty to age sixty-five a Pap test should be done as well as the new HPV test (Human papillomavirus) yearly. The presence of HPV can put you at risk for cervical cancer. The HPV test is preferred, but optional.

- Testing is not recommended for women over sixty-five who have had negative results until then. For serious cervical precancerous condition, testing should continue for twenty years even if those tests are past the age of sixty-five.

- For women who have had hysterectomies with their cervix removed, testing is not needed; however, they should still be seen yearly for routine GYN exams to examine all the parts that are still intact. Yes, you can get cancer anywhere.

Lung Cancer Screening

For those who are at high risk for lung cancer, there is a new test that can detect lung cancer up to five years before a tumor is visible. High-risk includes:

- anyone who was or is a smoker

- those who grew up in a smoking household
- family history of lung cancer
- exposure to radon or asbestos

Screening may seem like a waste of time, but it isn't if cancer is caught early.

This blood test—EarlyCDT-Lung tests—tests for the presence of autoantibodies to lung cancer proteins that form at the earliest stages of this disease. It's a simple blood test that is covered by most insurance. For more information go to www.HelloHaveYouHeard.com.

Cancer Gave Me a Great Excuse to Shop

Three weeks after my sixth and final chemo, I finally felt well enough to get back into shopping mode. I think I may have gone a little hog wild though, spending my "hundreds" like there was no tomorrow. It all started with a new Nikon camera, which I decided to gift to myself for Christmas that year. My boyfriend Shawn gave me "the look" and said, "Darlin', are you really going to pay that much money for a camera?"

And my somber response was, "Now Shawn, I could be dead this time next year, so I am not depriving myself of a good camera!" (Not that I really thought I wasn't going to be around the following year, but it kept him quiet for a while.)

Next it was off to The Bath Shop. As I loaded the packages onto Shawn's arms he said, "What are you going to do with all of this stuff?"

And my response was, "Shawn, after everything I've been through the past six months, I think I deserve a treat." He could not argue that logic.

Did I really need another pair of black boots? Well, I figured I deserved an "end of chemo" gift!

There's nothing like a shopping buzz to lift a weary spirit.
If you feel well enough to shop, treat yourself to something new.

HEALTH TIP #39
Treat Yourself to a New Snack

Do you have the guts? Pumpkin guts, I mean. More specifically, the seeds that are contained in the guts?

With or without their shell, pumpkin seeds have amazing health benefits. The pumpkin seed shell is just fiber and is sometimes hard to digest.
But the inside of the seeds are soft and flavorful. With or without the shell,
pumpkin seeds, or *pepitas*, as they are called, have been shown to:

- reduce inflammation (remember, inflammation causes chronic illness
  and is related to your risk of cancer)

- be high in protein: 1 ounce (28 grams) contains 7 grams of protein

- prevent kidney stones (they inhibit calcium oxalate—a common component of stones)

- supply your body with at least 30% of the RDA for magnesium, copper,
  and manganese

- prevent osteoporosis, as they are high in zinc; low zinc levels are linked
  with high rates of osteoporosis

- contain phytosterols, which lower LDL (the "bad") cholesterol

- improve bladder function and prostate health (for those of you that have
  one) as seen in results of a study being done in Europe

- contain L-tryptophan—which has a calming effect, but also can help
  symptoms of depression

- eliminate intestinal parasites (yes, bugs that live inside us like tapeworms
  as well as pinworms, which you can have without symptoms) when eaten
  with shell on

- contain a high level of iron; one ounce (about two tablespoons) of pepitas, or the shelled version, supplies you with more than 20 percent of
  what you need for the day

After you have prepared your pumpkin in an interesting and nutritious
recipe (or carved a face in the darn thing), separate the seeds and wash
them well in a strainer, removing all the slimy pumpkin insides. Lay them
out on a paper towel or paper bag and let them dry overnight. Then, spread
them on a cookie sheet and bake at 250°F for 30 to 45 minutes, stirring

once or twice. (Baking them longer at a lower temp preserves the nutritional value.)

If you want salt (and who doesn't?), you can toss the seeds with a *tiny bit* of cold-pressed organic extra virgin olive oil (not much—you don't want to fry them) and then sprinkle some sea salt over them before roasting.

Once roasted, you can eat them—husk and all—or you can shell them. I had read that there is a variety of pumpkin that has a "huskless seed," but the look on the produce manager's face at the supermarket told me . . . maybe not. Once roasted, I think the seeds taste fine with the husk on, but not everyone does.

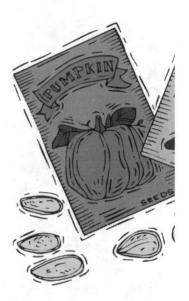

You can buy pepitas, which are shelled seeds, in bags. They are available in raw and roasted, salted or unsalted. Use pepitas in salads, oatmeal, cookie recipes, trail mix, or just eat plain as a snack. See what you've been missing all these years?

Try this Pepitas Brittle for a quick, sweet, healthy, high-protein snack: Combine one cup of raw pepitas and one tablespoon of pure maple syrup in a bowl and mix well. Spread in one flat clump on a parchment-lined cookie sheet. The clump should be flat, but not spread so far that the pepitas aren't all touching. Bake for 13 minutes in a preheated 350°F oven. Remove and let cool completely. Break into pieces like brittle.

A serving size is $^1/_4$ cup.

Calories: 196; Fat: 15.5 grams; Protein: 8.5 grams; Iron: 28% of RDA; Fiber: 1 gram.

(Courtesy of Healthful Habits Inc., www.facebook.com/healthfulhabitsinc.)

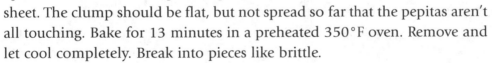

Include pepitas or whole pumpkin seeds in
your diet all year long for extra protein, iron,
and cancer-fighting anti-inflammatory effects.

Being Told How Great I Look

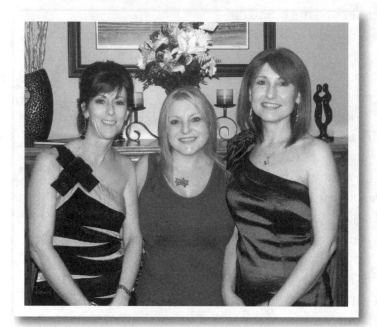

(left to right) Jackie, Juana, and Flo

I celebrated the end of my chemo by attending a Christmas dinner with my sister Juana and my BFF Jackie. Everyone was dressed in their finery and the compliments were whizzing by like bullets: "You look awesome." "Love your dress." "Looking great!" At one point, a lady turned to me and said, "You must be getting sick of people always telling you how great you look since you got cancer." I thought about it for a moment and said, "Naw!"

After being diagnosed, I began taking extra care with my appearance, particularly when I was heading out for a medical treatment or procedure. Before each chemo, for example, I would book myself an appointment at the spa to have a facial and a pedicure. On the night before each chemo, I did a special healing ritual, consisting of a candlelit bath, aromatherapy (a few drops of lavender oil in the bath), soft music, and meditation. On the day of my treatment, I would choose clothes that made me feel powerful, and I always wore my wig. The way I see it, when that nurse was headed at me with the "red devil," I wanted to look and feel like a formidable opponent, not some wimpy pushover in a baseball hat and pajamas.

Of course the aftereffects of chemo would leave me bedridden for several days, and during that time I allowed myself a break from my beauty rituals. However, even when I did not make a special effort with my appearance, I still got showered with compliments everywhere I went in my small town. Now come on folks, I know deep inside that when people said, "You look great," they meant "For someone with cancer," but hey, at forty-four, I was happy to take what I could get. Yeah, I kind of miss those compliments since my recovery.

If you have cancer, get used to people commenting on how good you look, and learn to graciously accept a compliment. A simple "thank you" will suffice.

HEALTH TIP #40
How to Build a Good-Looking Salad

You're trying to eat healthy so you decide to make a salad for lunch. You start with iceberg lettuce, and add tomatoes, croutons, and shredded cheese. Then you cover it with bottled ranch dressing and devour it. You sit back and say to yourself, *Self, you ate a healthy lunch, so go ahead and have that cupcake for dessert.*

Does this sound familiar?

Salads are your golden opportunity to eat a meal that contains all the ingredients that will provide you with extra protein and cancer-fighting vitamins, minerals, and phytochemicals as well as fiber and energy-producing carbs. While the salad above technically is "a salad," it could use a bit of fine-tuning. Let's give it a tune up, shall we?

Subtract: Let's start with the lettuce. Poor, pale iceberg lettuce has the lowest nutritional value of all the greens. Even celery beats it for vitamins and fiber! Just remember, the darker the leaf, the more minerals and vitamins the leaf contains. Compare the color of iceberg lettuce to spinach, Boston, or red-tip lettuce. It's not hard to spot the dud. (If only it was this easy on the singles scene, eh?)

Add: The abundance of different greens that you can use to form the base of your salad boggles the mind. Markets make it easy to take home a variety of mixed greens as they often come all together in one bag. Look for "mixed baby greens," which can contain tender crisp leaves of green leaf, red-tip, baby spinach, and arugula. Also consider other greens like watercress, dandelion, Swiss chard, kale, and French sorrel. (I know I'm leaving some out, but there are too many to list!) I also love to add fresh herb leaves like basil leaves, parsley, and cilantro to the salad, too, as it gives a little surprise to my taste buds and boosts the salad's nutritional benefits.

Subtract: While you don't necessarily have to subtract the tomatoes (although there are some who believe acidic foods like tomatoes promote cancer growth), you shouldn't stop at just one vegetable.

Add: Your tomatoes need company! Add veggies like diced raw zucchini, cucumbers, red peppers, summer squash, avocado, or red onion. Adding more colorful vegetables adds a good dose of fiber and antioxidant vitamins while "feeding" your eyes, too. To keep the tomatoes on the low acid side, choose varieties like yellow and purple, which are less acidic.

Subtract: Croutons don't add any nutritional value, but they do add unwanted fat and sodium. Processed croutons also contain preservatives and flavor enhancers like yeast extract, which is another name for unhealthy MSG (monosodium glutamate).

Add: Instead of croutons, get some plant-based protein into your salad by adding nuts and/or seeds. Walnuts and chia seeds provide disease-fighting omega-3 fatty acids. The Pepitas Brittle recipe found in Health Tip #39 is wonderful on salads. There are dozens of other nuts and seeds like sesame seeds and sliced almonds that provide protein, healthy fats, useful minerals, and an exotic flavor. Nuts and seeds are high in fat, so 1–2 servings is plenty.

Subtract: Shredded cheese provides protein and calcium, but like all dairy, it also can promote unwanted intestinal issues and slash your immune function. Dairy is also an "inflammatory-promoting" food and can lead to poor general health, and dairy protein, casein, may promote cancer growth.

Add: Here's your chance to power up the cancer fighting in your salad and add delicious sweetness, too. Throw in some dried cranberries, raisins, or dried cherries. Fresh fruit provides pleasure for your mouth and medicine for your immune system. The brighter the color, the stronger the health benefits. Fresh blueberries, strawberries, apples, or pears turn boring into *badda-bing!* (That's slang for "Yeah, baby!") You get extra health points if you have every color of the rainbow in that bowl. (Color-blind folks, please ask for help.)

Subtract: Now about that bottled ranch. Out of the twenty or so ingredients in most bottled ranch dressings, I could only find two that I wouldn't wince at: dried garlic and water. The rest of the ingredients came from dairy sources, food thickeners, and chemical flavor enhancers.

With a little tweaking, your salad can become the most powerful cancer-fighting meal of the day!

Add: Little-known fact: Salad dressings don't have to come from a bottle. Here's where you can be creative! Mix your own dressings using plant-based ingredients like extra-virgin olive oil, lemon, lime or apple juice, fresh garlic, chopped fresh herbs, sea salt, or whipped avocado. Fresh salsa makes a great salad dressing, too! Try the blueberry dressing recipe found in Health Tip #20. Mix up some extra to have on hand for tomorrow's salad.

Build a better salad and your salad will build a better you!

Cancer Shook Up My New Year's Resolutions

Before getting cancer, my New Year's resolutions were pretty much predictable:

A. Exercise more/get in shape

B. Eat healthier

C. Drink less

D. All of the above

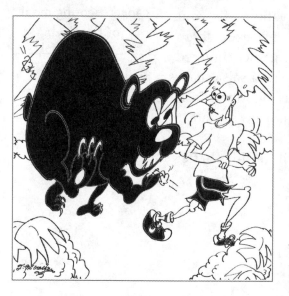

Boooorrrring! Even though I don't actually smoke, sometimes I would add "quit smoking" to my list, just because I'm pretty sure that is one resolution I can really stick to. Come February, when all of the other ideals have fallen to the wayside, and my friends are moaning about breaking their New Year's resolutions, at least I can hold my head high and say, "I haven't had a smoke so far this year!"

In 2012, for the first time in my life, I was starting a new year with cancer. The perk was, after twenty or more years of broken resolutions, I knew that THIS was the year I would honor them. Here was my list: A. Stay alive (which encompasses all of the old resolutions regarding eating, drinking, and exercising).

That was pretty much all I was going to commit to that year. How could I be sure that I would really do it? Well, just imagine that your resolution is to be able to run a mile. But it is hard to train for that because, you know, you get your period, your knees hurt, it rains, and so on, rendering it impossible to stick to your goal. Then one day, you are walking in the woods and suddenly a bear pops up behind you. Voila! The adrenaline kicks in and you run a mile back to your car. Well, cancer is that bear, and I was running for my life, so I was pretty sure that was all the motivation I needed. But just in case the healthy living thing didn't pan out that year however, I added:

B. Quit smoking

I am very happy to report that the healthy living thing did pan out, and I no longer have to fake quitting smoking.

Cancer is a great wake-up call. Even if you are like me and have been living a "healthy-ish" lifestyle, there is always room for improvement.

HEALTH TIP #41
Three Quick and Easy Resolutions to Shake Up Your Life

We all want fast and easy, right? Well it doesn't get any easier than this. By doing these three simple things, you will make incredible strides in the quality of your life and, quite possibly, the quantity of your life as well.

1. Stand Up

Are you sitting down for this? Well, don't! Several large population studies indicate that sitting is the worst thing you can do for your health. Two major studies looking at the activity profiles of almost one million people indicate that the more time you sit, the more likely you are of dying from heart disease, diabetes, and other factors. Even if you are a marathon runner who exercises three hours a day, if you spend the rest of the time sitting, either at your job, or in front of the TV, you still have the same higher risk of illness and death. The more hours you sit, the bigger the risks. Four to six hours seems to be the maximum sitting time per day. Standing for long periods did not show the same negative risks (which might be the reason for the gaining popularity of *standing* computer workstations).

Standing while on the phone, or putting your laptop on a file cabinet so you can stand to work, are ways to reduce long periods of sitting.

I wonder . . . could this mean the eventual end to chairs in doctors' waiting rooms?

Think about it: how long do you sit per day?

Stand up for you health!

2. *Breathe Deeply*

I'm gonna go out on a limb here and assume that you are breathing right now. In any event, I invite you to go ahead and take a really deep breath and hold it for two seconds before you release it. Feel good? Feel your cells getting a jolt of energy and your brain waking up?

Breathing is something that we all take for granted. We do it every day, but are we really getting the most out of this automatic body function?

Every cell in your body needs oxygen to survive. But daily stress can cause you to take short and shallow breaths. Deep breathing not only delivers a burst of oxygen to your body and brain, it also stimulates your diaphragm—that muscle in your gut that pulls your chest cavity open when you breathe. Your diaphragm is directly connected to the autonomic nervous system. That's the system that gives us extra energy when we're running from danger, but it's also the system that slows your body down and helps you to feel calm. Deep breathing stimulates the "parasympathetic" body response that tells our brain "everything is fine, all is well." As soon as this system is stimulated, your muscles begin to loosen, your heart rate slows down, and you feel more relaxed.

Oxygen is the first of the three vital necessities of life (the other two being water and food). Without breath, there is nothing else.

You can practice deep breathing anywhere. Just breathe in slowly, making sure your belly pushes out as you inhale, hold it for two seconds, then release the breath slowly. As you release try to imagine the stress leaving your body. Repeat this three or four times comfortably. Try this exercise when you really need it, like in the airport when your flight is delayed or if the person in front of you at the "ten items or less" line has eleven items.

Proper, efficient, deep breathing is an art that should be practiced. It might sound crazy to take a class on what you've been doing since you were born, but I encourage you to explore it. There are many different kinds of breathing, such as mindful breathing, meditative breathing, and *Ujjayi* breathing. You can check your local yoga studio or meditation center for breathing classes or look online for therapeutic breathing tapes that will help you get started. Become a professional breather!

3. *Install a Chlorine Filter*

We all need water to drink, and, in most cases, that means turning on the tap. But among the dozens of nasty substances in tap water, chlorine and its byproducts may be the most harmful. Lucky for us, they are the easiest to eliminate.

Chlorine is used in water purification. It's one of the chemicals that disinfects the water and is very effective at ensuring that the water we drink is "bug-free." The problem with chlorine occurs when it reacts with other natural contaminants in the water to form a group of toxins called trihalomethanes (THMs). The chemicals known as THMs have been linked to a variety of illnesses like asthma, heart disease, eczema, and cancer. Chloroform is one of the THMs that is causing concern.

A report by the World Health Organization on the safety of drinking water (*Trihalomethanes in drinking-water*, WHO, 2004) indicates there is clear evidence that the chemicals known as THMs are linked to bladder and liver cancers in animal models. Other studies have linked THMs to high risks of cancer and reproductive problems in humans. For this reason, the U.S. Environmental Protection Agency continues to reevaluate and set new limits on the levels of THMs that are allowed by law in the public water supply. Unfortunately, THMs are also absorbed through the skin when taking a shower, and you breathe in harmful vapors from the steam. Chlorine and its byproducts can cause dry, itchy skin and worsen skin conditions as well. This is why I like to call chlorine "the *other* Big C."

Luckily, an activated carbon filter will remove a large percentage of chlorine, THMs, and other harmful contaminants from your drinking and bathing water. Filters can be mounted on your kitchen faucet, hidden under your sink, or attached to your refrigerator water source. You can buy a water pitcher with a built-in filter, and there are even carbon filters that attach to a water bottle for travel! (Visit www.Brita.com.) Activated carbon filters can also be purchased for your showerheads. They are simple to install and maintain and come in many different styles and colors.

Stand up and hold your chlorine-free water high while you take a deep breath. It's healthy multi-tasking at its best!

The levels of filter power vary, so check the specifics on any filter you plan to purchase. You'll want to check for the maximum percentage of THMs, chlorine, and other contaminants filtered, but you also want to look for a filter that lasts, which would be indicated by the "manufacturer's rated capacity" or the number of gallons of water that the carbon could effectively filter.

Installing a water filter at your drinking water supply and in your shower is a fast and easy way to remove chlorine and THMs from your body, and add to your health.

Packing Light

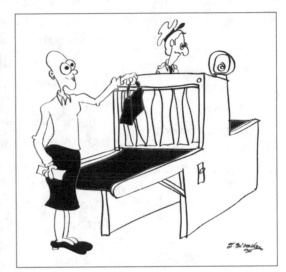

With the cancer clinic nearly 240 miles from my home and being in a long-distance relationship, I often found myself packing and unpacking my suitcase. Packing is a chore that I have never enjoyed, and it seems that I always manage to forget something. However, once I had lost my hair from the chemo, I was amazed at how much lighter I could pack. No more shampoo, conditioner, hairspray, mousse, hair dryer, straight iron, or Velcro rollers! All I needed was my well-groomed "mock hair" and some clothes.

Leave the hair-care products at home
and pack more shoes and purses.

HEALTH TIP #42
Don't Mock the Tuna

If you've started swapping animal-based foods for plant-based foods to reduce your risk of cancer, you may think some foods are just plain unswappable. Well, think again. I assure you, for every food that you love that contains meat, chicken, fish, or dairy, there is a combo of vegetables, fruits, nuts, or seeds that will satisfy your taste buds while providing you with the tools you need to reduce your risk of cancer and other illnesses.

Sometimes, you will see replacement recipes for chicken nuggets or egg salad that are vegan, called "mock" food—mock chicken nuggets, mock egg salad, and so on. To mock something is to make fun of it. Food choices should be respected, regardless if they're plant-based or not. Don't be a food meanie.

Occasionally, I like a good tuna salad sandwich. And until recently, I have just been "doing without" because of my plant-based eating style. However, even before I started limiting seafood in my diet, I tried to avoid large fish like tuna because of their high level of contaminates. Larger fish, because of the amount of food they consume and their size, have higher levels of mercury in their flesh. When you eat the contaminated fish, the mercury, in the form of methylmercury, accumulates in your body and can cause neurological damage over time. Fetal risks are greater. Your size determines the amount of mercury that is considered safe for you to consume. For example, according to the Environmental Protection Agency (EPA), a child weighing twenty pounds should only eat a sandwich made with white albacore tuna every ten weeks! Someone weighing one hundred and twenty pounds should wait eleven days before eating tuna again. Knowing that just reinforces my decision to eliminate tuna from my food choices, but I still liked the way it tasted.

> Exciting new recipes don't have to be "substitutions" for old favorites. They can just be exciting new recipes.

So How Do You Get the "Tuna" Without the "Fish"?

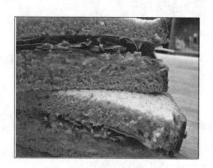

Here's the beauty of plants: There are tastes and textures to match anything in the animal world. In this case, seeds and chickpeas are used to get the texture and color, and flavorings are added for taste. When I found this recipe, I was skeptical, but after tasting it, and after seeing my husband (an anti-vegite) find the bowl of this in the fridge and devour it, I became a believer. I make this all the time because it's so easy. It's great as a dip, too.

Recipe and photo by Trish Cowper. For more great recipes like this, go to: www.infinebalance.com.

CHICKPEA OF THE SEA

YIELD: ABOUT 2 CUPS

1 cup cooked (or canned, but cooked is healthier) chickpeas, rinsed and drained

$1/2$ cup raw unroasted sunflower seeds

$1/4$ cup sesame seeds

1 tablespoon soy sauce

2 tablespoons lemon juice

2 teaspoons olive oil

A pinch or two of sea salt

1 to 2 stalks celery, finely diced

$1/4$ cup finely diced red onion, or less

$1/4$ to $1/2$ cup Vegenaise or any vegan mayo

A good pinch of fresh black pepper

If you're cooking your chickpeas to avoid the BPA in canned, cook this way: Place 1 cup of chickpeas in a bowl and add enough water to cover them. Let soak overnight. Drain, rinse, and transfer to a pot with a lid. Cover with water that is twice the amount of the chickpeas and bring to a boil. Cover, reduce heat, and simmer for 1 hour. Remove from heat and drain (This can be done up to 3 days in advance and kept in the fridge.)

In a blender or food processor, add chickpeas, seeds, soy sauce, lemon juice, olive oil, and sea salt. Add a tablespoon or two of water if you need to get the mixture to move a bit, but only if necessary. Blend until relatively smooth, but not pasty. It should have some texture to it. Transfer to a small mixing bowl and add celery, onion, mayo, and black pepper. Let it sit in the refrigerator at least 30 minutes or overnight. (This step is vital.) Makes enough filling for about 4 hearty sandwiches. Great with celery sticks and on salads, too.

NUTRITION IN $1/4$ OF THE MIX:

Calories: 319; Fat: 23 grams; Protein: 10grams; Fiber: 5.5 grams; Iron: 19% of the RDA; Calcium: 12.8% of the RDA; Vitamin C: 8.5% of the RDA.

A Free Trip to Florida

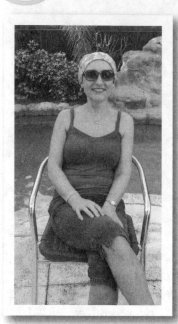

I was on a real high after surviving chemo and finally starting to feel like my old self again by Christmastime. I thought, *Life doesn't get any better than this.* Ah, but I was so wrong . . . life did get better! When I opened my Christmas gift from my sister, Lynette, and her generous husband, Jeff, I was surprised to find plane tickets to Florida! (To be accompanied by my boyfriend Shawn and my parents.)

The surprise vacation could not have come at a better time. It allowed me to recoup after my chemo treatments and prepared me both mentally and physically for my upcoming mastectomy. While my colleagues in Canada were trudging to work through several feet of snow, I was lounging by the pool, soaking up the rays, with a warm breeze blowing through my stubble. Without a doubt, that was one of the nicest perks of having cancer!

> There is nothing like a good dose of sunshine to lift your spirits when you are undergoing cancer treatments. If you are not able to fly off to a tropical destination, just get outside and enjoy the sunshine.

HEALTH TIP #43
Take a Vacation in Your Own Backyard

Contrary to what we might think, our natural habitat is not on a couch or in a cubicle. It's outdoors among the trees, grass, and fresh air. We keep forgetting that we belong to the "wild kingdom" and we are programmed by deep-seated, million-year-old genetics before anything else to realize that nature is our true home. You don't have to go farther than your own backyard to enjoy the benefits of green space, fresh air, and sunshine!

In line with this thought, recent studies show that humans are healthier when they have access to parks and green spaces. The connection between nature and health, both physical and mental, has been studied for years. Researchers at the University of Illinois are compiling fact-based evidence that shows we experience a "feeling" of well-being when we are exposed to the outdoors, but we also experience better blood sugar control, and we have an increased immune response, which can be translated into a reduction of cancer risk. They also found that simple exposures to green landscapes were associated with shorter recovery times from surgery.

On the flip side, those with no access to green spaces had a higher risk of obesity, cardiovascular disease, and death. The data results were independent of the person's amount of exercise and socioeconomic status.

> Exposure to the green spaces of the outdoors benefits your body, mind, and spirit—and best of all, it's free!

Scientists relate these human studies to what they see in the animal world. Animals taken out of their natural habitat and placed in concrete ones have higher rates of sickness and death, reproduction problems, and an odd phenomena called "soiling the nest," where animals destroy their man-made homes because of an inability to cope.

The same holds true for us. Comparisons were made of residences in urban areas. The neighborhoods with direct access to grass and trees had a lower rate of crime and vandalism regardless of socioeconomic status. Those living in these green areas also had more job satisfaction, better moods, less violence and aggression, and showed better impulse control when they had access to some form of nature, even if it was just a visual one.

Worldwide studies confirm this. In the Netherlands, for example, it is found that the general health of residents is directly related to the proximity of their green space. In Japan, longevity can be predicted by the same measure.

Research published in the journal *Science* compared postsurgical patients who had a view of trees with those who had a view of a brick wall. The nature-gazers needed fewer pain meds, suffered fewer minor complications such as fever, nausea, and constipation, and stayed an average of nearly three-quarter fewer days at the hospital.

Do your own experiment. The next time you feel tired, have a headache, or feel like punching a wall, get a big dose of trees, birds, flowers, and grass in your system and see what happens.

Perks for Parents

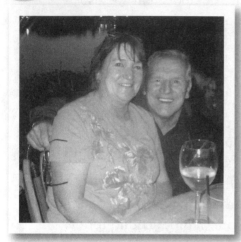

My parents, Len and Madeline Strang

I recently received a very moving message on my blog from a woman who said, "Our world came crashing down just after Christmas when our mom, our best friend, the woman who holds everything together, called and told us she was diagnosed with breast cancer." This statement brought home to me the reality that cancer truly is a family disease. When I was diagnosed, my whole family was grief stricken, none more so than my parents. However, just as cancer had its perks for me, it turns out that my cancer held some perks for them as well.

Dad has lived most of his life with chronic back pain, among other health issues. For many years he existed in the sick role, with Mom and his five daughters caring for him. After I was diagnosed, there was a big change in Dad. All of a sudden he started showing up at my house with his little tool kit asking if I needed anything fixed. (That is a man's way of nurturing, by the way.) While I was undergoing chemo, my sister Sherry experienced serious health issues as well, requiring emergency surgery. While Mom was at my home taking care of me, Dad was at Sherry's, nursing her back to health. What a reversal of roles!

At the age of sixty-eight, Dad got his first passport to travel outside Canada in order to accompany us on my surprise trip to Florida. Mom had been traveling to Florida for years to visit my sister, but she long ago gave up hope of ever getting Dad to go with her. It took everyone by surprise when he agreed to go with us, and I have to say, despite the discomfort he experienced during our travels, he was a real trooper. Dad still lives with chronic pain, but the experience of seeing his daughters through illness seems to have given him a new lease on life.

Another perk is the deeper closeness that seems to have developed between my parents. Pulling together in a time of crisis has taken them to a new level of intimacy. This is apparent, not only to our family, but to others as well. On the flight back from Florida, as my parents were chatting and laughing, the flight attendant asked them if they were on their honeymoon. Mom, a practical, no-nonsense person, laughed heartily at that comment. For her, it was a real knee-slapper! I think Dad took it as a compliment.

> It is sometimes difficult to allow ourselves to be nursed and nurtured by others. Keep in mind, however, that this blessing is a gift as much for the giver as the receiver.

HEALTH TIP #44
Keep in Mind—Colorful Means Healthy

If colorful means healthy, it's not hard to find the foods that you should avoid: White ones. White potatoes, white rice, white pasta, and white bread.

Let's compare sweet potatoes to white potatoes. Gorgeous, bright-orange sweet potatoes have 14,185 IUs of vitamin A, which is an antioxidant and powerful cancer fighter. That's 284 percent of your recommended daily allowance. White potatoes have 0 percent. Remember, inflammation equals disease. Certain foods promote an inflammatory response based on their nutritional content. One noted nutritionist has assigned inflammation points to foods, giving them either a positive or negative rating. Positive foods are anti-inflammatory, and the higher the number, the more potent the anti-inflammatory effect. Negative-numbered foods cause an inflammatory response. The higher that number is, the more the response is. For more information about this rating system, visit www.InflammationFactor.com. I am using the factor ratings here for comparison's sake only.

Sweet potatoes have an inflammation score of 124 (anti-inflammatory). White potatoes have a score of -66. That's a *negative* 66, which means that white potatoes cause a mild inflammatory response in your body, causing your body to react. Of course, one spud won't do you harm, but if white potatoes (or potato salad, potato chips, French fries, home fries, mashed potatoes . . . you get the idea), and many other inflammation-promoting foods find their way to your plate every day, and the foods that inhibit inflammation don't find their way there too, over time it could spell trouble.

How about pasta? White pasta has an inflammation factor of –302!

Negative 302 for a bowl of macaroni or spaghetti! If you choose to eat the pasta, you should balance it out with fresh veggies to make it a "pasta primavera." That way, the broccoli, red peppers, yellow squash, and garlic will balance out the negativity of the white stuff. (By the way, the inflammation factor for three cloves of raw garlic is +322.)

White bread comes from white flour, which is highly processed. White flour begins as wheat flour, and wheat flour begins as a whole grain. If you take that grain, crush it, strip it, run it through chemicals, and bleach it, you are left with a white powder called "all-purpose flour." Take the flour, add dough stabilizers, preservatives, high fructose corn syrup, and yeast. What you get is highly processed brand-named white bread that contains very little natural nutrition. (There are vitamins and iron in the bread, but they're added after the flour is processed.)

> Eat all the colors of the rainbow. (Hint: there's no white in a rainbow.)

White rice is just brown rice that's butt naked (or is it buck naked?). Yep, they stripped it of its nutritious high-fiber coating, and you're left with just the sticky, starch insides.

Potatoes, rice, pasta, and bread are all high-starch foods. Starch turns to sugar even before it hits your stomach. The enzymes in your saliva start the conversion process immediately. As the starch moves through the digestive tract, it is further metabolized into sugar and enters the blood very quickly. Experts agree: Sugar feeds disease.

These starchy, sticky foods also do a number on your intestines once they get there. White foods are like glue, gumming up the works. Think about what foods your doctor tells you to eat when you have diarrhea: white rice, white toast, white potatoes, and pasta. That's because they will stop runny stools in their tracks. But if you don't have diarrhea, all that glue will slow things down and can cause bloating and constipation.

Healthy bowels not only make you feel better and allow you to successfully zip up your jeans, but they are a necessary part of important vitamin and mineral absorption and have a lot to do with your body's detoxification system, ridding your body of unhealthy free radicals that damage cells and lead to disease.

I can't help but think of a typical fast-food meal—white-bread bun filled with meat, fried white potatoes . . . and if you add a vanilla shake—Okay, I'll quit there.

Home Alone

While I thoroughly enjoyed my Florida vacation, for me there's no place like home. I love solitude. However, a hectic work schedule combined with three children left very little "alone time" for me. Most nights I would drop into bed shortly after tucking Ben in for the night and fall asleep mid–"Hail Mary." Following my diagnosis, however, I had more time to myself than ever before in my life. And I was lovin' it!

Once the kids left for school, I had six glorious hours to myself every weekday. Sometimes I preplanned my day, as I had to be sure to include the boring stuff, like doctor's appointments, picking up prescriptions, and paying bills. Many days, however, I would awaken to a blank slate, which I could fill in any way I wanted. Here are some of my favorites:

- go for a walk

- do a meditation

- cook a pot of healthy soup

- sit in my sunroom with a cuppa and bird-watch

- read

- garden (in season)

- catch up on e-mails to my friends

As I continue to pursue these stress-relieving activities, I know that I am creating an environment that is most conducive to my continued health.

"Learn to enjoy your own company. You are the one person you can count on living with for the rest of your life."
—*Ann Richards*

HEALTH TIP #45
Another Thing You Can Count On:
BPA Is B-A-D

Plastic and its byproducts are all around us and found in places they shouldn't be (like your urine—more on that later). Just look around and you'll agree that pretty much everything you see is made of some form of plastic. But some plastics are "better" and "safer" than others.

The 1950s were great, weren't they? They brought us the Chevy Corvette, the Rat Pack, and a new, lightweight, fun-filled plastic: polycarbonate. Polycarbonates and PVC plastics are made from a substance called bisphenol-A, better known as BPA. BPA can leech out of the plastic and into your body. Polycarbonates containing BPA were widely used in food containers and bottles, but are mostly found today in other places like cash register receipts and canned-food linings. And unfortunately, recycling these materials is reintroducing BPA into more places, including toilet paper, napkins, and newspaper. It is harmful in many ways, despite what the chemical companies and mega manufacturers tell us, but it is still manufactured at a growing rate of 3.6 million tons a year! It is inexpensive to make and widely available for many uses. It's a manufacturer's dream!

But for us it's a nightmare because our body reacts the same way to the BPA in these plastics as it does to hormones, more specifically, the sex hormones. Exposure to endocrine disruptors, or chemicals that mimic hormones, potentiates the risk for hormonally related cancers like breast, ovarian, uterine, and prostate. But the harmful effects don't stop there. Here is a growing list of all abnormalities linked to BPA exposure:

- ovarian cancer
- prostate cancer
- miscarriage
- obesity
- infertility

- breast cancer
- premature birth
- liver disease
- diabetes
- erectile dysfunction

- feminizing male organs in utero

- heart disease/lipid abnormality

- attention-deficit disorder (ADD) and attention-deficit/hyperactivity disorder (ADHD)

BPA is one of the hundreds of chemicals found in newborns' umbilical cord blood and has been for years.

According to the Center for Disease Control (CDC) more than 90 percent of the American population over the age of six has detectable BPA in their urine. A recent study done at the University of Harvard showed a 1,221 percent increase in BPA levels in the urine of those who ate soup from cans three times a week, as the can linings are potent BPA leechers. (Some can linings and water-bottle linings are clear, so you don't even know they're there.) And don't think that avoiding plastic can liners will get you out of harm's way. Paper products, like copy paper, paper money, and airline tickets, contribute approximately thirty-three tons of BPA to the environment every year in the United States and Canada. We are exposed to those papers every day, and the employees that handle those papers every day are at an even higher risk of exposure.

> Be aware of the dangers of plastic exposure and make small changes to reduce it.

Lately, with increased interest in the dangers of BPA, there is more research being conducted on how BPA causes such clear changes in the reproductive hormones. We know that BPA binds with the estrogen receptors when we are exposed to it and disrupts hormone function. But now researchers have discovered that it is the metabolite of BPA, MBP, which plays a bigger role in the estrogen response by grabbing it with not just one receptor, like the BPA, but with two receptors, doubling the potency of the abnormal hormone response.

We know about BPA and the harm it's doing. We know BPA can get into our bodies by eating and drinking contaminated foods stored in BPA-lined cans and food containers, but it also easily passes through our skin and into our bloodstream from direct contact. Studies show it can remain on your skin for up to two hours. It is impossible to avoid all plastics in your life, so try to avoid plastic exposure as much as you can. Here are some general guidelines:

- Avoid eating canned food and choose frozen or fresh to avoid the BPA exposure in the can lining. This is especially strong in acidic foods like tomatoes and tomato soup.

- Choose plastics marked with #1, #2, #4, or #5, as these numbered plastics do not contain BPA. (Plastic marked #7 is categorized as "other," which can mean safe plant-based cellulose or unsafe BPA combo plastics. Check with the manufacturer for specifics.) However, even plastics that are marked "BPA-free" may still have BPA if they were recycled from BPA containing plastics. There's just no way of knowing.

- Reheat all foods in glass or ceramic containers, as heat tends to increase the leeching of the chemicals from plastics into your food. Don't use plastics for hot beverages or food.

- Avoid containers marked "PC" (polycarbonate) if the container is clear plastic.

- Don't reuse single-use plastics as they can break down and leech chemicals.

- If you work with cash register receipts, money, or thermal paper in other areas, wear gloves to protect yourself from BPA exposure.

- Avoid plastic teethers and toys and stick to cloth, cotton, and uncoated wood.

- Choose natural flooring instead of vinyl.

- Cover food with paper towels instead of plastic wrap when microwaving.

There are many chemicals that go into making plastics, not just harmful BPA. Be mindful of the plastics that are in your life.

For more information on plastic safety go to www.ewg.org.

Cancer Forced Me to Brush Up on My Math Skills

Math has never been my strong point. So you can just imagine my confusion when I started to investigate breast cancer statistics. There were stats for incidence, survival rates, recurrence rates, and lots of other numbers that made little sense to me. I really wanted to understand what I was getting myself into with this cancer thing, so I asked my daughter, an honors math student, to do a little tutorial with me before I set off to decipher the numbers. To think, if not for cancer, I would have gone through life with less than adequate math skills!

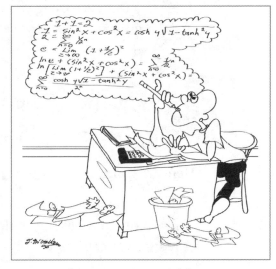

The first stat I found was rather daunting. Stage-3 breast cancer yields just over a 50 percent five-year survival rate. But wait, the news gets better. By exercising, I can reduce my risk of recurrence by nearly 40 percent. I'm a runner, so YAY for me! Believe it or not, the younger you are at the time of diagnosis, the lower your chances of survival, so being diagnosed after the age of forty ups my odds of surviving by another 3 percent. Yet another encouraging study found that a healthy diet resulted in as much as a 30 percent decrease in the risk of death following a cancer diagnosis. I am happy to report that I have fully embraced a healthy, cancer-fighting diet.

Now, bear with me while I do the math:

50% chance of survival overall

Plus 40% for exercising

Plus 3% for age at diagnosis

Plus 30% for a good diet

If my calculations are correct, my odds of surviving breast cancer are 123 percent. (Plus or minus 30 percent for drinking red wine. Scientists can't seem to agree on whether it is good for me or bad for me.)

DO NOT get too caught up in the stats when you have cancer; they can be misleading. You are not a statistic. DO everything you can to improve your health through exercise, a healthy diet, and maintaining a positive attitude.

HEALTH TIP #46
Try Crunching These Numbers

Here are some statistics (not to get caught up in):

- 30%—percentage of all cancer deaths in the United States that are caused by smoking. Quitting is the single most effective thing you can do to reduce your risk of cancer—above anything else.

- 30 to 40%—percentage of cancer deaths related to human behavior like poor diet and inactivity.

- 72,000,000—the number of people who are currently obese in the United States (2012).

- 54,304—the number of cancer deaths among women related to obesity in the United States this year (20% of all cancer deaths).

> Statistics can be sobering . . . and motivating.

- 95%—the number of umbilical cord blood samples that tested positive for DDT residue, a cancer-causing pesticide banned in 1972.

- 68%—the five-year survival rates for all cancers, up 18% from forty years ago.

- 93%—the percentage of all people, children included, who have detectable BPA (bisphenol-A, a chemical in plastic) in their urine.

- 83%—the number of cancers that are on the rise having to do with digestion and excretion (esophagus, pancreas, liver, bile duct, kidney). What did you have for lunch?

- 1,638,910—the number of new cases of cancer that are expected in 2012 in the United States alone.

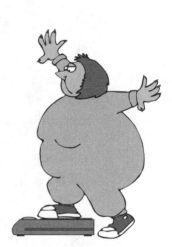

- 12,600,000—the number of new cancer cases that are expected worldwide in 2012.

- 5%—your chances of getting breast cancer in your lifetime in 1960 (1 in 20).

- 13%—your chances of getting breast cancer in your lifetime in 2012 (1 in 8).

- 234,580—new cases of breast cancer expected in 2013, an increase from 2012.

- 2%—The current amount of research money spent on stage-4 breast cancer (metastatic disease) even though 30% of all those diagnosed with any stage of breast cancer will go on to develop stage 4, and it is what ultimately kills.

- 800,000—the number of people who will die from heart disease in 2012 in the United States.

- 580,350—the number of people who will die from cancer in 2013 in the United States, which is an increase over 2012's figures.

- 100%—the number of people reading this who are literate.

Cancer Increased My Vocabulary

Invasive ductal carcinoma. Oncologist. Tamoxifen. Adjuvant therapy. Metastasis. Before getting cancer, I would have thought these words to be part of a foreign language. Now they are part of my everyday vocabulary. They are not pretty words, and some of them, I will admit, scare the living daylights out of me! There is one word, however, that I am happy to have learned from my cancer experience: psychoneuroimmunology. Ah, don't ya just love how it rolls off your tongue? Psychoneuroimmunology (pronounced "kale" . . . just kiddin', it is actually pronounced just as it is spelled) is the study of the interaction between psychological processes and the nervous and immune systems of the body. In other words, it is the study of the mind-body connection.

Many books have been written about the mind-body connection: *Love, Medicine and Miracles* (Bernie Siegel, MD), *The Power of Positive Thinking* (Norman Vincent Peale), and *You Can Heal Your Life* (Louise Hay) are among my favorites. Both Siegel and Hay propose that cancer can be caused by underlying psychological factors. Hay says that cancer is caused by holding on to resentment, which eats away at the spirit as cancer eats away at the body. I think she has a good point. One of the questions that Dr. Siegel asks his patients is "What happened to you in the two years leading up to your diagnosis?" He believes that traumatic life events can serve as precursors to cancer. That makes sense to me. In the two years leading up to my diagnosis, I was under stress, and lots of it!

Some people take offense to this way of thinking. "Are you saying that I caused my own cancer?" Well, not exactly, but according to this theory, how you live your life, how you cope with stress, and even your personality type can play a role in creating an environment in your body in which cancer can grow. Here is the good news: if your mind can play a role in making you sick, it can also play a role in healing you. BINGO! That's why I love this new word, psychoneuroimmunology (I just had to say it again). It is the reason why meditation, prayer, visualizations, affirmations, forgiveness exercises, and gardening are all important parts of my survival plan.

If you are going to read only one book on your cancer journey, make it this one. But if you are going to read a second, I would suggest *Love, Medicine and Miracles*.

HEALTH TIP #47
Here Are Some More Words to Add to Your Vocabulary

I don't know which is harder: pronouncing some of the ingredients on package labels or figuring out what they're doing there in the first place.

It seems like all labels—whether it's food, household products, or cosmetics—contain ingredients that leave us wondering if we are exposing ourselves to something harmful or harmless.

Ingredients like methylparabens, coco-glucoside, and sodium lauryl sulfate probably line your household shelves. Keeping in mind that there are entire books written about all the chemical agents that we are exposed to each day, the following are just a few that you may run across in your day-to-day activities and a brief comment on safety and what they do.

Parabens

Methylparaben, butylparaben, ethylparaben, benzylparaben, heptylparaben, isobutylparaben, and propylparaben. As a rule of thumb, if it ends in "paraben," it means the same thing: bad. Some cosmetic companies try to hide the parabens by using code names like Germaben II and LiquiPar Oil. Parabens are strong preservatives, and they are very cheap to manufacture and use, so big companies love them because they can make millions of bottles of their stuff and leave it on a shelf for years in some warehouse and it won't spoil.

Where is it? Parabens are used in all types of products, like cosmetics, lotions, shampoos, washes, some pharmaceutical syrups, and personal-care products like deodorant and toothpaste. Heptylparabens are found in non-carbonated soft drinks and beer.

Is it bad? While there is no conclusive evidence that parabens *cause* cancer, the evidence is clear that, in the lab, parabens fuel cancer cell growth and are estrogenic—that is, they mimic the hormone estrogen. The fact is, parabens have been found in breast cancer tumors, and there's a very good chance that you have parabens in your urine right now. (Remember, your skin is a *carrier*, not a barrier.) Parabens are synthetic chemicals and don't belong inside our bodies. Being exposed to so many personal-care products from multiple areas of our lives increases the exposure. You can avoid parabens by making different product choices, and it would benefit you to do so. There is evidence that when different parabens are combined in one product, they affect the growth of cancer cells exponentially. So if paraben A grows ten cancer cells and paraben B grows ten cancer cells, and you put paraben A and B together, instead of growing twenty cancer cells, they would grow one hundred!

So? Take a look at what you use every day and look for words ending with "paraben" in the ingredients. If you are using a large number of products containing these questionable chemicals, it's very easy to substitute some healthier options. Luckily there are many natural-based companies that are very happy to give you paraben-free products today, and larger brand-name companies are wising up to the fact that you are getting smarter by not only reading labels, but actually knowing what they mean.

Sodium Lauryl Sulfate

Sodium lauryl sulfate (SLS) is a synthetic foaming agent.

Where is it? SLS is found in a wide variety of shampoos, body washes, and facial cleansers. If the product needs to produce lather and suds, you'll probably find SLS.

Is it bad? It can be, but there is no evidence that SLS causes cancer and the Environmental Working Group's Cosmetic Database confirms it. Are you surprised? Most people have heard that SLS causes cancer and are avoiding it. So much so, that now natural-based companies are putting "no SLS" on their product labels. The fact is, sodium lauryl sulfate may have been confused with sodium *laureth* sulfate, which can contain 1,4 dioxane, a known carcinogen. That's not to say that down the line there won't be a problem with SLS, as many synthetics were first deemed "safe" only to find that they produced harmful effects.

So? SLS is a synthetic chemical, and it does get absorbed through your skin. It is a potent skin irritant so if you are avoiding chemicals, avoid it. Those with skin conditions like eczema and psoriasis or those prone to skin allergies would be smart to avoid it. However, there is no credible evidence to support the idea that SLS increases your risk for cancer. That said, you should avoid Sodium Laureth Sulfate.

Caramel Coloring

It sounds so yummy and is probably making your mouth water, but the name is very deceiving. Caramel coloring (as opposed to soft, chewy caramels) is a synthetic coloring agent often paired with ammonia in production and contains the chemicals 2-methylimidazole and 4-methylimidazole. We call this "ammonia caramel coloring," but it will probably only be listed as "caramel coloring" on the label.

Where is it? Found in anything that isn't dark brown but needs to be: cola-flavored soft drinks, beer, meat gravies, soy sauces, baked goods, and artificial chocolate-flavored products. I even found it in my "healthy" instant oatmeal!

Is it bad? In 2011, the International Agency for Research on Cancer concluded, based on current studies and research, that the chemical compounds in caramel coloring are "possibly carcinogenic to humans." Ammonia caramel coloring is also classified under California's Proposition 65 as a carcinogen. California warned that products containing 29 mcg of the chemical per serving would have to bear a health-warning label. In March 2012, testing done on two major name-brand colas found up to 150 mcg of the contaminant in every can—almost five times the level that needs to bear a warning.

So? Cola-flavored soft drinks colored with caramel coloring are one of the unhealthiest beverages existing today. The danger lies in the amount consumed. If you consume several cola-type soft drinks a day, not only does your diet need examining, but you are consuming a lot of caramel coloring in those soft drinks. To avoid it totally, just look for the "no artificial coloring" on the label, or check the label for caramel coloring.

Coco–Glucoside

I predict you will be seeing a lot more of this ingredient in the future. Coco-glucoside is a chemical foaming and cleansing agent produced by a reaction between glucose (sugar) and coconut oil–containing ingredients. Manufacturers love this synthetic ingredient because it sounds so natural. It really is an ingredient that has the best of both worlds. It was once "natural," but is made into a useful chemical.

Where is it? It is found in a multitude of cleansers and washes for your body and hair. Most of the companies that use coco-glucosides are "natural" companies (companies that offer alternatives to chemical-containing products) and may be using coco-glucosides as a replacement for sodium laurel sulfate.

Is it bad? There is no evidence that coco-glucosides are harmful in any way. That said, coco-glucosides are synthetic chemicals even though they are made from natural sources. If you are trying to go "all natural," you really can't include this in your playlist.

So? You can decide if this is something that fits into your personal-care product philosophy. If you are using a product that you love, coco-glucosides would not be a reason to switch.

Butylated Hydroxyanisole

Butylated hydroxyanisole (BHA) is a food preservative that keeps oils from going bad in processed foods and acts as a preservative in cosmetics. Often seen with its wicked stepsister butylated hydroxytoluene (BHT).

Where is it? Many processed items that sit on a shelf contain BHA: cereals, granola bars, cookies, crackers, gum, chips, and personal-care products like lipstick and lotion.

Is it bad? At first glance, it would appear yes, as the 2011 National Institutes of Health's Report on Carcinogens listed it as "reasonably anticipated to be a human carcinogen." But the controversy lies in the fact that the malignant tumors noted to grow in mice fed the stuff were located in the mouse's forestomach—an organ that humans don't have. The state of California does list it as a carcinogen.

> You don't need a decoder ring to decipher your labels; you just need some patience.

So? There is conflicting research on this chemical. Studies show that it does get broken down and metabolized in your body, so it is affecting your organs in some way. It is unclear whether small doses or large doses are unhealthy. If you're making an effort to eat more healthfully, and are eating more fresh foods, then you don't have to worry since only processed foods contain BHA and BHT. Which is yet another good reason to eat fresh.

This ends your vocabulary lesson for today. Don't be tempted to just skip over words you don't know in the ingredient list of your favorite products. There is a wealth of information out there to help you navigate through it. Check out these websites:

Center for Science in the Public Interest:
  www.cspinet.org/reports/chemcuisine.htm

U.S. Dept of Health and Human Services Product Database:
  http://householdproducts.nlm.nih.gov/index.htm

Skin Deep Cosmetics Database:
  www.ewg.org/skindeep

Cancer Helped Me See the World Through the Eyes of a Child

I was about four years old the first time I recall seeing a house lit up with colorful Christmas lights. I still remember the sound of the frosty snow crunching under my feet, and the feel of my mother's warm hand on mine as the snowflakes softly swirled about us that cool December evening. The sight of the lights reflected in the water filled me with such joy that it bubbled over to laughter.

At the age of forty-four I was blessed to experience, once again, the feeling of seeing Christmas lights for the "first time." I had just completed my last chemo session and my family pitched in to help with the decorating. It was just getting dark outside when I looked through the living room window to see my whole garden aglow. To everyone around me, it looked no different than it had for the past eight Christmases at this house. But lying on the couch in my chemo slumber, the sight filled me with such awe that it felt as if I was seeing these lights for the very first time. In that instant I understood what it meant to see the world through the eyes of a child.

I wish I could say that the feeling stayed with me, but the harsh realities of life with cancer soon replaced my feelings of joy and awe with those of fear and foreboding. While I strove to stay positive throughout my cancer journey, I am the first to acknowledge that cancer has more "quirks" than "perks." (I would have no trouble blogging "1,000 Quirks of Having Cancer.") The most troublesome of these is the worry that the cancer might return. For the first few weeks of the new year, this thought became more of an obsession to me than a worry, and I found myself frantically searching the Internet trying to find HOPE. I weighed the stats, analyzed my prognosis, and considered my odds. The more I researched, the more scared I became!

I soon discovered that the hope I was searching for was not to be found on the Internet, but in the form of a letter I received in the mail. Ireland is a seven-year-old girl who was preparing to make her first Holy Communion. Part of her preparation for this sacrament involved praying for the sick. After her mother showed her my blog, she decided to draw me a picture and send me a letter to help cheer me up. Ireland's letter reads in part:

> *You are very brave and strong, and you remind me of my very favorite horse in the whole world, Rosie O'Grady. One time Rosie hurt her foot and she couldn't walk very good but she tried every day to do her best. . . . I prayed for Rosie when she was sick and she got better. I will pray for you and soon you will be better and running and playing like Rosie.*

Ireland's letter lifted the veil of depression that had covered me for weeks. She was sure that her prayers helped Rosie O'Grady to get well. She was also certain that her prayers would make me well. That is the faith of a child. Those weeks I spent living in fear and doubt did nothing to help me on my road to recovery. Those simple words from a wise seven-year-old did. Thank you, Ireland, for reminding me of the gift of a child's faith.

Believe that your prayers will be answered.

HEALTH TIP #48
The Answer to the Deodorant Question

Does deodorant cause cancer?

The subject of antiperspirants/deodorants and cancer is muddy, to say the least. There were some Internet rumors that started around 1999 that antiperspirants/deodorants cause breast cancer and that you should stop using those products immediately. Fast forward a couple of decades, and we still don't have a conclusive answer, although the waters appear to be clearing. Here are a few of the facts.

We all hate to sweat and, more so, we all hate to smell—each other. Body odor is caused by bacteria that accumulates where we sweat: namely, our underarms. Sweating is a very healthy response to the body's becoming overheated. When we sweat, it keeps us cool, but it's not so "cool" to have pit stains on our silk blouses and T-shirts.

Body odor is normal. It's not always pleasant, but it's normal. Manufacturers decided it was time to make some money off our fear of "offending," and the antiperspirant/deodorant market was born. Your choices of weapons are antiperspirants, deodorants, or a combination of both.

Deodorants are odor neutralizing. Odor can be controlled by using certain substances and scents. Interesting and pleasant scents from "floral bouquet" to "sport" (whatever a "sport" smells like) have been developed.

The **antiperspirant** part of the product usually contains an aluminum base like aluminum zirconium tetrachlorohydrex glycine or aluminum chloride. There is usually a percentage next to the aluminum under the section marked "active ingredient," indicating what percentage is present in the product. The percentages for over-the-counter antiperspirants can range from 9 to 24 percent depending on how "strong" the antiperspirant is. Aluminum causes your sweat glands to swell, trapping the sweat inside your body and thereby keeping you dry. Not a very natural process, if you ask me, but it's practical when giving that presentation or attending that midsummer wedding.

Aluminum is a metal that is used to make cooking pans, cans, foil, and other products, but it also occurs naturally in foods. Beans, corn, and other foods contain traces of aluminum, especially when grown in clay-based soils or in places where the aluminum concentration of the water is high. You also ingest it with foods that have preservatives, artificial coloring, leavening, and anticaking chemicals added to them. Liquid and chalk-chew antacids like Mylanta are mostly aluminum based as well. Your body has no use for aluminum. The healthy human body has effective barriers (skin, lungs, gastrointestinal tract) to reduce the systemic absorption of aluminum ingested from water, foods, drugs, and air. The small amount of aluminum that finds its way into your body is excreted mostly in urine and, to a lesser extent, feces. No reports of aluminum poisoning from diet alone exist in the literature. However, aluminum is detrimental to those whose kidneys don't work well. Your antiperspirant is a daily source of aluminum exposure. Look at your antiperspirant label. It reads, "Ask a doctor before use if you have kidney disease." So we know that it gets into your body and goes through your kidneys, but does it cause cancer?

A study done in 2005 by Dr. P. D. Darbre in the *Journal of Inorganic Chemistry* shows a very definite danger in the absorption of aluminum through the skin in that the aluminum (specifically aluminum chloride and aluminum chlorhydrate) was noted to have *estrogen-like properties.* Alterations in hormones, like estrogen, have been shown to play a major part in breast cancer tumor proliferation as well as other hormone-sensitive cancers like ovarian, cervical, uterine, and prostate. This study showed that the absorption of aluminum through the skin had a direct affect on estrogen receptors and binders.

Dr. Darbre has been studying the effects on breast cancer from estrogenic substances in the environment for over ten years. Dr. Darbre's words are strong: "Given the wide exposure of the human population to antiperspirants, it will be important to establish dermal absorption in the local area of the breast and whether long term low level absorption could play a role in the increasing incidence of breast cancer."

Since the publication of this study, researchers have been trying to establish a definitive connection between the two; however, it's difficult to study the use of antiperspirants in a culture like ours where everyone starts using them as a young teen. Aluminum has been proven to have estrogen-like properties and remains on the "still-being-studied" list. Aluminum definitely enters your bloodstream from skin application, is capable of altering DNA, and has been shown to be a proven metalloestrogen, which is a metal that has hormonal influence in the body. The American Cancer Society will not state that the aluminum in underarm products is safe. They simply say, "More studies need to be done."

Then there are **fillers** in antiperspirants/deodorants; preservatives and chemicals that allow the product to "go on dry" and "go on invisible" so we can get dressed in five minutes in that little black dress and not have to worry about "white pits."

Some of these chemicals are harmless: sunflower oil, alcohol—but some cause concern.

Parabens, or PARAhydroxyBENzoates, are used as preservatives in many cosmetics and personal-care products. The paraben family, ethyl-, methyl-, propyl-, and butyl-, is mentioned in literature suggesting their links to all types of cancers. While parabens are being phased out of the antiperspirant/deodorant ingredient list of most manufacturers, it is still important to look for them and avoid them whenever you can.

Since 1999 there have been a handful of studies looking at the relationship between breast cancer and deodorants, but because they are conflicting and the antiperspirant/deodorant products are constantly changing, it's hard to say with 100 percent certainty that there is or isn't a relationship. The majority of breast cancers are found in the upper outer part of the breast right by the underarm. That's exactly where products are applied. Coincidence?

> Try a paraben-free, aluminum-free deodorant/ antiperspirant to see if this is something that will fit into your healthy lifestyle, but don't sweat it if you need the strong stuff once in a blue moon.

We want to smell nice and we don't like to sweat, but it is important to be informed and choose the best product. Since natural products without aluminum or parabens are widely available, why not use them? I'm not waiting for some large research study to tell me what I already believe. I use the natural salt crystal. The drawback is you have to wet it and then roll it on your underarm to activate the crystal. I have to use the blow dryer on my pits for several minutes before I get dressed, but once it's dry, it's fine and works very well on odor (so I'm told). One crystal lasts me over a year, so it definitely saves me money!

My opinion, for what it's worth, is that if you know that something *might* affect your risk, even if there is not 100 percent concrete proof, and you can avoid it painlessly, why not avoid it? I do think that we should avoid parabens at all costs (something I do). Aluminum-based products should be avoided as well. While there isn't 100 percent proof that aluminum causes cancer, the facts remain:

- Aluminum is absorbed into your bloodstream and is metabolized by your kidneys.

- Aluminum is found in breast tissue.

- Aluminum has been classified as a metalloestrogen, meaning it mimics estrogen in the body.

- Aluminum increases human breast cancer cells in the lab.

If you must use antiperspirants, choose the one without parabens and choose the one with the lowest percentage of aluminum on the label. I use the crystal most of the time, but if I am going out and dressed nicely, I will use the antiperspirant containing a low level of aluminum. It is not worth it for me to worry about wetness and have a crappy time constantly looking at my pits and being self-conscious for just one night of aluminum exposure. Because I don't get out much, I think this plan is a safe one for me.

The thought on chemical exposure, especially paraben and aluminum exposure, is that it's the long-term, low-level use that may increase risk for cancer. Think about making a change in your habit, as this is usually a product that you use every day of your life. A small change here might make a big difference on your health in the long run.

Cancer Motivated Me to Eat Healthier

By mid-January, with chemo behind me, I was gearing up for the next phase of my cancer treatments, a mastectomy. With this major surgery looming just around the corner, I needed to get my immune system pumped for another convalescence. It was time to make or break those healthy living New Year's resolutions.

Before getting cancer, I wasn't really motivated to eat healthy. I ate "healthy-ish" but indulged in junky foods and beverages whenever I felt like it. Most people I know eat a healthy diet in order to control their weight, but the truth is, I am just not prone to weight gain. Hey, don't hate me because I am thin! Once I was in cancer-fighting mode, however, I realized that I would have to trade in my diet colas for green teas and my potato chips for carrot sticks.

In keeping with my resolution, I set out on a trip to the supermarket to stock up on nutritious foods. I was obviously not the only person starting the new year with a promise to eat healthier. I couldn't help but snicker at my fellow shoppers pushing carts laden with fruits and veggies, while hungrily eyeing bins of marked-down Christmas goodies. I noticed one woman greedily fondling a half-price gingerbread house, then throwing it back in the bin and making a hasty retreat with her cart full of green beans and broccoli. I felt quite proud of myself as I checked in my groceries: sweet potatoes, zucchini, celery, quinoa (which I cannot even pronounce, let alone cook!), and some lovely green kale. I did have one question, though: what the heck is kale anyway and what am I supposed to do with it?

You are what you eat! For optimum health,
try to eat green leafy veggies every day.

HEALTH TIP #49
Then There's Kale (Pronounced "Kale")

Kale is definitely one of those vegetables that you look at and say, "Okay, it's green, so I know it's good for me, but what the heck am I supposed to do with it?"

Kale, being one of the leafy greens, has all the goodness you would expect from such a beautiful veggie. Use it as you would spinach or turnip greens by sautéing it in olive oil and garlic as a side dish, or tear up some raw leaves and mix it with your salad greens for a bit of healthy bitter. (Bitters aid digestion by increasing digestive enzymes.) Throw a handful into your favorite soup or stir-fry it. You can even give your morning shake a healthy boost and beautiful color by throwing in a handful of kale! (Blanch it in boiling water for 2 to 3 minutes first.)

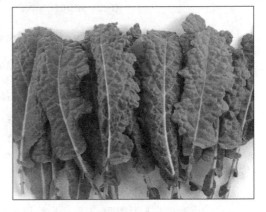

Curly or flat, kale has great nutritional value.

Kale is best when eaten soon after harvest, so this would be a great veggie to buy at a local farmers market, when it's in season.

With all of the health benefits of kale, it is little wonder that it is considered one of the new "super foods." If kale could talk, I am sure it would be boasting about its:

- **Anti-inflammatory properties:** Inflammation is the number-one cause of arthritis, heart disease, cancer, and a number of autoimmune diseases. Kale is an incredibly effective anti-inflammatory food, potentially preventing and even reversing these illnesses.

- **Iron content:** It is a common myth that vegetarians are anemic. In fact, the number of nonvegetarians with iron deficiencies is on the rise. Kale is a great source of iron and, per calorie, even has more iron than beef!

- **Calcium content:** Kale contains more calcium per calorie than milk (90 mg per serving), and the calcium is also more easily absorbed by the body than dairy products.

- **Fiber content:** Like protein, fiber is a macronutrient, which means we need it every day. Many people don't eat nearly enough and the deficiency is linked to heart disease, digestive disorders, and colon cancer, along with everyday annoyances like bloating and constipation. A one-cup serving of kale not only contains 10 percent of the recommended daily intake of fiber but as an added bonus, also provides over two grams of protein.

- **Omega fatty acids:** Essential omega fats (the "good" kind of fats) play an important role in our health. A serving of kale contains an impressive 121 mg of omega-3 fatty acids and 92 mg of omega-6 fatty acids, which is great when you're trying to boost your omega-3s.

- **Immunity properties:** Immunity is the key to cancer resistance. Kale is an incredibly rich source of immune-boosting carotenoid and flavonoid antioxidants that provide vitamins A and C. One serving of kale has 134 percent of the U.S. recommended daily allowance for vitamin C and an impressive 206 percent of the U.S. recommended daily allowance for vitamin A—that's 10,302 IUs!

- **Environmental sustainability:** Kale grows to maturity in fifty-five to sixty days. Kale can grow in most climates and is relatively easy to grow at home or on a farm. Just for comparison, raising one pound of beef requires sixteen pounds of grain, eleven times as much fossil fuel, and 2,400 more gallons of water than growing one pound of kale.

- **Low cal:** One cup of fresh kale has 30 calories and less than one milligram of fat per cup. Nuff said.

- **Cancer-fighting kick:** Kale belongs to the botanical family known as cruciferous, which has broccoli, cauliflower, and Brussels sprouts as its siblings. These vegetables are extremely high in phytochemicals, sulforaphane, and indole-3-carbinol. These are not just fancy words, they are also substances that have been shown to protect against cancer.

And I am pretty sure if kale were still boasting, it would have to add, "I offer many varieties to choose from like Redbor, Red Russian, Kamome Red, and Premier."

Unlike broccoli, cauliflower, and Brussels sprouts, kale can actually disguise itself as a junk food. Yes, folks, you heard it here first: kale chips! Just think of how cool it would be to sit in front of the TV, eat chips, and fight cancer at the same time. (Just to be clear here, it's the kale chips, *not* the sitting in front of the TV that fights cancer.) Kale shrinks to one half its amount with baking, which is great because you can eat twice as much without even knowing it. For this recipe, if you start with 12 cups, you'll have 6 when you finish, but you can really start off with any amount of kale, just know that you'll end up with half that amount when they're done.

> Kale, any way you make it, is a great addition to your healthy diet.

KALE CHIPS

YIELD: 6 CUPS

1 bunch kale (12 cups after stems removed), fresh from a farmers market if you can, as kale's flavor declines rapidly after it's picked; curly, flat, and Siberian varieties work well.

1 to 2 tablespoons organic extra virgin olive oil (or more depending on the amount of kale)

Desired seasoning: sea salt, Old Bay, cumin, garlic, or other seasonings, to taste

1. Preheat oven to 300°F.

2. Make sure your kale is well washed. I add about $1/8$ to $1/4$ cup of salt to the water in a full sink for extra cleaning as this helps remove any critters or dirt still clinging. Remove the stems and rip the leaves into large chip-size pieces. Not too small. Remember, they will shrink quite a bit.

3. Dry the kale extremely well. I can't emphasize this enough. They should be dry; not damp, not almost dry, but completely dry. Really, really dry. Bone dry. Am I making myself clear? I left mine to sit out on dry paper towels for a few hours.

4. Place leaves in a large bowl and drizzle with the olive oil. You want to coat each piece without drenching it. Work the oil into each leaf with your fingertips. (Then work the oil into your cuticles—it's great.)

5. Place pieces in a single layer on a cookie sheet and season as you like, or you can season the oil for a more uniform flavor.

6. Bake for 20 minutes.

7. Let cool for 10 minutes and pig out . . . er, veg out.

Store in airtight, firm bowls, not bags, as the chips are very delicate.

Hail to the kale!

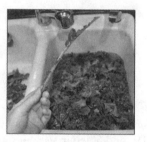

When boiling or sautéing kale or putting it in a shake,
use the stalks, as they hold additional nutrition.
However, when making chips, the stalks become sticklike,
so remove them (unless you are partial to eating sticks).

NUTRITION:

---

1 medium bunch raw (about 12 cups after stems removed) yields 6 cups of chips. Serving size: 1 cup; calories: 60; fat: 0; fiber: 2 grams; protein: 4 grams; vitamin A: 412% of the RDA; vitamin C: 268% of the RDA; vitamin K: 1368% of the RDA; iron: 12% of the RDA; calcium: 18% RDA; carbs: 14 grams.

Receiving Special Gifts

For me, one of the nicest perks of having cancer was being showered with get-well cards and gifts. Every gift, big and small, was special to me. Some gifts, however, in addition to being a thoughtful gesture, also had an interesting story behind them. The figurine of an angel holding a butterfly (pictured right), given to me by my friend Ronnie, is one such gift.

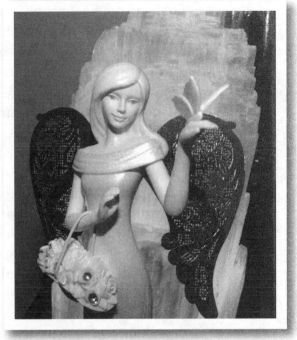

For many years, the angels have played an important role in my life. (You can get away with saying stuff like that once you have had cancer.) I call upon them on a daily basis for mundane things, such as helping me to locate lost items and keeping me safe on the highway. They have also helped me to weather the stormy times in my life. The angels have seen me through a painful divorce and my son's diagnosis of autism. I know they are about when I feel their peaceful presence and I get a sense of knowing that everything will be okay. The angels also let me know when they are at work with the symbol of a blue butterfly.

Never before have I needed reassurance from my angels as much as I did in the spring of 2011 when I was diagnosed with breast cancer. Even though I endured many uncomfortable and painful procedures, nothing can compare to the mental anguish of waiting for test results. Finding out about my diagnosis was not the worst part of this journey. The worst part of the experience was hearing my doctor say, "The scan shows something on your liver." At forty-four, I was relatively young, fit, and otherwise healthy. I knew that I had a good chance of beating breast cancer. However, if it had spread to my liver, I would be facing a much tougher battle.

It took six long weeks to hear the results of the tests on my liver. During that time, there was no shortage of messages from my angels. The blue butterflies were everywhere! They appeared on get-well cards, my computer monitor, and on other people's clothing and jewelry. Blue butterflies are not native to Newfoundland, and the chances of seeing one in real life ranked right up there with the chances of seeing a zebra walk out of the woods. So you can just imagine my surprise when I caught sight of one in my very own garden! (A blue butterfly, that is, not a zebra.) I was mesmerized by how it not only fluttered around my flowers but also seemed to dance around my body. I ran into the house to get Ronnie to witness this small miracle. As she and I talked quietly, the butterfly continued to dance around me for several minutes. It then landed on my left breast, the one with cancer, before flying off toward the water. Later that day, I cried tears of relief when I received the news that the spots on my liver were harmless.

The following day a package arrived in the mail, an unexpected gift from a colleague. When I opened the box, I was amazed to see a pendant of a blue butterfly, which was almost an exact replica in size and color of the one I had seen in my garden the day before. I immediately sent her an e-mail message to thank her for her gift and to ask, "How did you know the significance of blue butterflies to me?" She responded, "I didn't know that they are special to you. I was in a store in Florida when I saw this and it reminded me of you. I left the store with my husband, but felt compelled to go back and buy it for you." What an amazing "coincidence" that this gift would arrive the day after my blue butterfly experience!

I still had a long road ahead of me, but the angels continued to make their presence known on a regular basis, which helped me to remain calm. Yet on the day of my surgery, I had an uneasy feeling as I entered the operating room. I wished for one more sign, but as I looked around me at the steel doors, the sterile white walls, and the sea of green scrubs, I lost all hope of getting one. Just then the nurse reached for my arm bracelet and I saw it: a blue butterfly tattoo on the inside of her wrist! A wave of peace washed over me.

I believe that there is no such thing as coincidence; rather, these signs are heavenly messages. I do not know what the future holds for me, but these signs from the angels let me know that everything is unfolding according to God's plan.

> If you have not already done so, welcome the angels
> into your life. You can even get guided meditation
> CDs to help you use the power of your imagination
> to meet your guardian angel.

HEALTH TIP #50
Imagine This—Lucy in the Sky with Diamonds

The best example I can think of for popular guided imagery is the Beatles song "Lucy in the Sky with Diamonds." Whether you believe the myth that the title stands for LSD or not, the song is a journey that invites you to travel to a fairy-tale land and chill out:

> *"Picture yourself in a boat on a river . . .*
> *with tangerine trees and marmalade skies . . ."*

Doesn't that sound nice?

Guided imagery is that simple. It is the practice of closing your eyes, letting your mind go free, and picturing yourself in the stress-free place of your choosing. Through concentration and focus, you truly feel that you're there. You imagine the smells and sights of the place, which then elicits a physical relaxation response in your body. You can do this on your own, in a class, or with a recorded voice to help you. There are even special guided imagery sessions to help you "imagine" your immune system kicking the crap out of the cancer cells.

It is believed that through guided imagery, your mind can give your body signals to perform functions like cell repair, healing, and gaining strength.

When I was diagnosed with breast cancer, my five sisters chipped in and bought me an iPod. I filled that iPod with inspirational audio, guided imagery, relaxation sessions, and affirmations, and it came with me to every chemotherapy session. I found it very helpful to listen to a CD I had downloaded entitled *Meditations for Enhancing Your Immune System: Strengthen Your Body's Ability to Heal*, by Dr. Bernie Siegel. The audio is a guided imagery journey where you imagine you are injected into your own body so you can see what is going on and fix what needs to be fixed. By listening to Dr. Siegel's voice and allowing myself to be transported to my "inner self," it brought about a sense of self-awareness that was extremely useful and necessary for self-healing. The techniques I learned on the CD gave me some tools that I could use to get me through treatments as well. While the drugs were working on my body, I felt like I wasn't just sitting there doing nothing. I was actively helping those drugs to work by helping my mind to help my body to help the drugs to do their job.

Include guided imagery in your bag of survival tricks and take advantage of the mind/body relationship to perform self-healing.

There are many "journeys" you can take with guided imagery and many issues you can explore, such as health, love, stress, peace, and forgiveness. All it takes is the power of your mind.

Hundreds of Dollars Saved in Hair Care

They say be careful what you wish for. Lesson learned! Once my chemo treatments were done, I often found myself wishing my hair would grow in faster. I meant the hair ON MY HEAD, not my chin. I looked in the mirror one morning and thought I saw a bald dude with a goatee looking back at me. So I figure, one of the perks of having cancer was that I saved hundreds of dollars in hair care. Technically speaking, I had saved myself enough money to buy that new hair-removal gadget I saw on the shopping channel. Nontechnically speaking, the money was not actually "saved," but let's not split hairs, shall we?

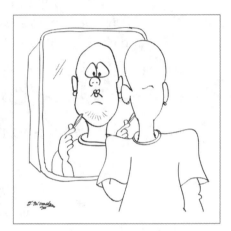

An average North American woman spends about $100 a month on hair care and hair removal. (Okay, I made that stat up. It is actually what I spend.) Calculate how much you saved due to chemo and treat yourself to something new.

HEALTH TIP #51
Treat Yourself to Chocolate Cupcakes

Hey, how did this tip find its way into this book? Everyone knows chocolate cupcakes aren't healthy. But wait a minute—these cupcakes are special. They're beetroot chocolate cupcakes! Betcha didn't know you could make dessert out of beets!

Beets are often processed for their natural sugar, so they are sweet by nature, and they give a gorgeous consistency and wonderful ruby red color to everything they touch (including your hands). This recipe is my own creation, but feel free to experiment with the recipe and change what you don't like. (Just don't change the beets, okay?) They don't really need frosting, but since the frosting is no sugar, no dairy, there's no need to say no.

Beets are high in fiber, vitamin C, folate, and potassium. The fact that this recipe is plant-based means you don't have to worry about animal fats and cholesterol. See? You can eat chocolate cupcakes with no guilt attached!

VEGAN CHOCOLATE BEETROOT CUPCAKES

YIELD: 10 TO 12 REGULAR-SIZED OR 24 MINI-CUPCAKES

Cupcakes:

$1^1/_2$ medium-sized beets (about $1^1/_2$ cups)

$1/_2$ cup pure maple syrup (real syrup, *not* Aunt Jemima's)

1 teaspoon pure vanilla extract

$1^1/_2$ cups unbleached all-purpose flour

$1/_2$ cup unsweetened cocoa powder

1 tablespoon aluminum-free baking powder

$1/_2$ teaspoon baking soda

$1/_2$ teaspoon sea salt

$1/_2$ teaspoon cinnamon

$1/_3$ cup low-fat coconut milk (or almond or rice milk)

$1/_2$ cup melted Earth Balance coconut spread or coconut oil

Chocolate No-Butter Buttercream Frosting:

11 Medjool dates (I've tried to use regular,
but they just don't compare; go with the Medjool)

1 ripe avocado

$1/_2$ teaspoon pure vanilla extract

$1/_3$ cup plus 1 teaspoon unsweetened cocoa powder

$1/_2$ tablespoon coconut milk

$1/_8$ teaspoon sea salt

Directions

1. Cut off greens and bottom "tail" of beets. Scrub beets under running water with a vegetable brush. Lightly peel any rough skin with a carrot peeler. Cut into small quarters or cubes and set in a steamer or place in a metal colander on top of saucepot filled with about 5 inches of water. Beets should not touch the water. Cover and boil water on medium-high heat. Steam beets for about 30 to 45 minutes. (Be careful that you don't steam all your water away!) Pieces should be very soft when pierced with a fork. Set aside to cool completely. This step can be done the day before. Store cooked beets in the fridge.

2. Place cooked beets, syrup, and vanilla in food processor and pulse to mix, then process on high for 3 to 5 minutes until very smooth (so pretty . . .)

3. Combine flour, cocoa, baking powder, baking soda, salt, and cinnamon in a mixing bowl. Add processed beets and coconut milk to dry mixture and stir to combine.

4. Melt coconut oil in a small pot over low heat for a minute or two until liquid. Add melted coconut oil to batter and stir well with a spoon.

5. Line cupcake tin with paper cups or with cooking oil spray and fill $3/4$ of the way full with batter. (It's okay to lick the bowl; there's no raw egg in there, and no one is watching.)

6. Bake at 350°F for 16 to 18 minutes (11 minutes for mini-cupcakes). Top should be firm to touch. Let cool for 15 minutes.

Frosting directions

1. Remove pits and skin from dates. This is a pain in the rump, but it affects the creaminess of the frosting. The skin of the date messes with the texture of the frosting. You can soak them overnight to make removing the peel easier, but you lose some of the sweetness that way. I place all 11 dates in a bowl of warm water for a few minutes, and peel them one by one using a pairing knife to start. Try to find dates whose skin is already loose to make it easy.

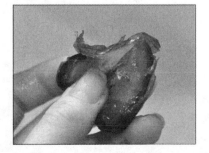

2. Wash and cut the avocado. Always wash fruits and veggies even if you don't eat the skin. When you drag your knife through to cut, you're dragging everything on the surface through the food.

3. Place everything in the food processor and process the bejeezus out of it on high until it's creamy smooth.

4. Frost cupcakes when they have cooled. Store frosted cupcakes in the refrigerator and eat within 3 days. I don't think you'll have them long enough for that to be a problem.

You can have your cake . . . and eat veggies while you do! Enjoy!

NUTRITION PER FROSTED REGULAR-SIZED CUPCAKE:

Calories: 300; protein: 4.1 grams; carbs: 33 grams; fat: 13.6 grams; fiber: 3.1 grams; iron: 15% of the RDA; calcium: 4.4% of the RDA; cholesterol: 0. (All nutrition is plant-based.)

A word about maple syrup: You might be wondering why I didn't suggest using "organic" maple syrup. Many brands of maple syrup come from maple trees that grow in the forest. It's pretty safe to say that trees in the forest aren't sprayed with pesticides. Because of the strict labeling, though, the syrup can't be labeled "organic" if it wasn't grown by the standards of organic farming. Check with the manufacturer to see where they harvest their syrup. Chances are, it's deep in a forest somewhere.

Eat your veggies as dessert and your mind will explode with endless other possibilities!

If your maple syrup does say "organic," that means they grew huge maple trees organically and that's pretty impressive.

Rockin' the Bandana

Until recently I thought that the right to wear hats and other headwear belonged to British royalty and certain ethnic groups. With the exception of my woolen toque, hats made me feel "pretentious," like I was trying to pull off a Kate Middleton. After losing my hair, however, I discovered a whole new line of accessories: hats, wigs, turbans, scarves, and my personal favorite, bandanas. I could coordinate my headdress to match any outfit, without feeling the least bit pretentious. In fact, I felt so confident with my new style that I continued to rock the bandana even after my hair returned.

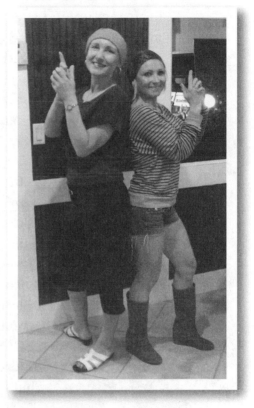

If you lose your hair due to chemo, try experimenting with different styles and varieties of headwear. You don't have to sacrifice comfort for style.

Flo rockin' the bandana with her sister, Lynette.

HEALTH TIP #52
Rock Out with a Different Kind of Exercise

Nobody puts Baby in the corner. Because that would keep her from getting her forty-five minutes of exercise for the day. And she does it by dirty dancing.

Dancing for fitness makes all the sense in the world. Everyone wants to dance, and, let's face it, sometimes the same old exercise routine can be boring. So why not dance your way to good health? (How does that saying go? Dance like no one is watching. . . .)

With so many forms of fitness dancing, there has to be one style that fits your personality.

Do you like drama? Try ballroom dancing. Not only will you get your heart rate up and stretch your muscles, but you can dress like a sparkly movie star and no one will say a word. Check the phone directory or the Internet for your nearest local dance studio. They will often have an open dance night where you can pay one price and learn a new step; no experience necessary! Ballroom dancing keeps your feet moving and also can include strengthening moves depending on the style of dance.

Do you own cowboy boots and know all the songs from the hit musical *Oklahoma?* Then square dancing might be your thing. Besides getting a great workout from the nonstop beat of the fiddle, you'll get to learn the meaning of terms like *promenade* and *star by the right*. Square dancing was part of the seventh-grade curriculum for phys ed, so don't worry that it's too hard to learn. Search online for square dancing lessons and events near you.

Never miss an *I Dream of Jeannie* rerun? Then you'll love belly dancing. You can take belly-dancing classes, but I think the best way to learn this is with a video or DVD in the privacy of your own home. That way you can put on your bells and bangles and bare your belly while you meet your exercise requirements. Go ahead . . . no one will watch . . . unless you want them to.

If you own a Wii, there's a great game called DanceDance Revolution. (The cool people call it DDR.) You stand on a mat that has four squares around you: forward, back, right, and left. By watching the screen, you have to follow what the dancer is doing by stepping on the correct square. As you get better, it speeds up, and when you get really good, it goes at crazy speeds. Even though it seems like your brain is getting the workout, your body does too by getting your heart rate up by marching, jumping, and moving your feet while you try to keep up with the dancer on the screen. You don't even feel like you're working out because it's so much fun! One downside: it's addictive.

Dancing has all the benefits of any other exercise, including more energy, stronger bones, increased flexibility and strength, and a reduction in your risk of illness. Plus it's lots of fun!

There are so many other kinds of dancing like salsa, line dancing, swing, or clogging. Or you can put on your favorite song and just move. Dancing is moving, and moving is exercise. No one ever said exercise had to be boring.

Dance your way to better health!

Cancer Cured Me of My Needle/Blood Phobia

When it comes to medical procedures, I have always been a bit of a wimp. In my early school days, I was renowned for my reaction to the public health nurse on "needle day." With a sense of shame, I recall actually biting a nurse and kicking a nun in the leg to escape my grade-one vaccination. While I no longer get physically violent with medical personnel (well, hardly ever), I have been known to get weak at the sight of blood and needles. As you can imagine, this proved to be quite an inconvenience during my cancer treatments. I am happy to report, however, that after being poked and prodded in places where no needle should ever venture, I have toughened up quite a bit and can now profess that I am completely cured of my needle/blood phobia!

The true test of my newfound toughness came with my left breast mastectomy in January 2012. I had conjured up images of how it would be when I saw my new physique for the first time. You know how it happens in the movies: the woman gently caresses her flat chest, her lip quivers, and silent tears flow down her face while violin music plays softly in the background. My experience was a little different. My cousin/nurse Lil was sitting in the room with me when I popped my head up and looked down at my green gown to check out my flat chest for the first time.

"Jeez, Lil," I said, "he went and took off the two of 'em !"

As it turns out, "rightie" had just slipped under my armpit, as is often the habit of saggy, middle-aged breasts, but she was still fully intact. Lil and I had a great giggle at my discovery. I wasn't sure if I was up to looking at the actual cut, but Lil is one of those old-school nurses, and she gave me little choice in the matter. As she cleaned the incision, we counted the staples together: One, two, three . . . twenty-nine.

"I guess I could round it up to thirty," I said to Lil.

"Or you could make like a man and exaggerate it up to sixty," she replied. We howled with laughter!

So there I was just days before my forty-fifth birthday, and my body had been forever altered. But ya know, I was okay with that. Like many women, I really struggled with the decision to have either a lumpectomy or a mastectomy. Unlike other types of cancer, breast cancer requires so many decisions by the patient: Do you want a lumpectomy or mastectomy? One breast or two? Prosthetic or reconstruction? I just wanted the doctor to TELL me what to do! What if I made the wrong choice? Well, "luckily" for me I did not have much of a choice in the matter. Even though I first opted for a lumpectomy, the cancer was so far advanced that I required a full radical mastectomy. Of course, losing any part of the anatomy can be traumatic, particularly when it is linked to sexuality and femininity. However, when I look in the mirror, I don't see a one-breasted woman. I see a strong woman who gave a breast to have life.

If you can face cancer head-on, nothing will ever have the power to scare you! (But if you are like me and really dread needles, it might be a good idea to get a port before chemo starts.)

HEALTH TIP #53
Fear Needles? Try Acupuncture

"So they stuck you with pins? What was *that* like?"

This is the question I got from my then ten-year-old daughter when I came back from seeing my acupuncturist. It's a reasonable question, and I have to say, while I was not apprehensive about my first treatment, I was curious.

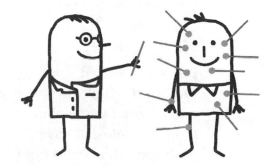

I was about halfway through my twenty-four week chemotherapy treatment when my stomach just shut down. The thought of eating any kind of food was just plain unappealing. (I can't even imagine the sick, nauseous feelings I had then, as I sit here sipping my delicious sweet potato soup now!)

I knew that I needed to keep up my strength if I was going to make it through another twelve weeks of this "treat"ment, and having tried all the tricks (and drugs) from the doctors, I decided to give acupuncture a try. I had nothing to lose, as there are no side effects to acupuncture. Nope, none.

What Is Acupuncture?

Acupuncture is an ancient Chinese method of treating a variety of conditions by stimulation of certain areas along your body. These linear areas, known as meridians, allow the "vital energy" to flow, allowing your body to function in a healthy way.

Just like a regular doctor would assess the blood flowing through your veins, an acupuncturist assesses the flow and distribution of vital energy within the meridians.

If there is restricted flow in a certain area, a very thin needle (I really shouldn't call them that, because they're not sharp) is inserted along the pathway to assist in the energy flow, much like if a stream is blocked by debris, poking a hole in it will reestablish flow. By inserting needles into the skin at varying depths, it is possible to stimulate nerves and release hormones to help that particular illness or condition.

I figured I would give it a try since millions of people use it, and it has been around over 2,000 years . . . (*umm*, conventional Western medicine was using leeches to treat headaches just 150 years ago . . . nuff said).

My First Visit

Being a registered nurse, I was careful about choosing an acupuncturist. I avoided the clinics that were in the back of nail salons. I did some asking around and I went online to look up the acupuncture centers in my area. I found a clinic that was started by an MD and certified acupuncturist, who graduated with honors from Emory Medical School (one of the most highly respected med schools in the United States). She headed the office, which consisted of three other certified acupuncturists and a massage therapist. Two of the acupuncturists were also certified Chinese herbalists. Herbalists are trained professionals who can suggest certain plants, roots, or teas to help with your particular problem.

I signed in as you would at any doctor's office and I took a seat in the waiting room. It was a regular, normal waiting room, with the local radio station playing and out-of-date magazines on the table. (I really expected to walk into a room with smoky incense, Far Eastern décor, and a gong in the corner. I have to admit, I was just a little bit disappointed.)

After filling out the usual paperwork, my therapist, David, came in and introduced himself. He was not Asian. He was from California and told me he had been practicing for fifteen years. He had a very calming nature about him, and I felt instantly relaxed.

He asked me all the usual health questions and about my medical history and why I was there. Then he looked at my tongue and took my pulse in both arms.

He told me that there was a good chance he could help me with the loss of appetite problem. He also said he could help with getting my liver to work better (since chemo is metabolized there and the liver gets overworked by chemo) and could work on getting my energy level up, which was one of my other complaints.

He instructed me to be very kind to my body while it was going through the chemo treatment and to try to eat cooked, soft, simple foods instead of raw to help my digestion and help my body retain the energy I needed to get through the next few weeks.

So far, he made a lot of sense to me.

He asked me to change into a cloth robe and he left the room. When I was ready, I was made comfortable on a soft table with pillows under my head and knees. David proceeded to insert a series of needles in my arms, head, legs, and stomach. Nothing was inserted in my back.

A bit about the needles:

● They are not sharp; they are rounded on the ends.

● They are hairlike in thickness; thinner than the smallest injection needles.

- They are single use—that is, they are discarded after each use and each person gets clean needles.

- There is NO blood.

- It does not hurt at all—in fact, I didn't feel a thing.

Once the needles were inserted, the lights were dimmed, some mild soft incense was burned, and a relaxing tape of gentle music was played. There I stayed for about thirty minutes while I "cleared my channels." This was probably the most relaxing thirty minutes I had experienced since my cancer diagnosis. I was in no pain, I was comfortable, and it was extremely pleasant and calming!

After thirty minutes, David came back and removed the needles, and I got dressed. The whole visit took about sixty minutes.

The Results

After the treatment, David asked me how I felt, and I told him, "Great!"

"How many treatments will I need before I feel like eating again?" I asked him.

"How long does it take you to get home?"

"About an hour . . . wait . . . what?" I was amazed, and a bit skeptical. "How often do I need to come back?" I asked. I really expected him to say something like "three times a week for the next ten weeks," but he said it was really up to me.

He suggested two more treatments over the next four weeks, but only if I felt I needed it. He didn't try to sell me anything (that was my other concern), and he actually said that he does not sell products out of the office, but he could tell me what to buy if I needed something and I could find the best price on my own. He also showed me the pressure point for nausea (about two inches up from my wrist on the inside of my arm in the center) and told me I could just press on this point if I felt any nausea coming on.

The cost of my initial visit was $150. Subsequent visits would be $100.

So off I went home. It took about an hour to get there.

When I got home I saw a can of vegetable soup in the pantry . . . I made it . . . and I ate it . . . along with two pieces of brown bread . . . and a little piece of dark chocolate. I was amazed and thrilled! I really couldn't believe it! My appetite was better!

I did end up going back to help with the liver clearance and to get a bit more energy. Although I couldn't "feel" my liver being cleared, I did feel a bit more energy and, since I was able to eat a little more, that helped my energy, too.

I have recommended acupuncture to a lot of my friends going through chemo. I have also heard of great results from people who tried it for chronic back pain and migraines. I asked about weight loss, and David said he really hasn't seen great results with using acupuncture alone for that. He also said acupuncture is not a cure-all. It is one aspect in a person's health along with proper, healthy diet, exercise, and meditation.

> Trying unconventional treatments during and after treatment can open up a new way of thinking and help you feel better at the same time.

Some skeptics told me it worked on me because of the power of suggestion. I don't think so, because it has been shown to work on animals and babies—so there goes that theory.

Aside from having to pay out-of-pocket for treatment, acupuncture has no "downside." While I didn't end up tossing my nausea medication, I loved the fact that my nausea was controlled without the use of (yet) more pills. I also was able to gain a lot of knowledge from David about diet and general health from a different perspective.

Cancer Made Me
Value Every Birthday

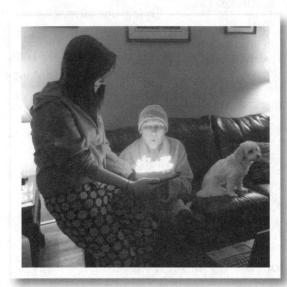

One thing cancer has done for me is make me really appreciate my birthdays! Never again will I complain about getting older, and these lines and wrinkles . . . I have earned every one.

While many women dread the big "Five-OH," I am sure it will be one of the happiest of my life. God willing, it will make me one of the just over 50 percent of stage-3 breast cancer patients who survives to the five-year mark. But I don't want to just stop at fifty! My greatest wish is to follow in my grandmother's footsteps. Nan Kearney, my namesake, is ninety-two years old. She lives on her own and is completely independent. She still gardens and cooks for herself every day. She is a great storyteller and has a memory that would put most twenty-year-olds to shame.

Nan raised twelve children over the years and has held more than fifty grandchildren and great-grandchildren. While I lose track of my growing family of cousins, she can call every one of them by name. So when I was blowing out my forty-five candles just days after losing my breast, I gave up on my usual wish (in case you are wondering, that would be a red, convertible Volkswagen Beetle). Instead, I wished to live long enough to see my children raised and to someday hold my own grandchildren.

Treasure every birthday, every day, and every breath. Party on!

HEALTH TIP #54
Forget the Toga Party . . . Have a Yoga Party

In the eighties, while Jane Fonda introduced us to aerobic workouts and striped leg warmers, a small group of "yoginis" were teaching an ancient form of exercise called yoga. Taken from Hindu culture and philosophy, and spanning back over five thousand years, yoga is a series of physical, mental, and spiritual exercises aimed at helping one to achieve a goal of health and happiness. There are many different types of yoga, but the one practiced most often here in the West is called Hatha yoga. Forty years ago, yoga might have been viewed as a "cult" or "fringe" activity, and, even if you wanted to practice it, classes and teachers were few and far between.

Luckily, with increased, widespread interest and increasing proof of the benefits of yoga (because we Westerners need proof, dammit), a growing number of people of all ages are engaging in this healthy practice and are enjoying significant benefits for their mind, body, and spirit. Just in the last ten years, the number of people practicing some form of yoga grew from 4 million to 20 million in the United States alone!

Practicing yoga can help you build a strong, well-toned body and a peaceful, balanced mind and also helps to deepen your spirituality regardless of your religious beliefs. Yoga sessions consist of a combination of breathing and relaxation exercises along with performing a series of poses. Some of them are as simple as just standing with your feet together as tall as you can. This pose is called "mountain pose." The poses are focused at building strength but are also meant to bring a better awareness of the connection between your body and your mind. The gentle flow as you move from one pose to the next helps your muscles to become strong and your joints to become active, and it also helps your internal organs to perform better.

An increasing number of people are turning to yoga as a way to help with the effects of cancer treatments and other illnesses. The proof is undeniable. Study after study proves that yoga helps to alter chemicals within the body that have a positive effect on anxiety, depression, and inflammation.

One study done at the University of Alberta looked at how yoga affected the quality of life in cancer patients, both during treatment and after. For two years researchers followed different groups of patients through a ten-week yoga course and then had them fill out questionnaires. At the end of the ten-week courses, 94 percent of them said they had improvements in their quality of life and said they felt better physically, were happier, and were less tired.

Another study measured the neurotransmitter in the brain responsible for relaxation (gamma-aminobutyric acid, or GABA). Those with anxiety disorders, chronic pain, depression, and post-traumatic stress syndrome have low levels of this biochemical. Sets of patients were assigned to either a walking group or a yoga group. At the end of twelve weeks, the neurotransmitter level was the same in the walking group, but in the yoga group it increased. The patients in the yoga group also reported a reduction in their symptoms.

Think you want to give yoga a try, but you have many reasons why you won't? See if any of the following match what you are thinking.

EXCUSE #1   I'm Too Old

There is no age that is too young or too old. If you're a beginner, then take a beginner's class. You'll probably notice all ages represented. And another thing: the oldest yoga instructor, Ida Herbert is ninety-six and has been teaching for sixty-three years, and she's still teaching! She also looks like she's fifty and competes professionally in ballroom dance with a partner who is thirty-one! Next excuse, please. . . .

EXCUSE #2   This Doesn't Look Like Exercise to Me

You're right: It doesn't *look* like exercise. But holding the various poses and moving from one to another strengthens every muscle in your body while it brings awareness to how you are feeling. Your heart rate and breathing will increase and your muscles will "feel it" the next day (in a good way of course). While there are risks with any exercise program, yoga's gentleness in achieving strength is more likely to promote healing than injury. And it is considered a "weight-bearing" exercise, so it helps to strengthen your bones as well. Keep going. . . .

EXCUSE #3   *It's Against My Religion*

Name one religion that is against health and happiness. While yoga is associated with Hindu and Buddhist culture, it is more of a spiritual philosophy, not a religion. You won't be asked to attend any kind of services, and, while there is a lot of breathing and meditation, there is no "prayer" to a certain "God" unless that is what you choose to do in your own head. There are many different ways to approach the spiritual part of the session, but it's up to you to decide what you bring to the session. There are even Christian-based yoga studios if that's what floats your boat. Got any more?

EXCUSE #4   *I Have a Bad Back and Can't Do All Those Twists*

Who doesn't have a bad back? A certified experienced instructor will be able to guide you through the sessions with complete comfort and safety. A bad back is why people *go* to yoga classes in the first place. Yoga has actually been shown to improve muscle and joint issues like pinched nerves and arthritis, and many of the poses are the same exercises physical therapists use to help their patients strengthen their backs when they are injured. Almost done?

EXCUSE #5   *Classes Will Be Too Far Away for Me to Attend*

Wrong again. For most, it's just a matter of finding a studio. Search "[your town] yoga studio" and I'll bet there are many. Try to find an instructor that you like, as everyone teaches a bit differently. What else?

EXCUSE #6   *I Have Cancer*

Perfect! Yoga can help with the symptoms you are having, like fatigue, pain, shortness of breath, and anxiety. And it can improve your immune system so you won't get sick during treatment. Still more?

EXCUSE #6   *I Don't Have Yoga Shoes*

No shoes needed. Just feet. On second thought, there are wheelchair yoga sessions, too, so I'm not sure you even need the feet.

So now that you're ready to try it, I suggest you go with an open mind and an open heart. For me, my biggest challenge was losing my competitive attitude. I was determined to contort my body into any and all the poses in exactly the way that the instructor (who had been teaching for twelve years) was demonstrating. But I learned that yoga isn't about who can be the downwardest-facing dog in the room; it's about your own personal experience and improving on that experience. Be gentle. There is no competition, just a total focus of mind and total awareness of body. After a good yoga session, you'll feel refreshed, calm, and rejuvenated. Also, after class, it's really hard to get mad and give someone the finger in the parking lot for cutting you off. Instead, you might find yourself adding that index finger and wishing them peace as you drive off.

> Yoga is more than just a bunch of sitting and breathing. It produces real healing, and it helps you find your stronger, more peacefully grounded inner self so you can handle your cancer, both during therapy and after.

Switching up your cardio exercise with yoga, alternating the two to get the most benefit and biggest reduction in cancer risk, is a great idea, as walking, cycling, and running offer their own health benefits.

Check your local listings for facilities that offer yoga. The best way to start is with a certified instructor so they can help you with the proper alignment of the poses and guide you through the breathing part of the session, but you can invest in some videos for use at home if you wish. Visit www.breastcanceryoga.com for yoga DVDs that are specifically targeted to breast cancer patients. Many spas and wellness centers, as well as most gyms and martial arts studios, offer yoga classes, too. Just make sure to get the 411 on the instructor to make sure they are certified and qualified to teach and that you're in the right level of class for your ability.

But be careful. That great feeling you get from yoga is totally addictive.

Cancer Taught Me a Lesson About Loving My Body

A couple of years ago I gave serious thought to having a breast lift. Even though the rest of my body was in pretty good shape, gravity (along with breast feeding) had not been kind to my breasts. My sagging bosom really bothered me. I thought, *If only my breasts were perkier, then I could really love my body.* Well, lucky for me I put it off until I could better afford it, which never came to pass. (I imagine I would be kicking myself now had I wasted all that money!)

Here is the irony: Now that I have only one breast, I see it as a beautiful part of my body. The same is true about my hair. I always hated my hair, complaining that it was too thin, too fine, or too mousey brown. When I looked in the mirror and saw the bit of black fuzz finally starting to come in on my head, I loved it! I had hair again, YAY! It took losing my hair to make me appreciate just having hair. Lesson learned. You will never again hear me complain about my big nose.

Love the skin you're in.

HEALTH TIP #55
Love the Skin You're In . . . by Using Proper, Healthy Sunscreen

Is sunscreen a part of your daily routine? The American Academy of Dermatology recommends that everyone apply sunscreen with an SPF of 30 or higher every day, even if it's cloudy. (UV rays can penetrate the clouds.) But less than 20 percent of us actually follow that rule!

There are mountains of sunscreen out there, but it's important to find a sunscreen that is free of chemical preservatives and substances that could affect your health, like "nano titanium dioxide" and "ultrafine titanium dioxide," especially when using sunscreen on children. The words are big, but the particles are supersmall, allowing them to pass easily into your bloodstream, invade organs, and even cross the blood-brain barrier and get "inside your head." That's great if the substance delivered is helpful medication to treat a brain tumor. But not so great if you're delivering potentially harmful chemicals like titanium dioxide to the same area. Titanium dioxide doesn't belong in the depths of my brain. (It might disturb the cobwebs.)

While there is no doubt that certain nanoparticles enter the bloodstream and can destroy DNA, the implications of what that means is still being debated.

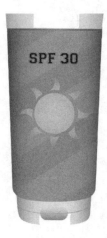

Look for plain zinc oxide and "non-nano" titanium dioxide when reading sunscreen labels. Try to avoid the microfine sprays and stick to the lotions when you can. "When you can" means "don't go crazy if you can't." It is healthier to apply the nano-sunscreen than to go without sunscreen because you couldn't find the right one.

We often don't think about applying sunscreen to kids unless we are at the beach, but just one burn to a child doubles their risk of developing skin cancer later in life. Kids need protection every day! It's a good habit to get into applying sunscreen before they go out to play or when getting ready for school. Children should be wearing at least SPF 30, and it should protect against UVA and UVB rays. Ideally, sunscreen should be applied every two hours when outside or after swimming if possible. Babies and toddlers should be kept out of the sun or covered as much as possible. Badger brand (www.badgerbalm.com) makes wonderfully safe sunscreen products for the whole family. (Nope, not getting a kickback from Badger. Just like 'em.)

What's the difference between UVA and UVB? (Other than one letter?)

UVA (ultraviolet A) rays penetrate deeply into your skin and do long-term damage like wrinkles and "leather skin." We've all seen the horrific effects of UVAs on older sun worshipers we see at the beach with elephant skin. UVA rays may also directly cause melanoma, the most serious kind of skin cancer.

UVB (ultraviolet B) are shortwave rays that are mostly responsible for causing painful sunburn and are also the main cause of basal and squamous cell skin cancer, as well as melanoma.

Needless to say, you should be wearing a sunscreen that protects from both.

What's SPF?

SPF means "sun protection factor." It indicates how long you can go out in the sun before you start to burn. An SPF of at least 30 is recommended for everyone. It is a little known fact that any SPF higher than 30 only blocks an additional 4 percent more UVBs. It won't hurt to use a higher SPF, though, and it adds a margin of error if you aren't applying the sunscreen as often or as heavily as you should, but the very high SPFs don't necessarily mean higher protection. In fact, the FDA is phasing out all products with an SPF over 50 because they offer no additional sunscreen protection when compared with the SPF 30 products.

But I want to look tanned!

I know we all want that "healthy glow," and you might want to believe that tanning beds are a safer option to sunbathing. However, tanning beds are just as dangerous (if not more so) than lying on the beach. One dermatologist refers to tanning beds as "suicide beds." (Move over, Dr. Kevorkian!)

In 2011, the World Health Organization's International Agency for Research on Cancer (IARC) concluded that indoor tanning does cause melanoma. You are 75 percent more likely to get melanoma if you use a tanning bed regularly, and the risk increases with more use.

Considering there are more tanning salons than streetlights in cities today, it's no wonder that melanoma is the fastest-growing cancer, increasing by the rate of 2 percent each year since 1997. It is also the most common form of cancer in people aged twenty-five to twenty-nine.

Ladies, there's nothing wrong with "faking it." There are wonderful, healthy self-tanning lotions on the market. There are even self-tanners with sunscreen built in. If you want to get a tan, get it the safe way. Lavera (www.Lavera.com) is one company that makes several wonderful products that are healthy and tan your skin beautifully without the sun's rays and without chemicals and preservatives.

Here are some more fun sun facts:

- The sun is strongest between 10 AM and 4 PM, so try to remember to take precautions during these hours: avoid direct sun, have children play in the shade, and don't take babies and toddlers out if you can help it.

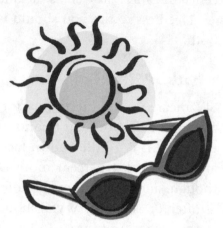

- Look like a movie star while you protect your eyes and prevent crow's feet by wearing UV-blocking sunglasses (attitude optional).

- Wear hats that shade your face and neck and make a fashion statement while you reduce your risk of skin cancer.

- Use extra caution near water, snow, and sand because they reflect light and can intensify the damaging rays of the sun. Sunburns don't only happen at the beach, ya know.

- Keep in mind that you still need protection in a car, as side window glass does not offer protection from UVA rays, which can cause deep skin damage and melanoma. Windshields usually provide full UVA and UVB protection, but check with your auto manufacturer.

Note: Even though sunscreens are more effective than ever, melanoma is one of the cancers that is on the rise. There is some growing controversy in the global community that has to deal with the efficacy of sunscreen *alone* to prevent melanoma. Some believe that the use of sunscreen gives people a false sense of security, so they feel safe spending extra time in the sun. Recent research advocates the use of sunscreen along with covering up (long sleeves, hat, and such) and avoidance of sun during midday (10 AM to 3 PM) to truly decrease your risk of skin cancers.

You can still have fun; just remember to respect the sun!

A Surprise Visitor

I am very fortunate to be one of five sisters. I am especially blessed that two of these sisters, Sherry and Juana, live close by. They have been an integral part of my support team. Although sister Lynette lives in Florida, she was able to come visit with me soon after my diagnosis, and I enjoyed an awesome stay with her the following January. However, sister Lessy lives in a land far, far away (Calgary), and I had not seen her in nearly two years at the time of my diagnosis. It is never easy to be away from your family, and this becomes even more true when you are facing cancer.

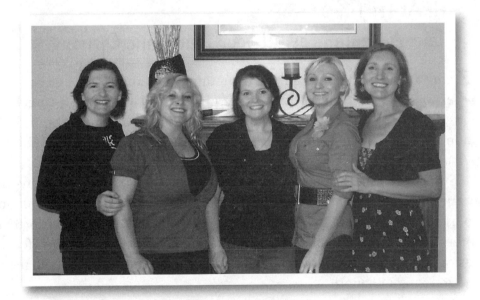

(left to right) Lessy, Juana, Sherry, Lynette, and Flo

One day, I got the surprise of my life when she unexpectedly strolled into my kitchen! Normally when Lessy comes to visit, I see very little of her, since she has so many other relatives and friends to see. But this time, she devoted her entire visit to spending time with me and transporting me to my medical appointments. What an unexpected and delightful perk! As an added bonus, Lessy is into various alternative-healing modalities, such as Reiki and craniosacral therapy, so I took advantage of a few freebies. My aura had never been cleaner and my chakras were completely balanced by the time her stay ended.

It is okay to take advantage of your siblings when
you have cancer. That is what they are there for.
(Besides, you would do the same for them.)

HEALTH TIP #56
Take Advantage of All Your Diagnostic Options

*B*eing a cancer patient, I can't help but think of all the radiation I've been exposed to over the course of my illness. And with Japan's nuclear power-plant mishap, and everything I am reading about radiation in cell phone use, I thought I would do some extensive research on the subject. (*Hmm*, I wonder if sitting in front of my computer is irradiating me?)

Surprisingly, radiation is completely natural. There is radioactivity all around us and even inside our own bodies. Our blood and bones contain potassium 40, carbon 14, and radium 226. There is also radiation that comes naturally from the soil and the air, which finds its way into our food. Basically, there are two types of radiation out there: nonionizing radiation and ionizing radiation.

Nonionizing radiation refers to waves that travel through the air but do not have enough energy to damage atoms and, ultimately, living cells. Some types of nonionizing radiation include electromagnetic (that is, from power lines), microwaves, radio waves, and infrared waves. This form of radiation can do damage, but it is in the form of heat damage (heat burns), not cell destruction and possible cancer.

Ionizing radiation includes x-rays, gamma rays, and UV rays (solar), and this is the type of radiation present when we think of nuclear radiation. Ionizing radiation causes damage to the body's cells and can cause cancer. We aren't aware of exposure to these types of rays unless we agree to a CT scan or nuclear medical test or we bake in our bikinis (and I don't mean cookies). This type of radiation is cumulative—that is, exposure adds up over your lifetime. It is also all around us in the environment.

So how much is too much? When we talk about "damage" and "harmful radiation," we want to know *how much radiation can I get and still be sure I won't grow another pinky finger.*

There are many ways of measuring radiation. For the purpose of continuity, I will use the unit "millisievert" or mSv. You may also hear of "rems" or "rads" when reading or hearing about radiation. They are all different ways to measure radiation, but it all means ionizing radiation.

We know from Japanese victims of Hiroshima, unfortunately, that sudden exposure (all at once, not over the course of a lifetime) to various levels of radiation produces the following effects:

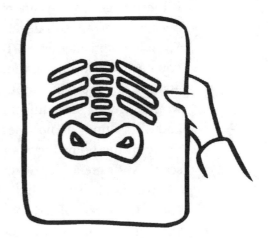

- 500 mSv—nausea

- 700 mSv—vomiting

- 750 mSv—hair loss in one to two weeks

- 900 mSv—diarrhea

- 1000 mSv—internal bleeding

- 4,000 mSv—death within two months

- 10,000 mSv—death in one to two weeks

- 20,000 mSv—death within hours

So we know what levels are harmful, but it's a bit trickier to determine what levels are "safe."

The general population is exposed to about 3 mSv/year through building materials, radon, soil, and foods grown in that soil. We know that these constant low levels of exposure are not harmful or the world's cancer rate would be 100 percent.

But what about diagnostic medical testing? I agree that safety must be a priority, but the risk has to be weighed against the benefit. When considering a medical diagnostic test, for example, is it really safer to forgo a mammogram (0.7 mSv) once a year because you are worried about radiation exposure?

CT scans can expose your body to 20 to 40 mSv at a time. If you have repeated CTs and have significant radiation exposure from other tests, this could put you at risk of developing cancers later in life. There are situations where repeated CTs are necessary, but unfortunately (in the United States) doctors are so "lawsuit conscious" that they often go overboard with diagnostic testing, checking and rechecking to make sure they haven't missed something that could lead to a lawsuit down the road.

Researchers found a population of 25,000 Japanese post-atomic-bomb survivors who were exposed to roughly the same amount of radiation as two CT scans. Based in part on those studies, the Food and Drug Administration estimates that an adult's lifetime risk of developing radiation-induced cancer from one CT scan is roughly 1 in 2,000. The risk for children is higher because kids are more sensitive to the harmful effects of radiation because they are still developing.

When considering a CT scan or any diagnostic test that uses radiation, you need to ask yourself (and ask your healthcare provider) "is this really necessary," and "is there another test such as an MRI or ultrasound tests that would give the same information as a CT scan without the radiation." MRIs and ultrasounds do not use any ionizing radiation, and when looking at soft tissue in the body, they can give the same information (most times) as CT scans. MRIs are a bit pricey, while ultrasounds are a bargain in comparison.

You can use a handy Radiation Risk Calculator at www.xrayrisk.com to check the levels of radiation of different diagnostic tests and to calculate your risk of cancer from the tests that you have had so far. Have fun!

Please note that any radiation treatment for a specific cancer tumor (excluding Hodgkin's disease, non-Hodgkin's lymphoma, or other cancers in which large areas are treated with radiation at once) may not be included in your lifetime overall cancer risk but may put you at risk for other conditions such as heart disease (if the left breast was radiated) or soft tissue cancers like sarcomas. You should check with your radiation oncologist for the specific risks that pertain to your cancer and area of treatment.

Cell phone radiation is composed of nonionizing radio frequency radiation. This is the type that can produce heat, like from a microwave. However a team of thirty-one scientists from fourteen countries, including the United States and Canada, after reviewing up-to-date studies on cell phones and cancer risk, found an increase in certain types of brain tumors in those with long-term cell phone use. You may see articles giving you the "SAR" or specific absorption rate for certain cell phone models. SAR is the unit of measure that was given to cell phone radiation. But it doesn't matter if you are using the lowest level phone because it all depends on the amount of time you spend with it pressed against your ear. Using the speaker option on your phone is always a healthier solution. (But using the speaker function around *me* would be very bad for *your* health.) Using a Bluetooth device is another good option as the radiation levels are up to one hundred times less than from a cell phone.

Since knowledge is power, you would be very powerful if you were aware of your levels of radiation so that you could make an informed choice before exposure.

The federal limits of radiation (above the natural 3 mSv/year) are as follows. These are just limit guidelines. It does not mean that you will get cancer if you exceed these limits. Exposure also is affected by a person's weight. A larger person would be less affected by 1 mSv than a smaller person (but that's *not* a reason to avoid losing weight if you need to).

- astronauts—250 mSv/year

- adults—50 mSv/year

- children under 18—5 mSv/year

- fetus—0.5 mSv/month (ultrasounds do not emit radiation)

Here is a list of common sources of ionizing radiation and the amounts of exposure:

- air travel—0.003 to 0.009 mSv/hour

- dental bitewing x-rays—0.01 mSv

- chest x-ray—0.1 mSv

- cardiac nuclear scan—40 mSv

- smoking—3 mSv/year (For one pack/day. Tobacco contains radioactive polonium 201 and lead 210. How d'ya like those cigarettes now?)

- airport backscatter (full body scan)—0.1 mSv (intentionally *not* getting into *this* controversy)

- airport scanner—0.005 mSv

- normal exposure from environment—3 mSv/year

- mammogram—0.4–0.7 mSv

- watching TV four hours/day for a year—0.02 mSv

Radiation could be the source of obsession if you consider all the radiation we come in contact with every day. Don't obsess or worry if you've already had three CT scans this year, but if there is an option for CT #4 that does not involve radiation, it might be something worth discussing with your healthcare provider. Obviously, if the benefits of having the CT scan outweigh the risk of having one, then you need to take that into account as well.

Please note: If you plan to do further research (and I hope you do), remember that 1 mSv is equal to 100 mrem. Some information sites have incorrect exposure reports because of the different units of measure.

Be aware of your radiation exposure and make
good choices when it comes to your health.

Handsome Doctors

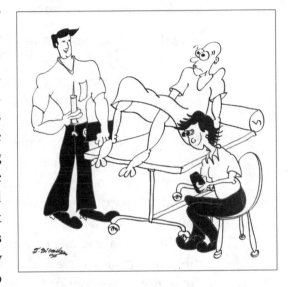

By mid-February, my ole mastectomy incision was not healing as well as expected, necessitating yet another visit to the hospital. I was feeling kind of flattered when my two sisters practically broke out in a fight over who was going to take me to this appointment. How sweet of these real-life Florence Nightingales to insist on holding my hand through another uncomfortable medical procedure. Yeah, right! The real truth reared its ugly head when I caught sister Lessy texting other sister Juana: "This place is crawling with hunks." And by "hunk," I am pretty sure she was referring to the surgeon who was coming at me with a rather large needle to remove fluid buildup from my chest.

While having to see so many doctors for my treatments was not a fun part of having cancer, the fact that some are easy on the eyes did make it a perk. With doctors nicknamed the likes of Dr. McDreamy, the Soap Opera Doctor, and Buns of Steel, I sometimes felt like I was in a real-life episode of *Grey's Anatomy!*

> Just because you have cancer doesn't mean you can't LOOK.

Health Tip #57
When Good Doctors Go Bad

Is it just me or are the number of great doctors dwindling? By "great," I mean one that has:

- intelligence without arrogance

- respect for what the patient wants

- willingness to listen

- a reluctance to pull out the prescription pad right away

- a good bedside manner

- updated magazines in the waiting room (this is probably asking for the impossible)

It seems that lately I am seeing doctors whose arrogance and incompetence factor is off the charts. I am seeing doctors who are much more interested in seeing as many patients as possible than in treating those patients properly. I'm sure a lot of it has to do with the restrictions and limitation placed on them by government regulations. The stress of trying to meet unrealistic requirements while dealing with insurance companies and malpractice leaves them little energy to do what they completed a lifetime of training for: taking care of you. Now of course, there are exceptions to every rule, and I'm sure there are those of you who have good doctors. (If so, keep the name to yourself or he/she will soon become too busy to see you!)

How can you spot a bad doctor? Consider these points:

1. **Competence: Has the doctor ever been sued for malpractice or does he/she have any outstanding legal issues?** For U.S. doctors, you can find this out by going to the state medical board website and typing in the doctor's name. Google this: medical board [the state the doctor is in].gov). This site will tell you about any lawsuits in the past or pending. It will also tell you where they went to school, how long they've been in practice, and any organizations that they belong to. Just because doctors get sued for malpractice does not make them bad doctors, but full disclosure sure feels right in this case.

2. **Common courtesy: When you call to make an appointment for your first visit, you should eventually be directed to a live person, not a machine.** You should be able to ask this person basics about the doctor, like how long has this person been practicing, when did they join the

group, and so on. If the person says, "I dunno," and is rude and doesn't deal with you professionally, think twice. If you're sick or need test results in the future, this is who you'll be dealing with. Quality doctors or doctors' groups hire quality office staff.

3. **Wait times: You can tell this is going to be bad if you walk in the waiting room and it is packed.** That means he/she probably isn't going to see you when your appointment time is scheduled. I take this as a direct form of disrespect for the patients and the value of their time. Certainly there are times when there are emergencies, and you just have to wait. But if you're waiting for no reason other than that the doctor can't manage time, that's an issue.

4. **Politeness:** Does the doctor greet you with "Good morning, Ms. Smith, nice to meet you," or is it "Okay, so why are you here?" If they're rushed, they are not thinking about the best way to treat you, just the fastest way.

5. **Cleanliness: Does the doctor wash his/her hands when he/she enters the room?** Is there even a sink to wash in the exam room? If you don't think this is important, think about what body part the doctor was examining in the previous room before he/she shook your hand. At the very least, they should use a waterless sanitizer on their hands in front of you.

6. **Attention: When you are telling the doctor your symptoms, are they engaged in what you are saying?** Or are they looking at their phone or reading your chart? Your past medical information should be reviewed *before* they go into the room so they can focus on the current problem.

7. **Defensiveness: When you mention an article that you read on the Internet, do they roll their eyes and get defensive?** Do they generalize by saying "you can't believe the stuff you read on the web!" They should be able to give their opinion on what you read without thinking you're a pain in the rump for trying to be informed about your own health. They should also be open, not instantly dismissive to alternative forms of treatment, or at the very least they should know what those alternative treatments are.

8. **Clear communication: If tests are needed, are they explained in detail,** giving the reason why the test is being performed, if there are any side effects, and when you should get the results? Or do they say, "I'm ordering some tests. See the receptionist on the way out for instructions."

9. **Follow up: Are you called with all your test results?** Whether they are normal or not? Don't accept the "if it's normal we won't call you" line. How do you know they even sent your test to the lab? Your blood tube could be sitting in the courier's car because it was impounded for too many parking tickets. There is no reason you should not be notified with your results by a qualified health professional who has the brains and knowledge to discuss the results with you. Here's a recent conversation I had with the office staff where my dad saw his doctor:

Not-old-enough-to-vote-girl staff (Noetvg staff): "I have your dad's blood work from last week and it shows something not right. The doctor wants him to take iron pills."

Me: "Ok, what did it show?"

Noetvg staff: "Um . . . the hem . . . hembloo . . . heem . . .

Me: "Hemoglobin?"

Noetvg staff: "Yeah! That's it! That was low."

Me (knowing full well what this means): *"What does that mean?"*

Noetvg staff: "Um . . . it has something to do with the blood."

Me (after having enough fun): *Can you have the doctor call me?*

Noetvg staff: Oh, no. You can't speak with the doctor! I can have a nurse call you.

Which brings me to #10:

10. **Accessible: Are you told you cannot speak directly with the doctor?** There is no reason that you can't talk to the person you have hired to manage your health. If you are directed to a nurse and still want to speak

with the doctor, ask the nurse to have the doctor call you in a reasonable amount of time. For nonemergencies, give it a day or two. If you can't get them on the phone in several days, ditch and switch.

11. **Too quick to prescribe: Does the doctor whip out the prescription pad before you even get out all your symptoms?** The drug companies rule the medical field these days. They fund the studies that say their drugs are the best and then sell the doctors on this idea. The drug companies have now turned directly to the patient through TV and Internet ads (if you haven't noticed), and they make it sound like you need their drugs to be happy. Sometimes drugs are necessary, of course, and they certainly have a place in treatment. But they are also the quick way to get you out of the exam room, and get the next patient in.

12. **Accepting of your choices: Does the doctor respect your wishes?** That is, if you choose not to take that drug that he/she wants to prescribe, do they shove it in your face, use scare tactics, or refuse to see you again?

Having confidence in who is treating you and being able to have a relationship with them in order to understand, ask questions, and challenge them can make all the difference in how well you do (or don't do) in treatment and recovery.

Of course with health care today, you may feel as if you don't have many choices. Get informed about your health-care plan. There may be only a few doctors you can choose from, but even in a small group there is one doctor that's the best choice. And whether you have confidence in your doctor or not, you should still be an active participant in your treatment.

> A quality doctor that you trust can make all the difference in your treatment outcome.

Trying to find yourself or your loved one a "great" doctor may take some time and a bit of effort, but it may also make things easier down the line when you need help making those tough health decisions.

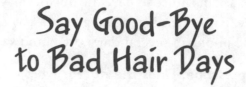

Say Good-Bye to Bad Hair Days

I dreaded going out into the heavy rain and wind to run my errands one winter day, but alas I had hungry mouths to feed. As I sprinted into the grocery store, I couldn't help but notice how many hair-dos had gone awry in the bad weather. There were flat dos, frizzy dos, and sticking-out-at-weird-angles-dos. I smugly grinned to myself, thinking how supersleek my hair would still look when I got home, despite the weather. You see, I had the advantage of being able to leave my hair at home on bad days like that one and wear a stylish hat instead.

If chemo has robbed you of your hair,
buy yourself a good selection of hats and
caps and say good-bye to bad hair days.

HEALTH TIP #58
Say Hello to Sea Salt

Salt, in its most basic form, is a combination of two chemicals: sodium and chloride. The way these two chemicals are put together and the other minerals that accompany them have a lot to do with how salt is used and how healthy it is.

Salt is the most widely used food seasoning. Not only do we cover most everything we eat with it, but it is also in virtually every processed food in the grocery store. (Look for the word "sodium" on the label.) Table salt and sea salt are both forms of sodium, but there are two basic differences: where it comes from and the added ingredients.

Table salt comes from underground mines. The salt is removed from the mine and undergoes extensive processing. The sodium and chloride are separated, and the other minerals it contains are weeded out. The sodium and chloride are then reassembled, refined, and ground down into fine grains. But the processing doesn't end there. Because any amount of moisture will cause clumping, a chemical anticaking agent is added. The agent is usually calcium silicate, but it could be ferric ammonium citrate, silicon dioxide, sodium ferrocyanide, magnesium silicate, magnesium carbonate, propylene glycol, aluminum calcium silicate, sodium aluminosilicate, sodium silicoaluminate (both of these contain aluminum), or calcium phosphate. And because the anticaking agent is bitter tasting, a form of sugar, either dextrose or glucose, is added to hide the taste.

Not exactly "salt of the earth" now, is it?

Further in the processing, iodine is also added because in the 1920s the U.S. government thought they would help rid the world of iodine deficiency. Iodine is necessary for proper thyroid function. (In their defense, because other countries adopted the idea of adding iodine to salt, the incidence of iodine deficiency has dramatically decreased.) Because all the other minerals are removed, and because it is ground so fine, a teaspoon of table salt contains a bit more "sodium" than a teaspoon of sea salt.

Sea salt, on the other hand, is harvested from the sea (there's a shocker!) and contains sodium and chloride in its natural mineral form as well as many other beneficial minerals like potassium, calcium, iron, and strontium. The salt is usually dried in the sun and then harvested. Natural sea salt has nothing added to it. It is not processed at all. It is usually ground into coarse or fine pieces. Sea salt can sometimes lose its flavor when cooked down, so it's usually added after the food is cooked. Some major manufacturers will take the sea salt, high-heat process it, or whiten it and still call it "sea salt." Unprocessed sea salt usually has a grey tint to it from the minerals. Look for the words "unprocessed" or call the manufacturer to verify.

Sea salt does not contain a significant source of iodine because iodine is not an abundant natural mineral in sea salt. However, humans need only 150 micrograms of iodine per day to maintain thyroid health. There are many other foods that contain iodine, like seafood (sea fish, seaweed, shrimp). Iodine is also found in vegetables and eggs. If you are a vegan (or even if you're not), it is a healthy habit to include some form of kelp or seaweed in your diet, if you can. Both seaweed and kelp are extremely high in iodine. One-quarter teaspoon of dried kelp contains 3,000 micrograms— we only need 150 micrograms per day. (On a side note: it is iodine that protects the thyroid from radiation in the case of a nuclear disaster. During the aftermath of the nuclear power plant accident in Japan, California stores and Internet suppliers of kelp pills and seaweed were sold out. For those "preppers" out there, I strongly suggest putting seaweed on your list entitled, "Supplies to Buy for the Nuclear Apocalypse.")

A Note About Sodium and Blood Pressure

It is estimated that 25 to 30 percent of all individuals (higher in blacks than whites) are "sodium sensitive." This means they retain fluid in such a significant amount that it raises blood pressure and puts them at risk for dozens of diseases like heart disease and organ failure. You wouldn't know you are salt-sensitive unless you check your blood pressure regularly. Humans only need 500 milligrams of sodium a day to live, but most people eating Western diets get more than 3,000 milligrams! A healthy diet generally includes a sodium intake of less than 2,300 milligrams per day. Your tongue becomes less sensitive to salt over time so it takes more salt to achieve the same flavor in your foods if you're overusing it. After about four to six weeks of gradual salt reduction, you'll be using less, and you won't notice it. Check your labels for sodium content and shoot for 2,000 milligrams per day. It would also help to take the saltshaker off the dinner table (sea salt or not) and replace it with a flavorful, natural spice replacement like Mrs. Dash or other salt-free seasonings (c'mon . . . there are thousands of other spices out there) if salt is the only seasoning you use.

To Review

Table salt is:

- highly processed (processed equals unhealthy)
- contains chemical anticaking ingredients

- contains sugar to mask the anticaking ingredient taste

- contains iodine which we need, but we can get elsewhere

- contains a bit more sodium per teaspoon than sea or other unrefined coarse salts

- has a very strong, pungent salt flavor when used for cooking

- is cheap

Sea salt is:

- not processed

- contains nothing artificial and nothing added

- contains dozens of necessary minerals that your body needs

- tastes great in and on food because it's pure

- does not contain iodine

> Get rid of unwanted, unhealthy chemicals and add some beneficial minerals and better flavor to your life by ditching the table salt and switching to a more natural one, like sea salt.

- has a slightly lower sodium content but you use less because of the flavorful mineral content and coarseness of the grain

- may lose some of the unique flavor when dissolved in cooking, but is great for added salt after

Other salts you might see are:

Dead Sea Salt: Because of the extremely high mineral content, you don't eat Dead Sea salt. Straight from the Dead Sea in the Mediterranean, bathing in it has been known to have healing and rejuvenating properties for centuries. Studies have been done using Dead Sea salt on skin conditions like psoriasis, and it has amazing healing power. It is also used on skin for blemishes, rashes, wrinkles, scars, and swelling.

Himalayan Pink Salt: This salt comes from the Himalayan Mountains and contains eighty-four minerals and trace elements, which give it its pink color and increased health benefits. This salt is delicious and is used in gourmet cooking as well as for cosmetic and healing purposes. Inhaled steam from Himalayan pink saltwater has been used for all respiratory ailments (asthma, bronchitis, sinus infections, and so on) with great success. Add several teaspoons to a bowl of steaming water, create a tent with a towel over your head, and breathe the steam for ten to twenty minutes.

Kosher Salt: Kosher salt contains no artificial preservatives or additives and is certified "Kosher" by authorities in such matters. Kosher salt can be mined or from the sea, and it usually a coarser grain than table salt. It is the coarse grain that makes it the chosen salt when "Koshering" meats. (Finer grains would run off the meat, whereas Kosher coarse salt sticks to it to draw out the blood and make the meat suitable to be prepared in a "Kosher" manner. That's where it gets its name.) Cooks like to use it because of the flavor, but it can't be used in baking because it does not dissolve quickly.

Fleur De Sel De Camargue French Sea Salt: Harvested from the south of France, it is sea salt for the snooty. This pure sea salt is collected in a very traditional way. A person known as a "raker" harvests the salt only from a certain place and only in certain weather conditions, places it in containers, and then seals the container with his signature. This salt is flakey rather than granular, is very expensive, and is used in gourmet cooking as a finishing salt that gets sprinkled over the tops of prepared foods (but probably not popcorn).

If you use a lot of salt in your home and you are using processed table salt, you may want to try some other options. If you've never tasted unprocessed sea salt, you may not know what you're missing—including healthy minerals!

A Five-Week Vacation

*C*hemo? *Check. Mastectomy? Check. Radiation . . .*

What would you call this: five weeks away from cooking and cleaning; away from packing lunches and helping with homework; away from all of the humdrum duties of running a household. A vacation? Yeah, that's how I chose to see it when I began my radiation therapy in late February. I was "zapped" every weekday for five weeks. Since the nearest hospital that offers this treatment was more than 200 miles away, I was forced to leave my small town and move to the city for the duration of my treatments. I wondered, *Whatever shall I do with myself for the next five weeks without my loveable kiddies and furry critter?* (I would still see them on the weekends.) Here's what I was thinking:

- take up yoga

- go to the movies

- dine out at nice restaurants

- visit a spa

- hang out at my favorite bookstore

- shop for some new workout clothes

- walk in the park

- visit a museum

- go to the flea market

- take in a dinner theater

I figured that would take care of the first week at least.

Each of my radiation treatments lasted about fifteen minutes, including getting me situated on the table. I made good use of that valuable time by using a visualization process that I had read about on CNN News. At the time, David Seidler had just won an Oscar for best original screenplay for *The King's Speech*. Six years earlier, Seidler had been diagnosed with bladder cancer. He attributes his survival to the use of his vivid imagination to visualize his cancer away! Whether or not the mind-body connection is strong enough to actually cure cancer is a topic that has been hotly debated for years. While there are many proponents of the mind-body connection, there are also many studies that show that it does not work. Seidler didn't care about the studies. He was convinced that he actually visualized away his bladder cancer.

Like Seidler, I didn't get all caught up in the studies. If one person says he cured his cancer through use of visualization, then that's all the proof I needed to give it a try. After all, what did I have to lose? So while that radiation was being beamed into my body, I visualized it as a golden, healing light. As this light entered my body, I imagined it making my healthy cells glow with vibrant health, while any remaining cancer cells shriveled up and disappeared. Imagine that!

Visualization is a great tool to add to your arsenal of cancer-fighting techniques. Whether or not it is proven to cure cancer is debatable. However, it HAS been proven to reduce stress and improve quality of life. What do you have to lose?

HEALTH TIP #59
Multivitamins . . . What Do You Have to Lose?

There are a boatload of studies that look at whether taking a multivitamin is worth it or not. But just like there is not one health routine that works for everyone, the same is true with multivitamins. The benefits depend on what kind of vitamin you take and your overall lifestyle. The latest (October

2012) study, which was funded by the National Institutes of Health, involved 15,000 men followed for ten years to look at cancer prevention. The study showed an 8 to 12 percent decrease in overall cancer incidence in those taking a daily multivitamin. So there may be some truth to the value of a multivitamin. But before you go out and buy a big warehouse-sized bottle, there are some things to know. Remember, vitamins are just puzzle pieces that complete a nutritional picture. The vitamin itself can't do anything. It needs proper overall nutrition and hydration to perform.

Food Vitamins Are Better Than Pill Vitamins

You could not survive on just water and multivitamins to live as they have no nutritional value. They must be used in conjunction with a healthy diet. The vitamins and minerals found in food seem to provide different benefits than just the vitamin pills alone. Vitamin A–rich foods are healthier and have more overall cancer prevention benefits than eating vitamin A poor foods along with popping a vitamin A pill.

You Still Need to Eat Healthy

Just because you can get 100 percent of your vitamin intake all in one shot does not mean you can fill the rest of the day with chips and candy. Because your healthy diet works in conjunction with the vitamins, your diet has more of an effect on your risk reduction than just taking a vitamin ever will.

Avoid the Megadoses

Look for vitamins that contain 100 percent of the recommended daily allowance (RDA) or less. High doses of the fat-soluble vitamins (A, D, E, and K) can do more harm than good when the dose is too high. Vitamin D is proving to be an exception to that rule, as daily recommendation doses are 600 mg/day, but cancer risk reduction doses can be up to 2,000 mg/day depending on what your blood levels are.

Break It Up

Water-soluble vitamins like C and the Bs, along with minerals, are most beneficial when they are available to your body's cells all day. But the fact that they are water-soluble means they aren't stored and they wash out of your body and down the toilet in a few hours. Breaking vitamin pills in half and taking half in the morning and half in the afternoon provides better availability to your system and a more efficient use of your pill.

Vitamins Are Not Replacements for Healthy Habits

Until they come out with an exercise pill, you can't omit your exercise because you took your vitamin. Sorry.

You Don't "Need" a Vitamin Pill

Look at multivitamins as an insurance policy. But realize there are far more important things you should be doing for your health.

If you eat a healthy, balanced, plant-based diet, you are getting everything you need. Just because there are studies that show increased benefit here or there, the bottom line is, you are an individual and only you know if a multi-vitamin is necessary. On the flip side, they certainly can't hurt when taken properly, but you may still need additional extra vitamin D and plant-based calcium based on your health history.

Families United

While at the cancer clinic awaiting one of my radiation treatments, I had the pleasure of meeting a lovely woman whose positive attitude shone through despite her stage-4 diagnosis. Somehow the conversation came around to my blog, and she was kind enough to share a perk with me. Sitting in a wheelchair with her mother by her side, she beamed as she told me about her three children and about how cancer seemed to bring her whole family closer together. As ugly as cancer is, I thought, it is beautiful how families unite in time of need.

My biggest fear when I learned that I had cancer was that my children might be left without a mother. This fear was magnified for Ben, as he is my youngest, he has autism, and his family spans two continents. My two older children, Kaitlyn and Donovan, are technically his "half" sister and brother (al-

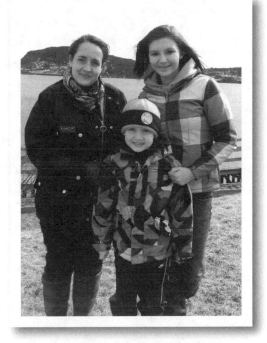

Ben with his British sister, Faye (left), and his Canadian sister, Kaitlyn (right).

though I do not allow that term in my house, as there is no such thing as halves when it comes to sibling love). He also has three "half" sisters in England from his father's side of the family.

I had the pleasure of witnessing Ben's joy when he was reunited with his British sister, Faye, as I was making ready for my trip back to the treatment center. Faye was kind enough to leave her "home sweet home" for two weeks to help her father take care of Ben during my absence. Although Ben is a boy of few words, I could tell by the way his face lit up that he and Faye share that special brother-sister bond despite not growing up together. I was so grateful that even the broad Atlantic could not keep this family from uniting in a time of need. It also gave me great comfort to know that when I do leave this world, at around the ripe old age of ninety, Ben will continue to be loved and looked after by his family.

Cancer has a way of bringing families together.
If you are separated or estranged from someone in
your family, reach out to them in your time of need.

 ## HEALTH TIP #60
Is Your Home Sweet Home Too Sweet?

How can sugar be bad? It grows on a cane and helps the "medicine go down"! If you haven't heard all the hullabaloo about how bad sugar is, listen up, because the evidence is mounting. (Go ahead and eat those bon-bons now, because you may not want to after you read this.)

But first, a brief (very brief) lesson about what sugar is and what happens to it in your body: When you consume foods containing carbohydrates (sugars are carbs), they are broken down and deposited in your blood as glucose. Glucose triggers the pancreas to produce insulin, which is a hormone that allows the glucose to be used in all your cells so you can think, move around, go to work . . . basically "live." If glucose couldn't enter the cells, they would die.

There are sugars that are naturally present in fruits and vegetables, and then there are "added sugars." Added sugars find their way into all processed foods: store-bought breads, cakes, cookies, cereals, granola bars—anything that was "made" by anything other than nature to make it taste good and make you want to buy it.

These "added sugars" are the problem.

Remember that pancreas that produces the insulin? That pancreas, which lies right next to its buddy and friend, the liver, works hard every day responding to the foods you eat. Foods that allow the blood sugar to rise slowly (vegetables, fruits, whole grains) give the pancreas ample time to produce insulin to effectively handle the sugar in your blood and get it into your cells so your body can function in a healthy way.

But eating added sweeteners like refined white or brown sugar, or man-made high fructose corn syrup, causes the blood sugar to rise very rapidly. When your system is flooded with such a large amount of glucose, the pancreas has to work extra hard. That's fine once in a while or for a short period of time, but like anything else, livers and pancreases included, if you over-work something continuously for a long time, it will wear out.

When your pancreas wears out, it is called "insulin resistance." Simply put, it means your body can't handle the amount of glucose you are shoveling into it, and because of the lack of insulin needed to get the glucose into the cells, your blood sugar remains high. Chronic elevated blood sugar is the definition of diabetes and can also lead to other illnesses, like heart disease, blindness, loss of limb sensation and chronic pain and/or numbness, and loss of limbs.

When the pancreas is in trouble, its buddy, the liver, wants to help out. When there is a very rapid rise in blood sugar, like with the ingestion of processed sugary foods, the liver metabolizes the "fructose" part of the sugar and then converts the rest of that sugar into liver fat. It's okay—the liver doesn't have a complex about being fat. Because as soon as the blood sugar normalizes, and with a little exercise from your muscles to work it off, the liver fat begins to go away. The problem occurs when the blood sugar *doesn't* normalize and there is *little or no* exercise. The liver stays fat and gets fatter. Fat livers can occur even if the person the liver belongs to is thin.

Fat livers are tired, sick livers. Fat livers also are part of a combination of symptoms known as "metabolic syndrome," which is related to obesity (in particular, apple-shaped, obese folks), diabetes, high blood pressure, and insulin resistance. It was also found that those with metabolic syndrome have increased serum C-reactive proteins, which indicates inflammation in the body. (The root of most major chronic illnesses is inflammation.) It is widely accepted in medicine today that metabolic syndrome poses a risk for many serious illnesses and is, unfortunately, on the rise.

Just like any chronic illness, high blood sugar and insulin resistance happen gradually over time. One candy bar or ice cream float won't send your pancreas and liver shouting for help. But if bad habits persist, with higher and higher amounts of refined, added sugar and high fructose corn syrup foods, this condition will eventually evolve. In the early 2000s with the explosion of high-sugar soft drinks and energy bars, the U.S. Department of Agriculture (USDA) estimated that the average person consumed 500 calories a day of refined sugar. (We're not counting the sugar that occurs in fruits and veggies here.) The increase in sugar consumption went hand in hand with the rapid rise in the incidence of diabetes and obesity, from **6 million** diabetics in 1980 to over **14 million** ten years ago, to over *25 million* today (and that's not counting the 7 million diabetics that don't even know they have it yet). I dare you to try and find a label of a processed food that doesn't have sugar listed in the ingredients. It's very hard to do, as sugar has found its way into peanut butter, bread, tomato sauce, ketchup, chips, even table salt . . . the list is endless. Our taste buds have grown so accustomed to everything tasting sweet that natural fruits and vegetables can taste bland in comparison.

So what does that have to do with cancer? It is a well-accepted fact that those with diabetes have an increased risk of cancer (as cited in the World Health Organization's International Agency for Research on Cancer). It all has to do with blood sugar and insulin. The more refined sugar there is in the blood, the faster the blood sugar rises, the more insulin must be produced to compensate. Tumors and many different kinds of cancers feed on insulin. Research is now shining a spotlight on the mechanism of this process in an attempt to understand how cancer develops and spreads.

One of the top researchers in this field is Dr. Craig Thompson, president of Memorial Sloan-Kettering Hospital in New York, and one of the world leaders in cancer research. Current research shows that insulin (and an insulin-like hormone that follows it, IGF-1) acts as the green light that tells precancerous cells to turn malignant and spread to other parts of the body.

Other researchers are building on this knowledge.

Stand Up To Cancer (www.standup2cancer.org) is an organization that funds cutting-edge research without an agenda—political or otherwise. They encourage teamwork instead of competition.

A huge Stand Up To Cancer grant was awarded to Dr. Lewis Cantley, former Harvard University researcher and current head of Weil Cornell Medical College's new cancer center. Since 2009, Dr. Cantley has led a "Dream Team" of talented researchers to study the effect of an insulin-signaling gene (PI3K) and its role in malignant women's cancers, specifically breast, ovarian, and endometrial.

Both Dr. Thompson, who also heads up a Stand Up To Cancer Dream Team, and Dr. Cantley agree that if excess sugar (and by sugar we mean "added" sugar) is the culprit in the development of insulin resistance, then they *can* truly say that sugar causes cancer. The evidence is pointing that way, and it looks like it won't be long before it's proven.

Of interesting note is that neither of these two brilliant scientists eats any refined sugar in their own diets. Dr. Thompson told *New York Times* author Gary Taubes, "I have eliminated refined sugar from my diet and eat as little as I possibly can because I believe ultimately it's something I can do to decrease my risk of cancer." Dr. Cantley simply said, "Sugar scares me."

How can something so sweet elicit such bitter thoughts?

Your added sugar is hiding from you. Manufacturers are getting very creative with their ingredients lists. Sugar can sound so harmless and natural when it's listed as "natural pure cane sugar" or "brown rice syrup." But alas, added sugar is added sugar. Here are some sugar aliases:

- date sugar
- corn syrup
- malt syrup
- maple syrup
- lactose
- molasses
- barley malt
- pretty much anything ending in -ose: dextrose, maltose, galactose, sucrose

- beet sugar
- invert sugar
- honey
- fruit juice concentrate
- maltodextrin
- refiner's syrup
- agave nectar
- and many others

There are several sweeteners that do not raise the blood sugar and are actually good choices when used in moderation. They are xylitol, stevia, and yacon syrup, and I'm sure more will be available as the demand increases.

A word about "natural sweeteners": Included in this list of "sugars" is honey, maple syrup, molasses, and agave nectar. While these are less processed and contain additional nutritional value by nature, they are still sugar and should be limited in your diet. I would certainly recommend switching from processed white sugar to a more natural form when using a sweetener for cooking, baking, and such. (By the way, a healthy diet does not include anything artificial, so I'm not even mentioning chemical, artificial, "no calorie" sweeteners here.)

> To help reduce your risk of disease, take note of where sugar is appearing in your foods and make a conscious effort to reduce it. Because you are sweet enough, don't you think?

Now that you know about sugar and cancer risk, just be mindful of the foods you eat. It's not the spoonful of honey in your herbal tea that you should eliminate. It's the morning donut with your coffee.

If you normally sprinkle sugar on your morning cereal, try berries instead. Just like salt, your taste buds actually develop a tolerance for sugar. One might say, an *addiction*. The more you eat, the more sugar it takes to satisfy your sweet tooth. Make the effort to reduce the sugar by substituting fruit or other flavorings like cinnamon, and, in about four to six weeks, your tolerance will decrease and you'll be just as satisfied with less sweetness.

Quality Time with My Girl

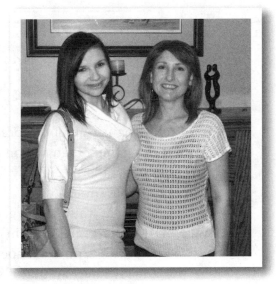

As a single parent, it is a rare luxury to find quality time to spend one on one with my three children. One day during my radiation treatments, I got to do just that: spend the whole day with my daughter, Kaitlyn. She was kind enough to take a day off school to come visit me and escort me to one of my appointments. We made the most of our time together in the city. The evening before my appointment, we got dressed up, met some friends at a nice restaurant, and enjoyed a delicious meal together. It was so relaxing to sit with our friends and talk about things other than cancer!

The next day, we started out with a walk through Bowring Park, where we stopped to feed the ducks and engage in a lively discussion on whether or not ducks have teeth. (Kaitlyn's friend, Haley, insists that one smiled at her, and she saw a distinct tooth!)

Next it was off for a healthy brunch, followed by a mini shopping spree. Finally, we made our way to the cancer clinic, and Kaitlyn waited while I was zapped with my daily dose of radiation. But alas, all good things must come to an end, and by 5:00 PM that day, I was abandoned for a "friend" who is a boy, but apparently not a "boyfriend."

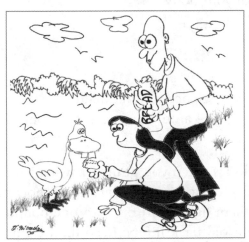

Hmm . . . it appears that Haley was right.

249

When you are fighting the Big C, it is even more important than ever to make the most of your time with family and friends. Watching a movie together, sharing a meal, or even just going for a walk are great ways to spend quality time with loved ones.

HEALTH TIP #61
How to Make the Most Out of Your Walking

Walking is one of the best exercises you can do. It doesn't require anything more than a good pair of walking shoes. (Just to be clear, walking shoes are made specifically for exercise walking; they're not just your most comfortable shoes.)

A regular routine of good, brisk walking can help shed unwanted pounds, relieve stress, aid in digestion, and strengthen your bones. Walking can help with arthritis, diabetes, heart disease, depression, and cancer. (But you already knew all that if you've been reading this book.)

Directions for walking:

1. Put on proper walking shoes.

2. Take right foot and put it in front of your body.

3. Take left foot and put it in front of your body.

4. Repeat.

C'mon, it ain't rocket surgery or brain science for that matter.

Here are eight ways that you can "up the ante" to get the most out of your daily walk.

1. **Use your arms.** You burn more calories when you pump or swing your arms, and no one will slow you down or stop you to chat. If you choose hand weights, remember to keep them light. Start off with one pound and don't exceed three pounds to avoid back injury. Keep the weights close to your body and your arm in an "L" position as you swing them.

2. **Take smaller steps.** Smaller steps mean you are moving more. If your goal is to take 10,000 steps a day, here's where you can get a big payoff. Keep up your speed as you increase the number of steps.

3. **Get some poles.** No, not Bob Polanski and his friends—Nordic poles. You'll burn 20 percent more calories by engaging the muscles in your upper body with poles. Plant the pole at a 45-degree angle behind you, then push forcefully against the ground to propel yourself forward. There are some great videos to show you how, or ask a knowledgeable person at the sporting goods store for help. (And I always thought those people I saw walking with poles were pretending to ski on pavement for fun.)

4. **Use your whole foot.** Roll through your step from heel to toe. When you get to the ball of your foot really push off. This will tone the muscles of your calf hamstring and glutes (translation: back of leg and butt).

5. **Stand straight.** Don't lean over. When your body is aligned, your back and butt muscles are able to work more powerfully, so you are able to walk faster and burn more calories. Leaning puts a strain on your lower back. Also, the stray dogs may not mess with you when you walk "like an alpha" or "top dog."

6. **Avoid steep hills if you can.** It's better to maintain your speed on a moderate hill or flat surface, than to slow down on a big hill. Steep hills are a strain on your back and can force you to work harder than you should, causing you to poop out sooner.

7. **Raise your heart rate.** Wearing a heart monitor is like having constant feedback. You will know when to speed up and slow down. If you don't have a monitor, you can use this formula to figure out where your heart rate should be during exercise: 220 minus your age multiplied by 0.7 or 0.8. This is 70 to 80 percent of your maximum heart rate for your age. You should be exercising so your heart rate stays within ten beats of this number. (Note: Taking certain medications that affect heart rates might change this number.)

8. **Add strength.** Consider pausing every five to seven minutes and do one minute of moves like push-ups (on your knees or hands) or lunges. If you're exercising with weights, here's the time to stop and do ten slow and controlled shoulder presses above your head or ten bicep curls. Do an Internet search to see the proper movement for these exercises. Then, check your form in a mirror before you head out to make sure you are helping and not hurting your muscles. Even if you stop walking to do these strength moves, your heart rate will remain elevated when the added moves are done correctly.

Working as a nurse in cardiac rehab, I saw people from the ages of thirty to eighty get great results in their fitness level, as well as success with their weight loss, with consistent proper walking. If you have never exercised before, start with just ten minutes, three times a week. Increase the time by two minutes each week until you get to forty-five to sixty minutes. Always begin and end with some muscle stretching to avoid injury and increase flexibility.

If you're going to walk, make the most out of it and get the full benefits for your whole body!

Be sensible and always check with your healthcare provider if you are just starting an exercise routine, especially if you are over the age of forty or have any chronic health issues, including cancer, or if you're on the mend from surgery.

I Haven't Been Sick Since I Got Cancer

One night, amid hacking and coughing, my boyfriend Shawn turned to me and said, "Darlin', maybe I should sleep in another room. I don't want you to catch this cold." To which I promptly replied, "Oh, don't worry about me. I haven't been sick since I got cancer." The words were already out of my mouth before I realized the irony of it! The truth was, I had not had a cold, flu, or stomach bug in nearly a year, despite being surrounded by contagious kids. Cold seasons came and went in my home, and I nursed each of my three children through the dreaded stomach flu, but for some reason, I was unaffected. Even my lifelong companion, irritable bowel syndrome (yes, it is as irritating as it sounds), took a hike.

Hmm. To what did I owe this reprieve from boogers and other unpleasantries? I chalked it up to a robust immune system. Before getting cancer, I took my immune system for granted, assuming that it would ward off the enemy fueled by the likes of diet colas and potato chips. While my killer T-cells snoozed, viruses and bacteria moved in and took up residence in my body. Then came the ultimate ambush: CANCER. What a rude awakening. I knew it was time to make friends with my killer Ts by feeding them nourishing foods and giving them some exercise. I even spent time each day pic-

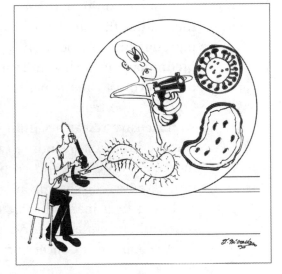

turing these little soldiers traveling through my body seeking and destroying the dreaded enemy. It paid off. Other than the adverse side effects of my treatments (which cannot be blamed on a lazy immune system), I was one of the healthiest cancer patients you'd ever meet.

Keep your immune system strong and healthy by feeding
your body nutritious, cancer-fighting foods, getting plenty
of rest, exercising, and reducing the stressors in your life.

HEALTH TIP #62
Load Your Immunity Guns with Curcumin

The spice that gives curry its beautiful golden color is turmeric. The active antioxidant ingredient in turmeric, curcumin, is the subject of studies all over the globe because of its potent immunity-boosting powers. The studies are very promising, but it's slow going because not many companies want to invest in studies that will confirm a cancer fighter that they can't get a patent for. (Natural spices and herbs can't be patented. No patent—no profits for big drug companies.)

But curcumin, in the form of turmeric, keeps making the news because the studies that *are* being done (mostly in university labs) are solid and reproducible. In laboratory studies at the University of Texas, for example, preliminary research found turmeric to be useful in preventing and blocking the growth of cancer such as melanoma tumor cells, breast cancer, colon cancer, and others.

Extensive research within the last two decades has revealed that most chronic illnesses, including cancer, diabetes, and cardiovascular and pulmonary diseases, are caused by the body's response to chronic inflammation. Suppressing chronic inflammation has the potential to delay, prevent, and even treat many chronic diseases, including cancer. Curcumin is one powerful anti-inflammatory!

The American Cancer Society states on their website:

Laboratory studies have also shown that curcumin interferes with several important molecular pathways involved in cancer development, growth, and spread.

Researchers are studying curcumin to learn whether it is an effective anti-inflammatory agent and whether it holds any promise for cancer prevention or treatment. A number of studies of curcumin have shown promising results.

Curcumin can kill cancer cells in laboratory (petri) dishes and also reduces growth of surviving cells. Curcumin also has been found to reduce development of several forms of cancer in laboratory animals and to shrink animal tumors. In studies of mice, curcumin appeared to help with blocking the plaques and proteins that cause problems in the brain during Alzheimer's disease.

It also has strong antiseptic properties, and some use it on cuts, scrapes, and burns for medicinal benefits.

Amazing stuff, right? Even though your bottle of turmeric is probably way in the back of your spice shelf behind the pumpkin pie spice that you use once a year. Yes, it is . . . remember? You bought it when you were going to make that exotic dish you saw on the cooking channel but ended up just making a peanut butter sandwich instead. (Okay, that was me.)

Turmeric is a very tasty spice alone, and it is also one of the spices found in curry. There are many different types of curry, but the yellow-colored curry that you see most often is made from turmeric, red pepper, cumin (no relation to curcumin), coriander, and fenugreek. I personally use turmeric in many day-to-day foods such as pea soup, in roasted vegetables, and in vegetarian chili. To get a good healthy dose and for a nice change from herbal tea, try turmeric tea.

Turmeric Tea

Bring two cups of water to a boil. Add $^1/_2$ teaspoon of ground turmeric. ($^1/_2$ teaspoon of shaved fresh ginger can also be added if you wish.) Reduce to a simmer for 10 minutes.

Strain the tea through a fine sieve or unbleached coffee filter into a cup; add honey, cinnamon, or lemon to taste. Sip slowly.

Turmeric, as curcumin, is also available in capsule form. When used as a spice in foods, the amount of turmeric you use is completely safe. However, if you plan to take curcumin in capsule form, you should note that it is *not recommended for people currently on chemotherapy* and also those:

● with kidney stones

● taking blood thinning agents (Coumadin, warfarin) or who have bleeding disorders

- taking drugs that suppress the immune system (because it improves the immune system)

- taking daily doses of NSAIDS (ibuprofen-type drugs)

- with diabetes; diabetics should use curcumin capsules with caution and check their blood sugar often when starting this supplement.

When you are undergoing chemotherapy treatment, you want to kill cells. Turmeric in the form of capsules provides such a large dose of antioxidant that it works *against* the slaughter. Once you've finished with chemo, though, it is worth considering.

As always, it is important to talk to your doctor about any herbal supplements you are taking. (There's no guarantee that they will have a clue about what to do with this information, but you should tell them anyway.)

Add curcumin in the form of turmeric or curry to your food. I can't think of a more delicious way to spice up your life and get rewarded for it!

Please note that you don't have to take a capsule to get the benefits of curcumin. Just include turmeric or curry spice in your favorite dishes. If you've never tried curry, I suggest you try it. The interesting exotic flavor is fun to use in many different Western foods. Or try blending turmeric with other flavors like onion, garlic, and rosemary when you use it on plain vegetables or in soups. Go ahead, and be exotic. It's good for you!

Cancer Forced Me to Forgive

Long before my diagnosis, I read a book that changed my life: *You Can Heal Your Life,* by Louise Hay. She believes that all dis-ease/disease in the body has an underlying emotional cause. In the case of cancer, the underlying cause is holding on to resentment, which eats away at the spirit as cancer eats away at the body. In order to free oneself of resentment, it is first necessary to forgive.

I believe in a holistic view of healing. I have taken a firm hand to healing my body, through my treatments, diet, exercise, and supplements. I realized, however, that true healing would not happen unless I also addressed the needs of mind and my spirit. I had some forgiving to do!

Every day for more than a month, I would visualize the people who have hurt me, and I would say in my mind, "I forgive you and I wish you well." Sometimes a little voice in my head would jump in and say, *"I forgive you and I wish you well—you bitch!"* But eventually I came to feel the truth of my words, and I was truly able to forgive. It does not matter that these people do not know that they are forgiven. Some of them may not even know that they have hurt me. This exercise was not about freeing them, but about freeing myself, since the only person I was hurting by holding on to resentment was me. Once I was able to release that energy, I opened a space in my spirit for true healing.

Although I was diligent in practicing this exercise, I still had a nagging feeling that I was forgetting to forgive someone. *Hmm . . .* my exes? Check. Friends? Check. Family members? Check. Coworkers? Check.

Then, one day, while waiting for a radiation treatment, I was mentally practicing my daily affirmation: *"I love and approve of myself just as I am,"* when that little voice in my head spoke up once again.

It said, *"How can you possibly approve of yourself just as you are? You are far from perfect. You are bossy, stubborn, and prone to anxiety."*

I then realized that the person I was forgetting to forgive was myself. I had never really forgiven myself for a failed marriage, and I harbored guilt for having hurt other people. I was also having trouble forgiving myself for Ben's autism. Deep inside I blamed myself for not creating him "perfect." So I was then forced to forgive the one person most in need of my forgiveness: me. Now when I say my affirmation, "I love and approve of myself just as I am," I really mean it, warts and all.

Repeat after me:
I love and approve of myself just as I am.

HEALTH TIP #63
I'll Take My Forgiveness in Pill Form, Please

I couldn't help wondering how I, a forty-one-year-old, exercising, optimal weighing, nonsmoking, low-fat eating, nonalcohol drinking, no family history, health-conscious woman could get stage-3 breast cancer. This same statement can be made for anyone with any illness. Why did I develop this disease, when the person next to me didn't?

I was aware of the mind-body relationship and the use of relaxation techniques to help with general health even before I was diagnosed. However, it wasn't until recently that I realized the vast amounts of clinical evidence that exists to support this idea.

Dr. Gabor Maté, a Hungarian-born medical doctor who resides in Canada, has written many books on the subject of linking mental stress to physical illness and addiction. His book, *When the Body Says No—Understanding the Stress-Disease Connection*, explains in detail how thoughts directly influence the nervous system, the immune system, and hormones. Just like the heart is a part of the circulatory system, your thoughts and feelings are part of the psychoneuroimmunoendocrinology system, or PNI system for short. "Mental stress is a major contributing factor to physical illness that we must understand in the prevention and treatment of disease," he wrote.

In the chapter entitled "Stress, Hormones, Repression, and Cancer," Dr. Maté points out the fact that if smoking caused lung cancer, then everyone who smokes would have lung cancer. But there are factors that come into play that allow the cancer cells, when exposed to cigarettes, to grow in some, and die in others. He states that your thoughts, feelings, and perceptions are a very real part of all the other systems responsible for keeping us illness-free. In explaining how all the systems of the body are linked and all "talk to" each other, he writes, "The PNI system is like a giant switchboard, always alight with coordinated messages coming in from all directions and going out to all directions at the same time. It follows, too, that whatever short-term or chronic stimulus acts on any one part of the PNI system, it has the potential to affect the other parts as well" (pages 88–89). "In numerous studies of cancer," he goes on to say, "the most consistently identified risk factor is the inability to express emotion, particularly the feeling associated with anger. . . . The person who does not feel or express 'negative' emotion will be isolated even if surrounded by friends because his real self is not seen. The sense of hopelessness follows . . . and hopelessness leads to helplessness, since nothing one can do is perceived as making any difference" (page 99).

Of course it's not as simple as "thinking" yourself well, and I do believe that environmental factors, diet, and lifestyle play a role in cancer diagnoses, too. However, there seems to be a missing piece to the puzzle to explain the rampant rise of this disease in younger and younger people, and this could provide that piece.

Women with families, in general (I am speaking generally here, with assumed exceptions), are the "pleasers" and caregivers in their family's lives. They make sure the ship is on course and everyone has their life jackets. They are responsible for seeing that everyone has what they need to be happy, often neglecting their own needs and expression of emotion in the process. In today's society, the stress of a working mom is multiplied tenfold with demands from two different directions, which leaves her very little downtime and, as a result, very little self-expression.

Women are often peacemakers, skilled at avoiding conflict and trying to make amends, sometimes for things she is not even guilty of. Today's "modern women" are taught by society to "hold things in" and keep things together without expressing too much emotion lest they be labeled "hysterical" (a term derived from the Latin word for "woman").

This repression wreaks havoc on the immune system!

Could this be one of the reasons why the incidence of breast cancer in this country has increased dramatically from 1 in 20 in the 1960s to 1 in less than 8 recently? It certainly seems possible. Some of the documented studies indicating this are as follows:

- Extreme suppression of anger was the most commonly identified characteristic of 160 breast cancer patients who were given a detailed psychological interview and self-administered questionnaire. Repressing anger magnified exposure to physiological stress, thereby increasing the risk of cancer. —*Journal of Psychosomatic Research*

- "(Holding a grudge over time) creates a state of chronic anxiety, and chronic anxiety has a predictable impact on a wide range of bodily functions, including the reproductive system, the digestive system, and the immune system," says Dr. Michael Barry, PhD, Cancer Treatment Centers of America, Philadelphia, Pennsylvania. "For example, stress hormones, including cortisol and adrenalin, have been shown to reduce the production of natural killer cells—the "foot soldiers" in the fight against cancer." (*The Forgiveness Project* by Dr. Michael Barry)

- "When you hold onto the bitterness for years, it stops you from living your life fully. As it turns out, it wears out your immune system and hurts your heart." —Stanford University Center for Research in Disease Prevention. (They even host workshops on forgiveness!)

- "I have collected 57 extremely well documented so-called cancer miracles. At a certain particular moment in time they decided that the anger and the depression were probably not the best way to go, since they had such little time left. And so they went from that to being loving, caring, no longer angry, no longer depressed, and able to talk to the people they loved. These 57 people had the same pattern. They gave up, totally, their anger, and they gave up, totally, their depression, by specifically a decision to do so. And at that point the tumors started to shrink." —Dr. Bernie Siegel, Clinical Professor of Surgery, Yale Medical School

- A study was done looking at 5-year survival and relapse incidences of women with breast cancer. It was found that those women who scored high in the "helplessness/hopelessness" category had increased incidence of relapse and death. —*The Lancet*, 1999

- A 2012 study at the University of Miami's Center for Psycho-Oncology Research has shown that a stress management program tailored to women with breast cancer can alter tumor-promoting processes at the molecular level. "The results suggest that the stress management intervention mitigates the influence of the stress of cancer treatment and promotes recovery over the first year." —*Journal of Psychological Biology*

There are hundreds of other examples of this kind of mind-body connection. So why doesn't the Western medical world recognize this and help patients to understand their role in prevention and cure? My feeling is, because there isn't a pill for it. There's no "forgiveness" pill. There is no "anger release" pill. There is no "empowerment" pill. It cannot be bought or sold. It has to be lived, learned, and practiced and is something we "Westerners" aren't exposed to. I want to be very clear on this: Finding repressed anger or uncovering unresolved issues does not mean *you* were to blame for getting cancer. But uncovering these feelings and dealing with them can influence your current state of mind and, in turn, can improve your current health.

> Examine your life and try to identify anger as well as helpless and hopeless feelings, and then try to chip away at them with professional help, stress-reducing techniques, or lifestyle changes.

For more information on the mind-body connection, check these out:

When The Body Says No—Understanding the Stress-Disease Connection by Gabor Maté, MD, and *Miss Diagnosed: Unraveling Chronic Stress* by Erin Bell. For an extraordinary story of forgiveness and healing, read *Left to Tell* by Immaculee Ilibagiza.

Cancer Motivated Me to Drop Some Bad Habits...

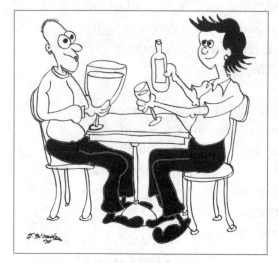

Cheers!

Before getting cancer, I considered myself to be living a healthy-ish lifestyle. I didn't smoke, I exercised on a regular basis, and I even ate the occasional green salad. But ya know, we all have our vices. For some it is chocolate (I couldn't be bothered); for others it's fast food (I'd much rather cook a leisurely meal at home); for me, it's wine. Nothing brings me more pleasure than sipping on a cold sauvignon blanc. First my taste buds spring to life, then I feel the warm sensation as it hits my belly, followed by the comforting feeling of wine-induced relaxation. *Ah . . .*

It is not my fault that I was born loving wine. What did mom expect by giving me a name like Florence? Obviously with a name that originated in Italy, I have a genetic predisposition to want wine with every meal. But alas, I have learned that alcohol in any form—even red wine, which can be good for your heart—is not good for cancer. Therefore, I have had to break my bad habit of having a glass of wine on a whim. While I still do engage in the occasional libation, I try to limit it to just ONE glass.

For optimum health,
limit your alcohol consumption.

HEALTH TIP #64
To Drink or Not to Drink?

That is the question with no solid answer.

Look hard enough, and you can find a study that supports your habits, whatever they may be. (I'm still on the hunt for one that says a messy desk will add years to your life.) But alas, if you are looking for solid hard evidence that says, "Alcohol doesn't affect your risk of cancer," you won't find it.

Every five years, the American Cancer Society publishes a document entitled "Nutritional and Physical Activity Guidelines for Cancer Prevention." Dozens of medical specialists and professionals get together and review hundred of studies with pages of data from the previous five years to determine if there have been any significant findings that they feel they want to share with us common folk.

Alcohol consumption is one of the topics studied. According to the most current (2011) guideline, the report states: "Drink no more than one drink per day for women or two drinks per day for men." (Damn that "high metabolic" Y chromosome.)

But why limit it at all? I know, you want the facts before you take such a drastic step. I hate to be the bearer of bad news, but . . .

It has been proven that alcohol is a risk factor for the following cancers:

- mouth
- throat
- voice box
- esophagus
- liver
- colon and rectum
- breast

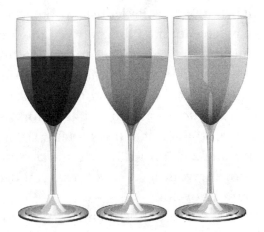

Alcohol is an irritant to tissue. (Ever get vodka in your eye? I have . . . don't ask.) So it makes sense that the area that alcohol "touches" as it passes through your teeth would be at risk. Irritated cells are damaged cells. When cells are damaged, they repair themselves. When they are repeatedly damaged, they are constantly building new tissue, which can increase the likelihood that somewhere along the line, a mistake will be made in the DNA. That mistake is a little thing we call "cancer." Furthermore, in the colon and rectum, alcohol and normal gut bacteria mix to form acetaldehyde, which is also a cancer-causing agent.

Alcohol is metabolized in the liver, so it should come as no surprise that it increases the risk of liver cancer. Also keep in mind that the liver is our "detox" machine. If you mess with the machine, and it malfunctions, it won't be able to rid our bodies of other harmful agents like pollution, plastics, chemicals, pesticides, and all the other dozens of impurities we come in contact with every day that threaten our health.

Breast cancer looks a bit out of place on this list, but it isn't. Alcohol raises your blood estrogen level. Estrogen is a hormone. Breast tissue is hormone sensitive. (Everyone "on the rag" right now can attest to this.) Your breast tissue will be affected by alcohol because it affects your hormones. Simple as that.

Recently, an interesting fact has been discovered that may have women lining up for a new test: a serum CYP2E1 test.

At a 2012 meeting of the American Society for Biochemistry and Molecular Biology, two scientists working out of the University of New Mexico may have found a link between the presence of a protein, CYP2E1, breast cancer, and alcohol. This protein is found in breast cells and actually breaks down ethanol, the alcohol part of a drink. While you might think "breaking down ethanol" is a good thing, it actually creates "free radicals" that are cell destructors and tumor activators. But not every woman's breasts have the same amount of this protein. Those with low CYP2E1 have a lower risk that the alcohol will create the destructive free radicals and cause harm. Knowing your level could help you decide if that glass of wine would be harmful or not.

But, on the other hand, alcohol in moderation may have the benefit of reducing your stress. For some, that glass of wine is the "off switch" when feeling stressed. Since stress is known to exacerbate many illnesses, the relaxation effect might just outweigh some of the risk from the alcohol itself. (At least that's what Flo keeps telling me.) Wine's relationship to stress levels seems an interesting subject, although I couldn't find that it has been studied anywhere. (If any scientist out there would like to conduct this study, Flo has volunteered to be a subject!)

Also, if your one drink a day is red wine, you are getting two important cancer-fighting agents: polyphenols and resveratrol. Both are the topics of current studies looking into their possible role in cancer prevention.

> Limiting yourself to one glass of wine is suggested for reducing cancer risk after treatment. But that doesn't mean you can't act like you've had three.

Bottom line: During treatment for cancer, you should avoid alcohol completely, but after you're finished with treatment, one drink of alcohol—one five-ounce glass of wine, one twelve-ounce beer, or $1^1/_2$ ounces of hard liquor per day—is fine as long as you and your healthcare practitioner agree. Sorry, you cannot "save" your one glass a day this week to drink seven on Saturday.

Cheers!

. . . And to Adopt Some Good Habits

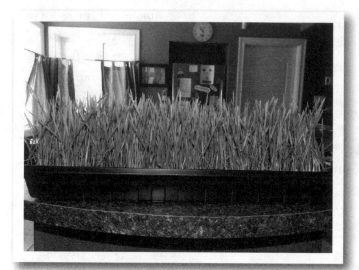

My son, Donovan, walked into the kitchen one morning and asked, "Mom, why does it smell like someone just mowed the lawn in here?"

"Well, son, that's my breakfast," I replied.

Yes, my friends, I was doing grass—wheatgrass, that is. In case you are wondering, it tastes every bit as good as it sounds (if you are a cow). However, along with kicking some old bad habits, cancer motivated me to adopt some new, healthy ones. Juicing wheatgrass was one of them.

I'd read a lot of good things about wheatgrass juice. I am no medical expert, but taking living grass, squeezing the green "blood" from it, and then drinking it has to be good for you. The fact that it ranks right up there with broccoli and raw cabbage in taste tests is further proof to me that it is healthy. Therefore, while it takes a lot of work to produce just one ounce of the juice I figured this new health kick was worth a try! While I have not kept up with juicing on a daily basis, I still do it from time to time. (My newest health kick is sprouting!)

Be open to trying new foods
for their health benefits.

HEALTH TIP #65
Get Keen on Keen-Wah (Spelled Q-U-I-N-O-A)

If you are trying to follow the most recent health recommendations and limit your animal product intake, you really should get to know quinoa (say KEEN-wah). Quinoa is cool and hip, and you can really tell that you're "in touch" with the health scene if you smugly smile as someone asks you, "Have you ever heard of Kwin-oh-a?"

"You mean *KEEN-wah*?"

"Oh yeah, I guess so. You are so cool."

(You nod in agreement.)

Quinoa is not new. It was considered the "mother of all grains" by the Incas thousands of years ago. But they were wrong. It isn't a grain at all. It's a seed. So it's perfect for those looking for plant-based proteins as well as those who need to eat gluten-free.

The United Nations has deemed 2013 as the International Year of Quinoa. Not sure what that means, but you'll be in step with the times if you include it in your diet no matter what the year. And that's very easy to do. Quinoa can be used in place of rice in most dishes or thrown into soups or salads. It can be ground into flour or flakes for use in baked foods and hot cereal. Quinoa has a natural coating consisting of saponins, a part of the seed that is bitter tasting, but most quinoa found in supermarkets has been rinsed to remove it. It's a good idea to rinse any quinoa in a fine strainer or cheesecloth under cold water for several minutes anyway and this will remove the saponins if they are present.

> Step out of your comfort zone to try things that you haven't. Quinoa is a healthy and easy way to start.

Quinoa has remarkable nutritional value. 1 cup of cooked quinoa has:

- 222 calories

- 4 grams of fat

- 8 grams of *complete protein*, which is the type of protein that has all the building blocks needed for cell growth and function. Quinoa is one of the two plant-based sources of complete protein. (The other is soybeans.)

- 0 cholesterol (Only animal products have cholesterol.)

- 5 grams of fiber (20% of the recommended daily allowance or RDA)
- 15% of the RDA for iron (for healthy blood)
- 58% of the RDA for manganese (important for strong bones)
- 30% of the RDA for magnesium (important for strong bones)
- 28% of the RDA for phosphorus (important for strong bones)
- 19% of the RDA for folate (an important B vitamin)

The following is my own personal response to my family wanting Sloppy Joe's and me wanting them to eat healthier. Since I don't bring red meat into the house anymore, I had to come up with an alternative that was not only "mother approved" but also tasted good. Quinoa to the rescue! I used the red quinoa to give them the whole visual "Sloppy Joe" experience, but the light color would work as well and taste the same.

HEALTHY JOE'S

YIELD: 8 (1/2 CUP) SERVINGS

1 cup uncooked red or light quinoa

1 acorn or buttercup squash

2 tablespoons extra-virgin organic olive oil

1 medium onion, diced

1 red or green pepper, diced

3 cloves fresh garlic crushed (let it rest 10 minutes before you crush it)

1 tomato, diced

1 teaspoon dried oregano

$1/2$ teaspoon dried basil or 1 teaspoon finely chopped fresh basil (fresh is always better)

$1/4$ teaspoon black pepper

1 (6-ounce) can or jar of tomato paste

$1/3$ cup water

1 to 2 teaspoons chili powder

$1^1/2$ teaspoons sea salt

Directions:

1. Prepare quinoa: rinse quinoa in fine strainer. Combine 1 cup of quinoa and 2 cups of water in a saucepan. Heat to boiling. Reduce heat, cover, and simmer for 15 minutes until water is absorbed. Set aside.

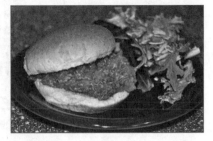

2. Bake whole green acorn or buttercup squash on foil in a baking dish or baking sheet in 350°F oven for 1 hour. Allow to cool so you can handle. Cut open and remove seeds. Scoop out of skin, discard seeds, and place flesh in a bowl. (This can be done ahead and refrigerated for 2 days.)

3. Heat 2 tablespoon of olive oil in a large saucepot over medium-high heat. Add onion, chopped red or green pepper, and crushed garlic and sauté for about 7 minutes until onions are translucent. Stir often to avoid browning.

4. Add chopped tomato, oregano, basil, and pepper and heat well, 1 to 2 minutes, stirring. Add 6-ounce can of tomato paste and $1/3$ cup water and heat well, 1 to 2 minutes. Reduce heat.

5. Add cooked squash, 1 $1/2$ teaspoons sea salt, 1 to 2 teaspoons chili powder, and quinoa and mix well. (Add sea salt or chili powder to taste. Some like it hot!)

This recipe makes about 4 cups. If you have some left over, it is great over brown rice, in a wrap with other veggies, or just by itself as a side dish.

Enjoy!

NUTRITION:

Calories: 139; Fat: 3.5 grams; Fiber: 5.3 grams; Protein: 5 grams; Carbs: 22 grams; Iron: 15% of the RDA; Vitamin A: 18% of the RDA; Vitamin C: 42% of the RDA

There are entire books dedicated to cooking quinoa. Explore recipes or substitute quinoa for rice in your boring rice recipes.

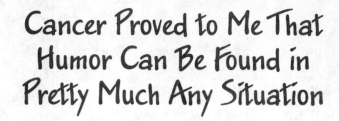

Cancer Proved to Me That Humor Can Be Found in Pretty Much Any Situation

One of my boyfriend Shawn's friends, whom I've never met, once said to him, "I read Florence's blog. She must be hilarious!" To which he replied, "Naw, she's not that funny in real life." And it's true! Maybe it is something about having cancer that makes me see that humor can be found in pretty much any situation, if I look hard enough.

Perhaps the most stoic example I have ever heard about humor in the face of hardship was told to me by my friend who is a social worker. A man in his thirties, after being told that he was terminally ill, said to her, "The doctor told me I only have two weeks left to live. I told him I would take the first week in July and the last week in August."

That is a true story and a shining example that laughter and joy come so naturally to the human spirit. Even on the toughest days, there is always something to laugh about.

LAUGH!

HEALTH TIP #66
That Clown Is Not Funny (You Know Who I'm Talkin' About)

Hurry up!

How many times do you find yourself rushing here or there, late for a meeting or your kid's soccer practice? When life squeezes your time into no time, you may be tempted to hit the drive-through for a quick meal.

Eating drive-through once or twice a month is fine, but getting your dinner in a paper sack as a habit could contribute to you and your family developing chronic illnesses. It seems that "habitual takeout" can become a lifestyle, as in 2011 Americans alone spent over $110 billion on fast food, and every day about one quarter of the U.S. population eats some form of fast food. Americans spend more money on fast food than all other forms of media: books, magazines, newspapers, video, and music . . . combined. Fast food has wormed its way into current society's habitual behavior.

What's the problem with fast food? Plenty!

1. **Nutritional value:** Most menu items have calories, total fat, and sodium that is off the charts. I took the top three most popular fast-food chains and averaged the nutritional value of their most popular adult meals. A meal was a sandwich or main plate (for chicken), fries, and a soft drink. I did not include condiments or desserts. Here are the results:

    Average calories for one meal was 1,453 calories. The average person should consume approximately 1,800 to 2,400 calories a day based on their size, age, and activity level. This meal does not leave much wiggle room for the other two. (Let's hope breakfast wasn't fast food either . . . yikes!)

    Average fat for one meal was 66 grams. Fat intake per day should be below 55 grams. So sorry, no more fat for you today (and you're 11 grams in the red for tomorrow). Excess fat not only leads to obesity (which is at an all-time high, encompassing 30 percent of the entire U.S. adult population) and heart disease but is a risk factor for cancer. And choosing chicken won't help as popular fast-food chicken meals are higher in fat than the popular burger meals.

    Average sodium (salt) content for one meal: 1,453 milligrams of sodium. Daily limit should be 2,300 milligrams. Excess salt in the diet can lead to high blood pressure and heart disease in some.

    Fast food restaurants are now required by law to list the calorie content on the menu for customers to see. *Hmmm* . . . somehow, I doubt that hungry customers will be walking out or choosing salads because of the calorie number next to their favorite burger.

2. **It's hard to avoid animal products:** Okay, I'm not a dim bulb. I know I'm not going to find a vegan meal in the drive-through. While some restaurants are adding plant-based sides and breakfasts, it's pretty safe to say that if you're eating drive-through, you're eating animal products: meat, chicken, cheese, sour cream, bacon, butter, and such. Both the American Institute for Cancer Research and the National Institutes of Health encourage limiting animal products to reduce your risk of all cancers.

3. **Manner of eating:** Hello, it's *fast* food. It's not called sit-down-and-relax-and-eat-like-a-human-being food. Even the décor is stressful as restaurants know that eating around the colors red and yellow have been shown to make diners eat quickly and leave.

> It's okay to have fast food once in a while. But try not to let it be a habit and jeopardize your overall health.

Speed eating is unhealthy in general as good digestion relies on a good blood supply to the stomach and intestines. If you eat and run, which is the idea with fast food, then you are not allowing enough time for your food to digest properly, which can lead to gas, bloating, constipation, diarrhea, and acid indigestion. Increased acid production can promote the development of certain types of colon cancers, and poor bowel habits promoted by fast food reduce the effectiveness of your colon and liver to detox your whole system.

4. **Kids' meals:** One of the top fast-food chains estimates that they will serve one hundred million kids' meals in 2013. That's 100,000,000 (in case you were wondering what that looks like in numbers), and that's just one company. (For comparison, one hundred million equals about three times the entire population of Canada.) Real kids need real food.

Once in a while, fast food is a necessary convenience, but make it a once-in-a-while thing, not a routine.

Cancer Introduced Me to Many Phenomenal Women

Through my journey with cancer and my experiences with blogging, I have had the privilege of meeting other strong and inspirational women who are living happy and fulfilling lives while facing cancer. The person who has most inspired me through my journey is a former student of mine, nineteen-year-old Beck. Due to an oversight in reporting her initial test results, Beck's cancer has advanced to stage 4 and is considered incurable. Rather than become bitter about this unfair twist of fate, Beck strives to make the most of every day with her family, friends, and fiancée. She shared this message with me:

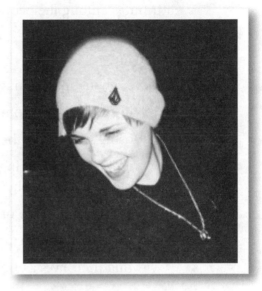

Meet Beck: An amazing young stage–4 cancer warrior who is inspiring me to live each day to the fullest.

I fight because I'm finally happy. I love living life. . . . A lot of people when they're diagnosed look at it as "I'm dying," the way I look at it, I'm living until the day I die. I'm trying my hardest to stay strong and keep the people that matter to me happy. You just have to live each day to the fullest.

Being diagnosed was the best, but worst thing that's ever happened to me. It made me open my eyes fully and realize how important the simplicity of life is. It's not about money or fancy things; it's the simple things like watching my brother grow older, teaching him about the things I've learned throughout my lifetime, making my mom smile, and making the best of every day so that when the day comes that I pass away, my loved ones are left with the best of memories.

When people say half the battle is your attitude, it's so true! When a lot of people are diagnosed, they give up. They're discouraged, fearful, and it's completely understandable. But if you keep a positive attitude, I believe anyone can beat this, even if the doctors say there's no chance of curing the illness. There ARE miracles!

In her book *From Incurable to Incredible: Cancer Survivors Who Beat the Odds*, Tami Boehmer shares stories of people who created health in the face of seemingly insurmountable odds. Tami recognized a common group of attributes among the people she interviewed. These are:

- refusing to buy into statistics and the death sentences many of them were given

- never giving up, no matter what

- relying on support from family, loved ones, or support groups

- choosing to look on the bright side and see the gifts cancer brings

- giving back and making a difference in other people's lives, whether it was fund-raising, lobbying, or supporting other survivors

- having a strong sense of faith

- being proactive participants in their health care

- viewing their lives as transformed by their experience

These characteristics define what Boehmer calls miracle survivors. Yes, Beck, there are miracles.

BELIEVE IN MIRACLES!

HEALTH TIP #67
The "Miraculous" Vitamin D

Try searching "vitamin D" on the Internet and you will get over 20 million entries! Vitamin D is the "hot" vitamin these days, partly because of the remarkable discoveries made about it in just the last decade.

Vitamin D is one of the fat-soluble vitamins found in many food sources. (Fat-soluble means it needs to be metabolized with fat to make it work. The other fat-soluble vitamins are A, E, and K.) Vitamin D is unique in that your body can actually produce the stuff just from a day at the beach. Sunlight exposure causes a process in your body that turns the sunlight into vitamin D. Because the body can manufacture vitamin D, some say it should be labeled a "hormone." I think we should call it a "vitamone" because it does the job of both.

One major biological function of vitamin D is to regulate normal blood levels of calcium and phosphorus that are necessary for healthy bone and muscle. The latest research also shows that vitamin D plays a huge role in preventing inflammation, helping to control hypertension (high blood pressure), and even plays a role in cavity prevention. Vitamin D has strong ties to preventing cancer and several autoimmune diseases, including multiple sclerosis, diabetes, and rheumatoid arthritis. There is a definite link between vitamin D and a healthy immune system. As you can see, there is good reason for its popularity! I'd want this vitamone at *my* next party.

Being a cancer survivor, I am particularly interested in the role of cancer prevention. It turns out that vitamin D plays an important role in the management of "cell elimination" or *apoptosis.* When cells don't belong, there is a mechanism in the body that arranges to have them stop reproducing. If this "cell-subtraction" function is lacking, abnormal overgrowth of cells can occur, which is the definition of cancer.

Recently, it was noted that a significant number of breast cancer patients, for whatever reason, had very low levels of vitamin D. (I was one of them.) While there has not been proof that the low levels *cause* the cancer, there definitely seems to be a relationship between the two. And the low levels don't stop there. A study of over 1,400 randomly selected healthy women showed that over 50 percent of them had low vitamin D levels too. Children and the elderly are also coming up short as well. It is unknown what effect the low levels are having on their general health, but when found, a low vitamin D level is, luckily, an easy fix with supplementation.

So how can you get some of that "D"-lightful stuff? There are several ways to get it.

Naturally: Skin will help produce vitamin D by exposure to sunlight without sunscreen. Five to ten minutes a day, three times a week is sufficient to produce adequate levels of vitamin D in your system. This small amount of sun should not be enough to put you at any increased risk of skin cancer, but the Skin Cancer Foundation still warns of excess exposure and warns that "more is not better" when trying to boost vitamin D levels this way.

Foods: It is hard to eat enough foods to get the levels of D needed to satisfy the new suggested higher daily intake levels. Vitamin D is contained in eggs, fish and fish oil, fortified dairy products, and (dare I say it?) beef liver (*ugh*). Those on vegan or low-fat diets can get their vitamin D by consuming fortified foods like cereals and plant-based milks.

Supplements: Here is where it gets tricky. Initially, the RDA (recommended daily allowance) of vitamin D was 200 IU/day. (IU stand for international units and in the case of vitamin D can be interchanged with mg or milligrams.) But we now know that 200 IU/day is just not enough based on the widespread deficiencies discovered. So the U.S. Food and Drug Administration (FDA) raised the RDA intake level to 600 IU/day. But with ever-evolving research, the consensus among the health community is that every adult should be taking 1,000 to 2,000 IU/day, especially the elderly, dark-skinned people, those who live in colder climates (and don't get sunlight exposure), those who are overweight (vitamin D is prevented from absorption in overweight persons), and those who have inflammatory bowel disease like Crohn's (ingested vitamin D is absorbed in your intestinal tract). In order to obtain these higher intake levels, a supplement is probably necessary. Vitamin D is supplied in two forms: Vitamin D2 and D3. Vitamin D3, in supplement form, seems to be the better absorbed and is the form you will most commonly see in supplements. How much you take should ideally be based on your vitamin D blood levels and adjusted to keep the level within a normal range of 35 to 60 ng/dl. Of course, any supplement that you decide to take should be discussed with your healthcare specialist. And if your healthcare specialist says you don't need extra vitamin D, please have them call me and we'll have a chat.

Some bits of info about vitamin pills:

- Since vitamins are not regulated by the FDA, there is no guarantee that because the bottle says "Vitamin D3, 1,000 IU," that it contains what it states. Use a reputable vitamin company. Look at their philosophy. Look at who *really* owns the company. How long have they been around? Any of their claims about certain products should have data to support it.

- Vitamins lose their potency so check expiration dates.

- Look for a descriptive label. Does it say just "Vitamin D," or "Vitamin D3, 1,000 IU"?

- Look at the fillers. Are there yeasts, preservatives, bulking agents, binding agents?

- Does the company "do good" for the community? Do they donate a portion of sales to research?

Toxicity: Initially, there was not enough evidence to put a number on the upper limit for vitamin D intake. Blood levels are routinely measured, and we can see how supplementation affects these levels. Knowing that blood levels should be maintained between 35 and 60 ng/dl led the Food and Nutrition Board to initially establish *very* conservative maximum upper-intake levels of 4,000 IU/day with a serum blood level of vitamin D not to exceed 60 ng/dl. The maximum used to be 2,000 IU/day but was recently raised based on new research. Who knows where it will go in the future.

> Taking a vitamin D supplement may be one of the easiest things you can do to boost immunity and reduce your risk for a handful of illnesses, including cancer.

Vitamin D toxicity can further be avoided by taking it in conjunction with vitamin K. When taken with vitamin K, vitamin D is less likely to reach toxic levels. Certain companies are now combining vitamin D with vitamin K. The RDA for vitamin K is 150 mcg/day. I would not be surprised if you start to see more supplements that contain a combo of vitamins D and K in the future. If you choose to take a multivitamin, it would be a good idea to take your extra vitamin D with it as most multi's contain K. (Or you can just take your vitamin D with a big dose of high vitamin K kale or any other dark green leafy vegetable.)

Speaking of multivitamins, if you plan to take extra vitamin D, check your multi and your extra calcium (if you take it) to see if there's any vitamin D in those. You may not need extra D if it's covered elsewhere.

If you get your blood levels checked, and your levels are low, you may be prescribed 50,000 IU/week for several weeks until your levels are corrected. There is no danger of toxicity from taking 50,000/week for a few weeks under a doctor's supervision to get your serum D up to normal. Toxicity symptoms are rarely seen when intake is less than 10,000 IU/day; they include muscle cramping and heart rhythm problems due to high blood calcium levels. Again, getting your blood tested is the best way to find the perfect amount of vitamin D you need for your body.

I would strongly suggest (and I don't usually *strongly suggest* anything) that you ask your doctor to check your vitamin D level (ask for the vitamin D 25-hyroxy blood test) and treat accordingly.

Cancer Allowed Me to Feel Like a Movie Star

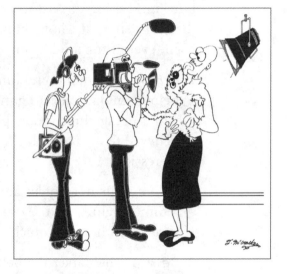

*A*nd the Oscar for best supporting actress in the role of dog lover goes to *(drum roll please . . .)*

When I first started my "Perks of Having Cancer" blog, I was interviewed by the NTV Evening News, and, believe it or not, it made me feel like a real movie star! Although they aired only about a three-minute clip on the program, the whole production took well over an hour to film. The interview part was real, but I will let you in on a secret, I was pretty much acting for the rest of it. Me gazing out the window with a wistful look on my face: acting. Me holding up a smoothie and saying "cheers": acting. Me playing with my dog, Patches, and looking lovingly into her furry face: big-time acting. Now don't get me wrong, I do love and appreciate Patches, but I certainly didn't appreciate her licking at my face (especially after seeing what she was licking before my face). But I must admit, I looked like a real natural in the news clip! Which is why I think I should be nominated for an Oscar. Oh, gotta run, I think that might be the paparazzi outside my door . . . never mind, it's just the paperboy.

If cancer is getting you down, let your imagination go wild! Pretend you are a famous actress or a country superstar, whatever turns your crank. Whether you have these experiences for real or just imagine them, the same "feel-good" hormones will course through your body.

HEALTH TIP #68
And the Winners Are . . . Envelope Please

Knowing that you probably love lists as much as I do, I've compiled my favorite list of cancer-fighting foods. There are many more I could add, but I'm keeping this list to ten. Keep in mind that eating a well-balanced diet consisting of whole, unprocessed, colorful foods is cancer-fighting in itself, even if the food is not on this special list.

1. **Lemons:** Vitamin C and limonene in lemons strengthens immunity and helps stimulate cancer-fighting cells in the body. Lemons and lemon juice, while being citrus foods, promote alkalinity in your body. It is widely believed that a more alkaline system prevents cancer and may even cause regression.

2. **Garlic:** Allicin, a potent antioxidant and anti-inflammatory, and allixin, a tumor fighter, are the reasons this delicious bulb made the list. Just be sure to eat it raw as much of the benefits are reduced in cooking.

3. **Berries:** The darker the better, although all berries have cancer-fighting properties and contain ten or more cancer-fighting plant chemicals. Get black and blue (berries, that is) for the most benefit.

4. **Avocado:** Great for your liver, the organ responsible for cleaning toxins out of your system, avocados provide plenty of potassium and beta-carotene and are rich in glutathione, a powerful antioxidant.

5. **Chile peppers:** The hotter the better as it's the "hot stuff," or capsaicin that is thought to attack cancer-causing substances in your body.

6. **Broccoli:** Lutein and zeaxanthin are the powerful cancer-fighting sub-stances found in all the cruciferous veggies: broccoli, cauliflower, kale, Brussels sprouts, and cabbage. Not the most loved group of veggies, but they should be!

7. **Raw Carrots:** Beta-carotene, a vitamin A precursor and a potent anti-oxidant, and falcarinol, a cancer preventative, are abundant in carrots. Eating them raw gives you the most benefit. Shred them in your salads or use them to dip into something healthy like hummus.

8. **Mushrooms:** Specifically shiitake, maitake, reishi, and turkey tail, which are strong immunity builders and potent cancer fighters because they are are high in beta-glucans and polysaccharide-K (PSK).

9. **Red grapes:** Loaded with bioflavonoids and ellagic acid, which helps prevent cancer, as well as resveratrol, which is an immunity booster.

> Think of foods as your medicines to fight and prevent cancer, and take your medicine every day.

10. **Olive oil:** While a diet high in fat was shown to be a risk factor for colon cancer, those who ate a diet high in fat that consisted of olive oil showed no increased risk, suggesting that it provides some protective factor. Organic extra-virgin olive oil is the best of the best.

Be creative and see how many of these foods you can eat today!

I Could Finally Admit
I Believe in Angels and Fairies

Having cancer allowed me to feel comfortable being the REAL me. I even came out of the "spiritual closet" and admitted that I believe in angels and fairies, without people calling me crazy . . . well at least not to my face.

My name is Florence and I am a Certified Angel Therapist. There, I said it. Not only do I believe in angels, but I also talk to them, and they communicate back through signs and symbols (such as a butterfly or a white feather). Before getting cancer, I would never have admitted this publically for fear that people would think I was cuckoo. After all, I am a professional psychologist with a reputation to uphold. However, once I had cancer, it didn't really bother me if people thought I was weird. In fact, it was kind of a relief to show my true colors.

Up until about five years ago, I figured that angels, like Santa and the tooth fairy, belonged to the realm of childhood imaginations. Then one day, while browsing a bookstore in England, I came upon an interesting book called *The Psychic's Bible* by Jane Struthers. As I flipped through its pages, I stopped upon a picture of a white, fluffy feather with this caption: "Angels often leave a white feather as their calling card." Although I didn't believe in the existence of angels at that time, I was intrigued by this little book, and so I decided that it would make a good read on my return flight home to Canada.

Just the next day, I got the opportunity to put my angels to the test! My friend and I were gearing ourselves for the grueling journey through Heathrow Airport with my four-year-old son, when we discovered a mix-up in our departure time. Anyone who has ever visited this busy airport will know that at least two hours is required to check in, clear security, and make it to your gate. However, we found ourselves at our hotel with only one hour to departure and a half an hour drive to the airport, with no cab in sight. Even if we did manage to get a cab, I knew that it would be practically impossible to navigate the long lineups of Heathrow in less than thirty minutes! Suddenly I remembered what I had read in *The Psychic's Bible*, and in desperation, I whispered a prayer to enlist the help of my angels. Soon after saying the prayer, I was surprised to see a white, fluffy feather on the ground at my feet. *An amazing coincidence*, I thought. However, through what I can only describe as a series of small miracles, we made the flight. From then on, I have been a believer.

Now I talk to my angels on a daily basis. My angels have also become an important part of my survival plan as I call upon them to administer healing to my body and spirit. As I listen to my guided angel meditation CDs, I can actually feel the energy of their presence (*Angel Therapy Meditations*, by Doreen Virtue, 2008).

You don't have to wait to get cancer to be the real you, but if you have been holding back, now is a great time to start. Who cares if everyone thinks you're nuts?

HEALTH TIP #69
Did Somebody Say "Nuts"?
Good Reasons to Grab Your Nuts and Go!

Not those nuts!

Nuts are giant seeds that are covered in a hard shell. They supply all the compact nutrition of any other seed and also are an excellent source of protein, fiber, and healthy fats. Tasty and great to eat "on-the-go," nuts are an easy way to ensure that you're getting everything you need nutritionally.

Most nuts are great by themselves, but you can also go nuts by adding nuts to your salad or smoothie, blending them into your soup, or adding ground nuts to your hot or cold cereal in the morning. In many plant-based recipes, nuts are used to add creaminess and richness. You can even make cheesecake using cashews in place of the cream cheese.

Here is a rundown of the top varieties, their calorie content, and what makes them so special. I could go on and on about the health benefits (I am a little nutty about nuts), but these are the highlights.

All the nuts are relatively high in total fat, but the fat contained in nuts are beneficial to your body instead of settling in your arteries. Still, if you're watching your calorie intake, just stick to one or two serving sizes per day.

Walnuts

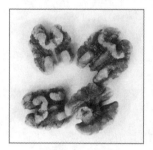

Serving size: 14 halves (that's 7 whole in case you don't do numbers) • calories: 185

Omega-3: 2.6 grams—the only nut to have high omega-3s, an extremely important fatty acid for overall health. One serving of walnuts has as much omega-3 fatty acid as 4 ounces of canned salmon.

Walnuts are great in muffins and cookies and truly belong in every bowl of oatmeal on the planet.

Special fact: The type of omega-3 fatty acid found in walnuts provides all the benefits that other omega-3s do, but it is high in alpha-linoleic fatty acids, which has brain-boosting power that can help to prevent dementia and Alzheimer's.

Always store your walnuts in the fridge as they can become moldy.

Almonds

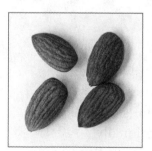

Serving size: 23 nuts • calories: 163

Almonds are the favorite nuts of dieticians as they are low calorie and high fiber.

Special fact: Almonds lead the nuts in fiber content, vitamin E, and calcium. A $1/4$ cup serving of almonds has more calcium than $1/2$ cup of ice cream (95 versus 85 milligrams), and it is the only nut that you can sliver. (Go ahead and try slivering a pine nut . . . I dare you.)

Due to a past salmonella scare, almonds sold commercially in the United States are processed by pasteurization, even if they say "raw" on the bag.

Macadamia

Serving size: 11 nuts ● calories: 204

Notoriously hard to shell and expensive, but oh so exotic and tasty.

Special fact: Macadamia nuts are high in thiamine, which helps keep your nervous system healthy. They also make us think of Hawaii, and that feels nice.

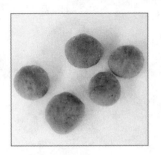

Pistachios

Serving size: 49 nuts ● calories: 162

Pistachios are related to the mango.

Special fact: Pistachios are rich in lutein, an antioxidant for healthy vision and skin. They also have as much potassium as a small banana (287 mg). Notice that natural pistachios are beige, not red. The red dye added after harvest that turns your fingers a pretty shade of pink is used to hide imperfections. (And I always thought they grew on pink trees.)

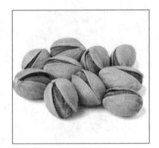

Cashews

Serving size: 18 nuts ● calories: 163

One of the favorites to eat on their own.

Special fact: You can get 10 percent of your daily RDA of iron in one serving of cashews. They are also a great source of folate (a cancer fighter) and vitamin K (which helps blood to clot normally and is vital for normal vitamin D absorption).

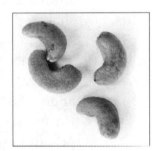

Brazil Nuts

Serving size: 6 nuts ● calories: 186

Brazil nut trees can live 500 years!

Special fact: One Brazil nut contains more than the required daily allowance for selenium. Selenium is the subject of many studies that suggest it can prevent cancers. While it is essential for thyroid health, too much selenium can cause hair loss (yikes!), so limit your servings to one and don't eat Brazil nuts every day.

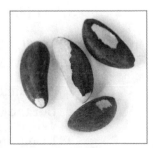

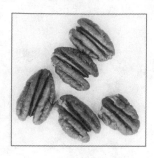

Pecans

Serving size: 19 halves • calories: 196
There's more to pecans than PIE.

Special fact: Pecans are rich in beta-sitosterol, a type of plant sterol found to lower cholesterol and aid in prostate health as well as fight cancer. They're healthy no matter how you say them—PEE-cans or pi-CONS.

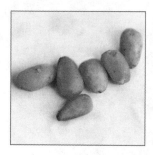

Pine Nuts

Serving size: $1/4$ cup • calories: 228
The smallest of the nuts is big on nutrition.

Special fact: Pine nuts are high in manganese, a mineral that helps metabolize carbs and proteins and also increases hormones that help you to feel full, which makes it a great "weight-loss nut." They are also high in iron (3 milligrams per serving). Pine nuts are soft when raw but have a wonderful flavor when toasted. Place on an oven-safe pan and bake for 15 to 20 minutes in a 350°F oven, stirring every 10 minutes. Pine nuts are great for adding creaminess to shakes.

Notice I didn't include peanuts in this list of nuts because peanuts are technically not nuts at all. They are part of the legume family, as in beans, and while they aren't unhealthy, they don't rate high enough in nutrition (in my snooty opinion) to belong to the special nut family. If you like peanut butter, try almond butter, which packs a bit more nutrition (fiber and calcium) and tastes just as good with grape jelly. Here are some tips when making your nut selection.

- When buying any nut, read your labels to avoid hydrogenated oils and added salt, which can sabotage your healthy eating plan.

- "Roasted" nuts are heated in oil, while "dry roasted" nuts are heated without the use of oil.

- In nature, nuts have a natural enzyme inhibiter coating to prevent the nut from sprouting too soon. This enzyme inhibiter also can affect our digestive enzymes and cause stomach upset. Some nuts, like cashews and pistachios, are heat processed and this enzyme is removed. Almonds, by law, are heat pasteurized even if the label says "raw." Some still advocate soaking all nuts for eight to twelve hours in water and then dehydrating them or slow roasting them in the oven at 170 degrees Fahrenheit for twleve to twenty-four hours to aid digestion. (Higher than 170 degrees seems to destroy some of the beneficial nutrients.)

- It's a good idea to store nuts in the refrigerator. Nuts freeze very well for long-term storage.

The bottom line is: roasted or raw, walnut or pine, nuts are an easy option for adding nutritional value to your diet.

But for-the-love-of-all-that-is-clean, don't eat the nuts in that wooden bowl at the bar! Do you know the number of people who reached into that bowl that didn't wash their hands after using the restroom?! It's disgusting!

> Think "nuts" when looking for a snack or when your meal needs a little nutrition boost.

Cancer Made Me the Preferred Sister-Wife

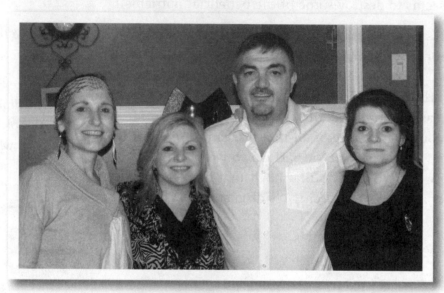

Bob with his sister-wives, Flo, Juana, and Sherry

I am very fortunate to have two of my sisters, Sherry and Juana, living so close by. They were a tremendous help to me during my cancer treatments. Juana and I are both single, and, for a long time, Sherry's better half, Bob, was the only man on the scene. So Bob shared his time between our three houses in terms of doing general repairs and maintenance, putting up Christmas lights, digging snow, and other manly chores. We fondly came to refer to ourselves as Bob's sister-wives. (However, unlike REAL sister-wives, we don't do sleepovers.) After my diagnosis of cancer, I got more than my fair share of sister-wife time with Bob. As soon as anything needed fixing, a message was dispatched: Code red—Florence's fridge is leaking. Send Bob STAT . . . and the repair was done.

> It is perfectly okay to use your cancer to get stuff fixed around your house.

HEALTH TIP #70
Prepare Your House for the Apocalypse . . .
or Just Have a Tasty, Healthy Snack

Freeze-dried food. It sounds unhealthy and unnatural, doesn't it?

The reality is, freeze-dried food makes perfect sense for anyone wanting to eat healthier and for those stocking their fallout shelters for the end of the world.

Ask any astronaut and they'll tell you that freeze-dried food has the same nutritional content and appearance as fresh food, but without the water. Which means the food can be stored for up to twenty-five years! These light-weight, brightly colored morsels can be rehydrated, used in cooking, or eaten right out of the bag or industrial-sized drum.

Freeze-dried are not the same as "dehydrated" or "dried" foods. Here's the difference in case you were wondering.

Dehydration is a process where the water is removed from the food by slow heat. This can be in an oven, by the sun, or by the wind. It can be done at home with a dehydrator, but it is time-consuming. Dehydrated foods are lightweight but contain a bit more water than freeze-dried, so their texture is a bit chewy (we've all had raisins, right?). Some commercially dehydrated foods have added sulfur or preservatives in them—and do you really need those? Dried food is a bit more compact than freeze-dried, but the rehydration time is longer. Dehydrated foods look very different from their origins.

Freeze-drying is a process where the food is flash frozen and then placed in a vacuum chamber where the water is removed by evaporating the ice at temps as low as -50 degrees Fahrenheit. This retains the foods' appearance and shape. Freeze-dried foods rehydrate in minutes—much faster than dehydrated, and the food regains its original texture and flavor. Foods like cheese and ice cream can undergo this process too, as can pre-pared foods like pasta and casseroles. But because of the manufacturing process, freeze-dried foods are more expensive. But the flavor is far superior to dried, and your choice of foods is endless. (Imagine taking "freeze-dried" lasagna on your next camping trip!)

Here are some brief facts about freeze-dried foods:

- Freeze-dried foods have a shelf life of up to twenty-five years in a sealed can, and up to six months after opening if the lid is kept tightly sealed when not in use.

- Freeze-dried foods usually contain no additives, preservatives, or extra ingredients (but check your manufacturer).

- Unlike canned foods, there is no added salt and no leaching of BPA from the can lining.

- Freeze-dried foods are practically weightless so they're great on a hike or when traveling.

- They are compact so they store nicely.

- To rehydrate, just place in hot water for a few minutes or cold water for 20 to 45 minutes.

- They are identical to fresh foods in antioxidant and nutritional value.

- Organic choices are available.

- You can cook simply with freeze-dried foods. For example, if you make soup, you can throw in any vegetable at the very end as they are already cooked.

Strawberries, for example, may look expensive at first glance because a 1.2-ounce bag of these sweet nothings is $4.00 U.S. But that's about the same price as what a pint (16 ounces) of fresh would cost at the local market, and rehydrated would yield about the same amount (13.2 ounces) given the 11 to 1 rehydration ratio, which is also about the same price as frozen. And frozen won't last when that asteroid takes out all the electricity in the world and your freezer becomes just a big heavy bookshelf with doors.

I don't think freeze-dried foods are meant to replace fresh, but for a snack idea, for your emergency stash, or for hiking or traveling, it's pure genius.

Consider it just another option you have when looking at nutritious, low-calorie foods. It's convenient (and a little magical) to think that you have six pounds of strawberries sitting in your pantry, for you to use in recipes or slip in your pocket.

And admit it . . . you secretly want to be an astronaut.

> Freeze-dried foods are a great way to keep healthy food choices close at hand.

Here are some suppliers:

- Mountain House: www.MountainHouse.com

- Nitro-pak: www.nitro-pak.com/products/freeze-dried-foods

- The Ready Store: www.theReadyStore.com

Treats in the Mail

Before cancer, my visits to the post office normally yielded only unwanted flyers and even more unwanted bills. After being diagnosed, however, I emptied my mailbox each day like a child would empty a stocking on Christmas morning. Many days embedded among the flyers and (sigh . . .) bills, I'd find a gold nugget: a card, a note, or a gift sent to cheer me through my recovery. One particular day, I was very fortunate to find not one, but two of these nuggets in the mail, both very personal and thoughtful gifts. Then later in the day, some of my former colleagues showed up at the door with a big bouquet of flowers to share a cup of tea and a few laughs. It really made me appreciate having so many kind and thoughtful people in my life.

If you are fortunate enough to have people in your life who send a card, a gift, a wish for your recovery, a prayer, or to visit with you, REJOICE!

HEALTH TIP #71
REJOICE! Chocolate Is Actually Good for You!

Chocolate is healthy! Yay!

Yes, all that money we pump into scientific studies has finally paid off! It turns out that chocolate, more specifically, dark chocolate containing 70 percent cacao or more has many health benefits.

Besides lowering your risk of heart disease and stroke, the substances found in chocolate can also reduce your risk of cancer by acting as antioxidants and anti-inflammatories.

And more important than fighting any disease, dark chocolate reduces aging effects on your skin, giving you a more youthful appearance. Does it get any better than this?!

The secret lies with the seeds of the cacao tree. Cacao is one of the main ingredients in chocolate. The cacao seeds contain high levels of polyphenols and flavanols (a class of antioxidants), which are the healthy compounds that help fight disease and aging. Cacao seeds are one of the world's most concentrated sources of these powerhouse antioxidants.

But you must eat your chocolate dark. Milk chocolate and white chocolate don't have the same benefits. The darker the better, as the darker chocolates have higher levels of flavanols and lower levels of added sugar. As you might expect, adding lots of sugar defeats the beneficial action of the cacao. Look for chocolate that is 70 percent cacao or more because that will provide you with the most healthy benefits and it will contain the lowest amounts of sugar.

Also choose organic dark chocolates that don't use preservatives or artificial flavorings. Using natural organic unsweetened cocoa powder has even more benefits than bar chocolates, as the powder is pure cacao with nothing added. You can use pure cacao/cocoa powder to make healthy goodies where you can control the type and amount of sugar you use. (Check out my Beetroot Cupcake recipe in Health Tip #51.) Sorry, processed and packaged hot cocoa just has the cocoa name, but it does not offer the same antioxidant benefits as dark chocolate products.

> When you want a treat, reach for dark chocolate to boost health and happiness.

As a side note: cacao and cocoa are the same part of the plant, but some use cacao to mean powder from the raw bean and cocoa to mean powder from the roasted bean. Others say the tree is called a cacao tree and the beans and their powder are called cocoa. Either way, look for a high percentage of the stuff in your dark chocolate product.

I wish I could say that more is better in this case, but alas, there is a suggested limit to your chocolate intake. One to two ounces per day seems to be the magic number to keep you healthy and avoid too many extra calories. But even with this limitation, you have to agree, this is the best news you've heard in a long time.

Cancer Made Me Reevaluate the Relationships in My Life

People expect that when you get cancer you suddenly get great insights into life. Well, they are right. When I am asked about my great insights, I have only one: The only thing that really matters in life is people. You already knew that, right? Yeah, so did I, intellectually. But knowing it and really believing it are two different things. And cancer has the perk of allowing you to really feel the truth of that statement, as it helps you to truly appreciate the people in your life.

One relationship that I have come to feel more grateful for is with my children. My teenagers, Kaitlyn and Donovan, really stepped up to the plate following my diagnosis. I am the type of mother who does everything for her kids (some would say "spoils them") so it wasn't easy for me to let my kids become my caregivers. However, I had never been more proud of them. I realized that giving them more responsibility did not make me any less of a mother, and it gave them valuable skills to carry into adulthood.

When Ben, my youngest child, was diagnosed with autism at the age of three, that became my obsession. I have read hundreds of books and articles, attended numerous workshops and training sessions, been an active participant in his therapy, and even became trained in alternative healing modes so that I could administer therapy. I figured that if I tried hard enough (and spent enough money!), I could fix Ben's autism. After getting cancer, it suddenly dawned on me: "Ben has autism. No big deal! He is healthy and happy and that is what really matters." My goal is no longer to fix his autism, but rather to help him reach his greatest potential.

The biggest relationship metamorphosis occurred between my family and me. We have always been close, but being the independent (okay, some would say "stubborn") personality that I am, I would sometimes shut my family out. It is not easy being a single parent, particularly with Ben's challenging behaviors. However, I would rarely ask my parents and sisters for help. If they offered, I would often refuse, figuring that this was *my* responsibility. When cancer knocked me down, I had no choice but to accept their help. I suddenly realized that I was not burdening them with my problems. They *wanted* to help, and by allowing them into my life and Ben's life, I was actually giving them a gift.

My relationship to Ben's father, my "second ex," also changed after my diagnosis, as he became the main caregiver in Ben's life. It allowed me to see his unending patience with our son and the genuine love that they share. When I was away for treatments, I was content in the knowledge that Ben was in good hands.

Finally, I have been blessed from a very young age with meaningful friendships. My friends are my soldiers. These phenomenal women have been in the trenches with me for more than a decade. They have cried with me, laughed with me, and drank wine with me through divorce, new relationships, breakups, Ben's diagnosis of autism, and then the Big C. I can depend on them for anything. I thank God for this wonderful gift of friendship, and I thank these friends for sharing my life—the good, the bad, and the ugly. (As an added perk, cancer helped me to find a new friend, my smart and funny cowriter, Susan!)

When you are battling cancer, your time and energy become
more precious to you. Don't waste it on toxic relationships; instead
nurture those relationships that allow you to be your best self.

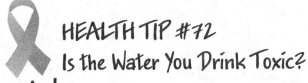

HEALTH TIP #72
Is the Water You Drink Toxic?

Water, water, everywhere . . . but which one should you drink?

You know you should be drinking more water, but there are just so many darn choices out there: purified, tap, artesian, mineral, coconut. It is enough to drive you to drink! But then you're back to where you started.

Listed here is a rundown of all the different waters and all the assorted details about each one, so you can determine which is right for your health.

Tap Water

In the United States, tap water falls under the jurisdiction of the Environmental Protection Agency (EPA) and is federally regulated and locally enforced. Frequent testing is mandated, checking for many contaminants on a regular basis, and reports of the findings are required to be posted publicly once a year. As a comparison, in the United States, bottled water falls under Food and Drug Administration (FDA) jurisdiction and the safety testing is much less strict. For example, local tap water is required to test for bacteria over 100x/month, whereas bottled water is required to test for bacteria only 4x/month.

Source: Depends on your local area. Some sources could be from rivers, lakes, and streams, or wells. Rainwater and groundwater can also be used. Check your local treatment facility to see how yours starts out.

Cost: $0.00125/16 ounces or $0.01/gallon.

Contains: In the United States, you can go to: www.water.epa.gov to see what your local drinking water contains. You can get somewhat of an idea what's there, but it may not tell you the whole story. The report will list minerals, bacteria, and other substances like mercury and lead, along with the reported amounts measured in the test sample. However, the water described in the report posted on the Internet doesn't mean that's what comes out of *your* faucet. Each home has different pipes, and different water flows—therefore, different contaminates. The county won't test the water from inside your home, but you can have a private testing company do it if you choose. Take a minute to find out what's in your water.

Filtering your tap water is a no brainer. There is no disputing that drinking chlorine and its byproducts in your tap water is harmful and unhealthy. Activated carbon filters are great at removing these

Fun Fact: It might surprise you to learn that 25% of all bottled water actually comes from tap water. Some is further treated by additional filtration and some is not.

contaminates. Recent testing done by *Good Housekeeping* in an independent lab showed that common household fridge filters actually do a good job of filtering out chlorine and pharmaceuticals from the water as well. Pharmaceuticals? Yes, there are probably drugs in your water. Prescription medications are peed out and flushed into your water supply, and water treatment plants are not required to test for them or remove them. While they exist in very small amounts, any amount of hormones, painkillers, or Viagra is too much for me. Generally speaking, the refrigerator-type and water-line type filters (activated charcoal) were able to filter 40 to 92 percent of these contaminates. The pitcher-type charcoal filters were fair in what they filtered, but many of them didn't last as long. There are hundreds of in-home water filtration systems available, from simple one-step filters to complex, expensive multistep systems. Check to see which of them fits your needs and the types of contaminates they remove.

The one thing fridge (carbon) filters do *not* remove is fluoride. Fluoride is a mineral that is found in nature, but since 1945 it been added to U.S. tap water (in most U.S. states and thirteen other countries). What started out as a crusade to make strong teeth has turned into the overdosing of a large part of the public with fluoride. Fluoride is toxic, plain and simple. Just look on your fluoride-containing toothpaste and it says, "If more than used for brushing is accidentally swallowed, get medical help or contact poison control center right away." And "the amount used for brushing" is supposed to be a pea-size . . . not the entire length of your toothbrush. Fluoride is also classified as a "treatment," which means it is a medication. Technically, the government is medicating you without your consent. (I know, I sound like a kook, but it's true.) Fluoride is supposed to prevent tooth decay, but because so many other products like toothpaste, mouthwashes, and gum are highly fluoridated, it is causing harm. Excess exposure to fluoride causes skeletal fluorosis, which is a weakening of the bones, and increases risk of fractures. Based on results of new studies and reported public health problems, the government agencies review the recommended fluoride levels and set new guidelines regularly.

A review of the literature done in 2006 by a panel of medical and environmental experts hired by the U.S. government stated, "The evidence on the potential of fluoride to initiate or promote cancers, particularly of the bone, is tentative and mixed and that, overall, the literature does not clearly indicate that fluoride either is or is not carcinogenic in humans." In other words, we just don't know if fluoride causes cancer or not.

If you aren't lucky enough to own a high level multistep filtration system designed to remove fluoride, then do your best to remove it in other areas of your life. Avoid toothpaste and mouthwashes that contain fluoride and "just say no" to extra fluoride treatments at the dentist. Bottled water may or may not contain fluoride, as they are not required to list that on the label. Contact the bottler for that info.

For more information on fluoride and the fight to get rid of it in the water system, visit www.fluoridealert.org.

If you plan to take your filtered tap water on the go, purchase a 100 percent stainless-steel bottle that resists bacteria growth and will keep your water cold. Make sure the bottle does not contain an inside plastic coating as the plastic might contain unhealthy BPA, a chemical that can leech into your water and cause health problems.

You would think that with the invention of indoor plumbing and tap water, we would be satisfied with the water that comes right into our homes for a few cents a gallon. But in 1977, someone saw that if you make bottled water a "trend" (some might even say "a fashion statement") and scare people into thinking their tap water is dirty, you could make a pretty sizable profit. Today, that profit is $4 billion/year. (Is that good marketing or what?) There are roughly 200 different bottled water companies in the United States alone!

Our eyes see a seal on the bottle and we perceive this product as "safe," "pure," or "healthy" when that may not be the case.

Purified Water

By definition, "purified" means it is treated with a process to remove solids (minerals) and bacteria. Water can be purified by reverse osmosis, distillation, or deionization. All of these simple methods separate the water (H_2O) from all the particles, bacteria, and minerals. Water that is used for product manufacture, like soft drinks, cosmetics, and cleansers, are made with "purified" water. Purified drinking water often has minerals added to improve the taste. When bottled water companies *add* something to your water, it must appear on the label.

You can also purchase distilled water, which is just H_2O and nothing else. The distillation process uses heat and steam to remove all the minerals and other contaminants. Distilled water is used in your car battery and in your iron because it won't leave any mineral deposit stains or residue. While distilled water is not harmful, it is not recommended to be your #1 choice for drinking unless there are minerals added. Minerals in your drinking water keep your blood healthy and also make the water taste better.

Source: Local tap water. Watch out for brands that just say "drinking water." This could be a brand that just bottles the water from the tap with minimal filtering, packages it, and marks it up 10,000 percent. (When a major nationwide chain-store brand of drinking water was tested, it had the exact same contents of all minerals and chlorine as the water from their drinking fountain in their store along with higher than allowed concentrations of pollutants.)

Cost: Similar to spring water: $0.40 to $1.50/16 ounces or $3.20 to $12.00/gallon.

Contains: H_2O plus whatever else the bottler has added.

Club Soda is purified water with carbonation. Sodium bicarbonate is added to counter the acidity of the carbon dioxide used for carbonation.

Soda water is plain purified water with carbonation added.

Spring Water

By definition, spring water is any water that is derived from an underground source that flows to the surface.

Source: From an underground spring. One company can have many different "springs" that they source from. The water can run from a glacier, or originate as rainwater that is absorbed into the earth at higher elevations and runs down to an outlet.

Cost: $.40 to $1.50/16 ounces or $3.20 to $12.00/gallon.

Contains: The contents of spring water are whatever happens to be in the spring. Usually this includes calcium, magnesium, fluoride, potassium, and sodium. Since all springs are different, each company should have a report of the water analysis on their website.

Mineral Water

Mineral water is obtained from a mineral spring and must contain at least 250 ppm (parts per million) of solids (minerals).

Source: Springs, aquifers, wells, or any other source that yields water having at least 250 ppm (parts per million) total solids. No minerals can be added to the water to reach 250 ppm. It must be in the water at the source. A few of the minerals found are sodium, calcium, potassium, and magnesium—all necessary minerals for good health.

Cost: Roughly $ 2.40/16 ounces or $19.30/gallon.

Contains: Each brand of mineral water has its own mineral content but must have at least 250 ppm of total solids. Usually, the main minerals are listed on the bottle, or you can go to the manufacturer's website or call them for more info on the content.

Mineral water is considered "healthy" water because it provides some of what your body needs every day. Someone who drinks over one liter of mineral water/day can get up to 15 percent of their recommended daily calcium intake. Most mineral waters are alkaline, or have a high pH. Many believe that ingesting foods that are alkaline reduces your risk of cancer by providing an unfavorable environment for the cancer cells to grow.

There are also benefits to bathing in mineral springs, both hot and cold, and many exist around the world for this purpose. Similar to using Epsom salts when you have sore muscles, the high mineral content of the mineral springs has soothing and medicinal healing properties. If you have money to burn, I suppose you could fill your hot tub with Perrier.

Artesian Water

Water that flows from an underground source under its own power to the surface. Picture a "water volcano" of sorts.

Source: There are many sources around the world. Although "artesian" sounds very exotic, it just means "coming from underground." Any water well that flows on its own without pumping, whether it's in Fiji or in your backyard, is also considered "artesian."

Cost: Approximately $2.20/16 ounces or $17.90/gallon.

Contains: Various minerals totaling less than 250ppm including silica, fluoride, and bicarbonate, among others. Check the manufacturer's site for specifics.

Well Water

Same as artesian, only you have to drill for it and pump it out. Where I live, and in many other places, well water is consumed regularly from a personal well that is accessed on the owner's property. There are a few companies that bottle their waters from wells.

Source: Well water is from an aquifer or water trapped hundreds of feet below the surface in the bedrock (not just from digging a hole down in the dirt like in a wishing well). There is no danger of groundwater runoff from fertilizers or other chemicals from true well water. Well water should be tested for bacteria and nitrates and other possible human health hazards regularly, but because the water source is millions of years old, once a year is usually sufficient for testing as that water doesn't flow and change like other water sources do.

Cost: Drilling a well and having a pump installed is costly, but once in place, all the water is free. There are some bottlers who sell well water and will label it "spring" water, because it technically may come from an underground spring, but it was obtained by drilling a well. Costs range from $1.00 to $2.10/16 ounces or $8.00 to $16.80/gallon.

Contains: Well water contains whatever is contained in the spring that was tapped and is very similar to artesian water.

Vitamin-Type Water

This really has no business being called "water" at all. It really is a sweetened man-made beverage. It sounds very healthy, doesn't it? But I know you're smarter than that.

Source: Processed, flavored product using any water source they choose.

Cost: $1 to $4/16 ounces, depending on the brand. Some popular brands are Vitaminwater, Powerade, Propel, Waddajuice, and SoBe Lifewater, among others.

Contains: Water, vitamins, coloring, sugar, or other natural sweeteners. It can also contain preservatives and artificial sweeteners, herbs, and caffeine.

In July 2010, a judge ruled that one of the main brands of vitamin water had to remove claims on their label that it is "healthy" as it contains 33 grams of sugar. (A can of cola has 39.9 grams.) It's no big shock that the major soda companies are the primary manufacturers of these "healthy alternatives to sugary soft drinks." Remember: vitamin-type water is neither.

Coconut Water

The newest member of the water family, coconut water has exploded onto the stage, making claims that it is healthier and more effective than any sports drink. In the last five years (2007–2012), the coconut water industry went from $0 in sales to $35 million in sales.

Source: From the young green coconut, this is the precursor to coconut milk. While coconut milk is high in fat, coconut water is high in carbs and minerals and is 95 percent "water."

Cost: $2 to $4 /11 ounces, $23 to $46/ gallon.

Contains: Coconut water is very high in potassium and also has some sodium and magnesium.

Despite the claims, testing indicated that coconut water does not rehydrate after exercise any better than plain water. It's not harmful, but if you read claims that it can cure cancer and prevent diabetes, that may be a bit of an overstatement. While I'm a big fan of coconuts, in the end, coconut water is just fruit juice without the fructose (sugar). Nutrition aside, if you feel oh-so-trendsetting to be seen with your coconut water bottle, I say go for it.

Beware of "coconut-*flavored* water," which is H_2O with natural or artificial coconut flavor added. This kind of water never saw a coconut in its life.

The Number of Bottles That Are Made to Meet Americans' Demands for Bottled Water

- Requires more than 1.5 million barrels of oil annually, enough to fuel some 100,000 U.S. cars for a year according to the Earth Policy Institute.

- About 86% of plastic water bottles in the United States become garbage or litter.

- Plastic debris in the environment can take between 400 and 1,000 years to degrade.

Our health depends on a healthy environment.

Bottom Line

Carbon-filtered tap water is the most economical and easiest way to get your healthy drinking water, although some contaminants will still remain. If you are lucky enough to own a reverse osmosis system (multilevel) in your home, you can filter out pretty much everything that's left. Think about where the bulk of your drinking water comes from, try to make adjustments to improve the quality, and then see if that fits into your healthy lifestyle.

Being healthy means drinking lots of water. Be informed about what kind of water you drink, and don't assume that because it has a sealed cap and high price tag, that it's good for you.

Cancer Brought Out the Family Resemblance to My Son

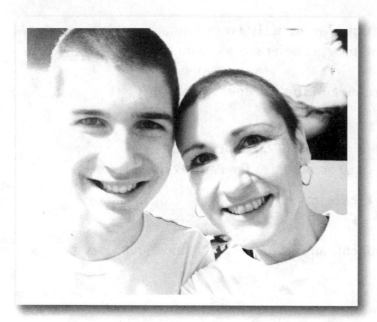

Ever since the day Donovan was born, I've been hearing the same thing over and over again, "He looks JUST like his father." However, following my cancer treatments, people started to notice my resemblance to my handsome son. Maybe it's the eyes? Could it be the nose? No, it was definitely the hair!

While not all chemo drugs cause hair loss, baldness is the universal telltale sign that a woman has cancer. Some women are quite comfortable with their lack of locks. I met a brave woman at the cancer clinic who told me that the only time she covers her head is when it is cold outside. If people stare at her in a rude way, she will say something like, "Excuse me, do I have a hair out of place?" That takes courage. For some women, on the other hand, losing their hair is more emotionally traumatic than losing a breast.

I fell somewhere in between those two extremes. I can honestly say that I did not shed a tear when my hair fell out shortly after my first chemo session. In fact, once it started coming out by the handful, I was like someone with obsessive-compulsive disorder. As one woman put it, "It was like plucking a chicken. Once I started, I couldn't stop." While I've never had the pleasure of plucking an actual chicken, I did give literal meaning to the expression, "I feel like pulling my hair out!"

Although I was personally comfortable with my own baldness, I was not comfortable enough to bare it to the world. At least not until my hair started to come in again. The only reason I was comfortable with my look was because I was told that I look JUST like Demi Moore from the movie *G.I. Jane*. Well, I was told that mostly by myself, but if you stretch your imagination just a little you might pick up on the resemblance. Is it the eyes? The nose? No, it is definitely the hair.

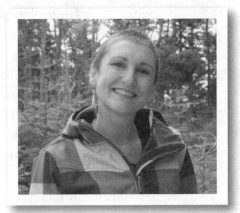

G.I. Flo

While being bald as a pumpkin has its perks, it is a joyous day when new hair starts to grow in. Be patient, it *will* grow back.

HEALTH TIP #73
While We Are on the Topic of Pumpkins

Native Americans introduced us to this beautiful orange vegetable, which is:

- rich in antioxidants
- cholesterol lowering
- anti-inflammatory
- cancer fighting
- healing
- and has powerful anti-aging properties

And what do we do with it? Do we make it a staple in our diet for its many health-promoting properties? Nope. Instead, we carve faces in it once a year.

It's a fact that a pumpkin is not only a cool Halloween prop but is a powerful health food as well. However, if the only food you can think of when I say "pumpkin" is "pumpkin pie," then you need a pumpkin lesson. So here it is: Pumpkins for Dummies.

Pumpkins belong to the gourd family, but they're not "gourdy" at all. Extremely nutritious and very high in beta-carotene (which is converted to vitamin A), pumpkins supply wonderful antioxidants, which help the body to slow down the aging process and fight disease. A diet high in beta-carotene is linked with lowering your risk of gastric, lung, breast, and colorectal cancers. One cup of pumpkin flesh contains 763 percent of the recommended daily allowance for vitamin A!

Pumpkin has it all:

- virtually no fat with 0 cholesterol (as do all plant-based foods)

- low in calories at 49 calories per cup

- moderately high in fiber: 11% of your daily requirement

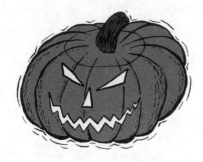

- 2 grams of protein per serving

- exploding with vitamin A: 38,135 IUs in one cup!

- bursting with potassium: 14% of your daily requirement

- a good amount of vitamin E: 13% of your daily recommended amount

- a good source of folate, riboflavin, iron, magnesium, copper, manganese, and zinc

- and it contains omega-3 fatty acids, which help with overall health and the reduction in the risk of chronic illnesses

Of course there are obvious ways you can eat pumpkin, like pumpkin bread, pumpkin cookies, and, of course, pie. But broaden your vision and cut the sugar. Try this soup to get your pumpkin the healthy way. It contains curry, which is largely made up of turmeric, another great cancer fighter.

CREAMY PUMPKIN SOUP

YIELD: 9 CUPS

1 small, whole pie pumpkin, which is 4 cups cooked
or 4 cups canned pumpkin

1 tablespoon extra-virgin olive oil

1 cup chopped white or sweet onion (1 medium)

2 crushed garlic cloves, peeled
(let them rest for ten minutes to release cancer-fighting "allicin")

$1/2$ teaspoon salt—use healthier sea salt if possible

$1/2$ teaspoon ground black pepper

1 tablespoon curry powder and 2 teaspoons olive oil
mixed together

4 cups (low sodium if you like) vegetable broth

1 cup toasted walnut pieces or 1 cup toasted pine nuts

1 cup low-fat coconut milk or rice milk, or almond milk

Coconut cream and chopped coriander sprigs, for garnish,
if presentation is important

Note: If nuts are not toasted, place in oven-safe dish and
bake for 15 to 20 minutes at 350°F.

Directions:

1. Place whole pumpkin on a cookie sheet or in oven-safe bake-ware dish, pierce it a few times with a fork, and bake at 350°F for about one hour until a fork can easily pierce the flesh. (You can do this ahead and refrigerate up to 2 days.)

2. In large soup pot, heat 1 tablespoon olive oil over medium heat. Add chopped onion and two crushed garlic cloves, salt, and pepper, and cook without browning, until tender and translucent, about 10 minutes. Stir in the curry powder and oil mixture. Stir in vegetable stock and bring to a boil over medium-high heat.

3. Add soft cooked pumpkin to pot and return to boil. Stir, and boil lightly for 5 minutes.

4. Transfer half of the pumpkin mixture to a blender and add half the nuts. Process until smooth (and then process 1 minute more—you don't want any tiny pieces of nuts—you want it to be smooth). **Be careful when putting hot liquid in a blender.** Leave the top open, covered by a clean dishtowel for venting steam, when blending. (I tried using a handheld blender for this recipe, but it didn't puree the nuts enough; however, I might not be proficient in the hand-mixing department, so you can give it a try.) Repeat with the other half of the mixture and the remainder of the nuts.

> Don't wait for Halloween to enjoy this wonderful and powerful cancer-fighting vegetable.

5. After entire mixture has been processed, return pumpkin-nut mix back to pot and whisk in your choice of milk. (I personally love coconut.) Heat over low heat until heated all the way through. Do not overheat or boil.

6. Optional garnishes: coconut cream and coriander sprigs. Place a can of coconut milk in the fridge for several hours. Open can, scoop out the thick cream that rises to the top, and place in a bowl and whisk until smooth. Ladle soup into bowls. Add a dollop of coconut cream to each bowl and add a sprig of coriander for garnish if you like.

NUTRITION PER 1 CUP SERVING:

Calories: 178; Fat: 13 grams; Protein: 3.5 grams; Fiber: 4 grams; Vitamin A: 343% of the RDA; Vitamin C: 10% of the RDA; Iron: 9% of the RDA.

Cancer Gave Me a New Way of Marking Time

On March 15, 2011, I sat in my living room with a few friends, celebrating my friend Sherry's forty-fourth birthday. Eventually the conversation came around to an acquaintance of ours who was dying from a very aggressive form of breast cancer. I said, "Look around you, ladies. With the stats as they are, there is a good chance that one of us could get breast cancer."

Hey, I didn't mean ME! I meant Sherry, Jackie, or Madonna. Surely I wasn't going to get breast cancer. I was young, healthy, fit, and had no family history. As if some creepy premonition were unfolding, I found it the very next day: a lump in my left breast. Life would never be the same. I do not remember the exact day that I received my diagnosis, or when I had my biopsy or lumpectomy, but I will always mark March 16 as the day cancer came into my life (completely uninvited, I might add).

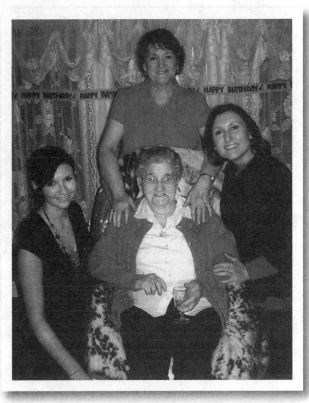

My Grandmother's ninetieth birthday, Dec. 2010 B.C.

People mark time by major life-altering events, such as when you get married, have children, or move to a new city. Cancer became my new way of marking time. It is as if a line was drawn through my life and everything became referenced to the cancer. When did I buy my Kia? February 2011 B.C. (before cancer). When did my boyfriend Shawn and I take our first

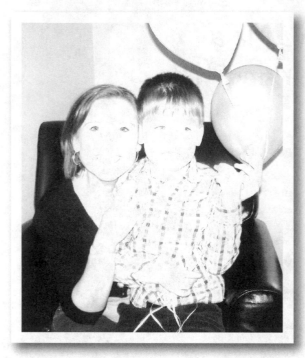

Ben's sixth birthday, May 2011 A.D.

vacation together? October 2012 A.D. (after diagnosis).

You may be thinking that life A.D. cannot possibly be as fulfilling as life B.C. But that is not necessarily the case. I believe that happiness and a positive attitude are choices that people make every day. After I had gone through the grieving process, which took about six months, I was faced with a choice. I could choose to focus on the pain, suffering, and utter devastation that is cancer. There is no denying that few things in life can rival a cancer diagnosis for the award of "worst thing that could ever happen to you." Cancer brings with it the terror of facing an untimely death; uncomfortable and painful treatments and procedures; loss of identity; coming to grips with a new body image; strained relationships; and financial setbacks or ruin. That is the reality of cancer.

But for some "fortunate" cancer patients, the diagnosis brings with it another reality. When faced with their mortality, some people come to realize what is really important in life, and then go on to make life-altering changes. I am one of those fortunate people. Having cancer forced me to evaluate my life and make some major changes. I ended some relationships that were not serving me well and put more of my energy into those that were. I identified work environments that were toxic to my spirit and embraced a change in my career. I started to feed my body nutritious foods and made exercise, prayer, and meditation an important part of my day. As ironic as it may sound, the year I battled cancer was the hardest but also one of the happiest times of my life.

Would I give up my cancer experience? Absolutely, in a heartbeat! However, I would not want to part with the changes that cancer forced me to make in my life. Some say that a positive attitude alone cannot cure cancer.

I agree. However, a positive attitude combined with positive action will give me the best chances of surviving this disease. If that means I have to make changes to my diet, I *will* make changes to my diet. If that means I have to exercise more, I *will* exercise more. If that means I have to stop drinking wine . . . well, let's not get carried away here. Wine is a plant-based beverage after all!

You did not have a choice in getting cancer, but you
do have a choice in the attitude you bring to it.

HEALTH TIP #74
Change Your Attitude Through Affirmations

The definition of the word *affirmation* is: the declaration that something is true.

Can you really make something true simply by saying it? Many believe that the answer is yes. Affirmations work great to change your beliefs and attitudes about yourself, but they don't always work on things outside of yourself. (For example, I've been saying, "My house is clean" for a week now and it doesn't seem to be working.)

When it comes to your brain, affirmations can be very powerful. We are often victims of "self-bullying" and negative affirmations that we aren't even aware of. How often have you done something forgetful and said to yourself, "You are always forgetting things! You are so stupid!" If someone else said these things to you, I hope you would defend your intelligence. But we let ourselves get away with it, don't we? Those negative thoughts and affirmations when repeated over time can actually make you more forgetful and "stupid."

Luckily, it works the other way too. We can use affirmations, or positive messages to ourselves, to help improve our attitudes and feelings about ourselves. Constant verbal suggestions, over time, can shape the way you think and, in turn, the way you respond to things and your decision-making. This power of suggestion works not only on your brain but also on your body.

Dr. Loretta J. Standley, FIAMA (www.drstandley.com), is a holistic healer, both physical and spiritual, with many areas of expertise. She is a firm believer and witness to the power of affirmations. She states:

> Our spoken word is our "command." When we speak, we are giving instructions on the invisible plane. It is the same as filling out a requisition, placing a food order or staking a claim on a piece of property. The purpose of affirmations is not about rattling them off as fast as you can so that maybe you will luck out and things will finally go right for you. The purpose of affirmations is to train your mind to think differently and to train your mind to speak differently, thereby being very clear with the Universe what it is you desire.
>
> The "conscious mind" is the Sergeant and the "subconscious mind" is the Soldier. The Sergeant directs, commands and orders the Soldier. Affirmations play the role of the Sergeant, so you are literally training the mind to think and react differently. When the Sergeant barks out a command, the Soldier instantly reacts to the command. In a nutshell—make certain you are barking out to the Universe the right orders!

Dr. Standley states that you can train your mind to help your body to be healthy. Controlling your words will control your mind. The conscious mind "acts," and the subconscious mind "reacts."

You can start reciting your positive health affirmations today, but according to Dr. Standley, it takes forty days to impress your desire upon the subconscious mind. You must recite the affirmations forty times a day for forty days in a row. Dr. Standley suggests putting forty beads or coins in a cup and taking one out each time an affirmation is recited so you won't have to think about counting them. If you miss a day in the string of forty days, you must start from the beginning. But not before you think about what it was that distracted you, and express gratitude for realizing it.

You should feel the statement you are making and concentrate on the words. Choose one or more of the following affirmations based on what you feel best fits your needs:

- God gave me a healthy body and, in gratitude, I take good care of myself.

- I eat healthy, nutritious, and digestible food every day.

- I have a healthy spirit, mind, and body.

- I drink large amounts of thirst-quenching water every day.

- I have a healthy heart and strong set of lungs.

- My strong body has fully recovered and healed.

- I AM living a long and healthy life.

- I AM miraculously cured by the touch of God's divine hand.

Since "I AM" is the name God gave when Moses asked what he should call Him, beginning your affirmation with "I AM" calls the conscience mind to embrace the God or divine presence within. "The repetition of an affirmation beginning with 'I AM' strengthens and supports clarity," says Dr. Standley.

My dad also believed in affirmations. When I was sick and just getting over my double mastectomy, he asked me to look in the mirror every day and say out loud, "Every day in every way I'm getting stronger and stronger." Yeah, I felt silly doing it, but hey, it was my dad asking me to do this, and I was not about to disobey. The first few times I tried it, I couldn't look in the mirror. I felt like I was lying to myself. I just muttered it quickly and continued on with my day. Eventually, after several weeks, I was able to look myself in the eye, because it was starting to come true. Pretty soon it was not only easy to say, it was fun . . . like a self-directed pep talk.

Later on, when I was using guided imagery during chemo, I would listen to Belleruth Naparstek's CD. A portion of the General Wellness CD contained affirmations. Belleruth's voice is totally relaxing, and it's easy to focus on what she is saying. According to her, for some, affirmations sometimes work better than guided imagery techniques. She asks you to listen to the affirmation, take it in, and repeat it if you wish. Some of Belleruth's affirmations are:

- I know that when I forgive myself and others for errors of the past, I help my body to be well.

- I call upon my intention to maintain good health and a strong sense of well-being. I engage my powerful will to assist my body in doing this.

- When I eat, I instruct my body to use whatever it needs and to reject whatever is unhealthy to me. I sense my body following these instructions.

- More and more I can let go of worrying about things I cannot control and focus on my own inner peacefulness.

I strongly recommend looking into using a CD to help with affirmations. For some, it helps you to get started, so that you can then take over the affirmations yourself when you are ready.

Affirmations are easy, free, and it's one of those "nothing-to-lose" actions. You can also use them to make improvements, not only in general wellness, but in other areas such as money, love, success, or weight loss.

Go to www.BelleruthNaparstek.com. Belleruth has wonderful guided imagery and affirmation CDs to help with lots of issues. There's even one to help with chemo and radiation.

Try affirmations to boost the
healing power of your brain.

Cancer Made Me a More Interesting Person

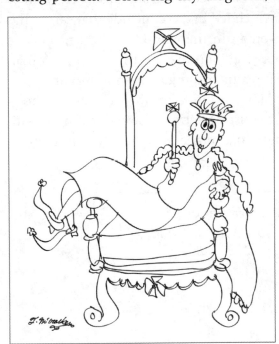

Have you ever seen those Dos Equis beer commercials featuring "the most interesting man in the world"? They are a riot! I have discovered that one of the cool things about having cancer is that it makes me a more interesting person. Following my diagnosis, any time I went out in public, I noticed people whispering and looking my way, and I am pretty sure they were saying the words, "Florence Strang" followed by "cancer." (Just mouth those words for yourself and you will agree, they are pretty easy to discern, even for the novice lip reader.) I don't know many of these people, but they all suddenly seem to be interested in knowing ME. Since my diagnosis, I have been asked to speak at fund-raising events, high schools, various group meetings, and even formal dinners. Not to mention, I have been interviewed on TV, the radio, and by several magazines. It is like cancer has turned me into some kind of a local celebrity!

I used to be introduced something like: "This is Florence, she is a psychologist." Or "Meet Flo, she is a fabulous gardener." However, that changed after my diagnosis. Now, I am likely to be introduced as "I would like you to meet Flo. She is a cancer survivor."

When my youngest sister, Lynette, came for a visit shortly after I was diagnosed, she insisted on taking me out for a night on the town. Lynette has the type of personality where she can light up a room just by walking into it. (It helps that she looks like a Barbie doll.) She is very friendly and will talk to everyone she meets. For example:

"Hi, I'm Lynette, and this is my sister Florence. She has cancer."

"No way! But she looks great!"

"Yeah, really. She's bald underneath that wig, though. Ya want me to get her to take it off and show you?"

"Ah, no, that's okay, I believe you. Can I buy you two a drink?"

And as we went from bar to bar, these people seemed to be truly interested in hearing my cancer story. Which led me to conclude that cancer has made me "the most interesting woman in the world." Well, if not in the whole world, I think I am safe in saying I am the most interesting woman in Newfoundland. Or at least the most interesting woman in Lewin's Cove. (Oh, wait a second, there is that lady who lives on the next street who is part-hoarder and has 100 cats . . . my sister Sherry.) However, I can say with 100 percent confidence that cancer has made me the most interesting woman on my street!

If nothing else, a cancer diagnosis
certainly makes you more "interesting."

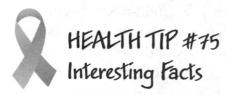

HEALTH TIP #75
Interesting Facts

Here are some interesting facts to go with your interesting personality:

- Besides being a cancer-fighting food, two weekly servings (about 1 ounce each) of dark chocolate (70% cacao or more) led to a 32 percent reduction in heart failure for women. Just to clarify—that's two *weekly* servings, not *daily*. (*Circulation Journal*: AHA)

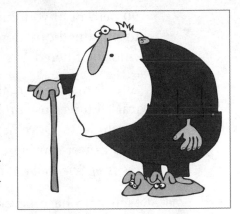

- A firm handshake and a brisk walking pace are accurate predictors of a longer life expectancy. (UK's Medical Research Council)

- Countries that celebrate full-figured Santas have higher rates of childhood obesity. (*British Medical Journal*)

- Americans take about 5,117 steps a day—far short of the expert-recommended and healthy 10,000 steps. (*Medicine & Science*) Wear a pedometer to check yours!

- Sleep-deprived people have higher levels of the stress hormone cortisol, which can lead to weight gain, diabetes, and depression. Six hours is the minimum amount of time for hitting the sack; seven or eight is even better.

- Daily alcohol (two servings a day for men, one for women) can benefit the cardiovascular system by preventing clots that can lead to heart attacks and strokes, and raising the HDL (the good) cholesterol. But there is no health benefit if you save up your daily intake for the weekend (damn), and drinking more than two drinks a day has a negative effect. (University of Berkeley *Wellness Letter*)

- Standing burns 50 calories in 45 minutes (but that's no reason to stand in line for donuts and milk shakes).

- In the 1950s doctors in America and the UK actually encouraged their patients to start smoking to improve their lung function. For the tobacco companies these were the "good ole days."

- It takes smokers three tries on average to quit smoking. Why not make it your New Year's Resolution—for the third year in a row? Never quit quitting!

- 90 percent of your lungs are composed of water, which is a good reason to put this book down and drink some. (USA.gov) Just make sure it's chlorine filtered.

- Americans eat more than 20 billion hot dogs per year. Nitrites are chemical additives used to preserve and add flavoring to hot dogs and other lunchmeats. Once in the body, they react with body chemicals and turn into cancer-causing carcinogens. (*Why Millions Survive Cancer: The Successes of Science by Lauren Pecorino*).

- Men who have never married are up to 35 percent more likely to die from cancer than those who are married. In terms of surviving cancer, women also benefited from being married, but to a lesser extent. (BMC Public Health 2011)

Statistics can be fun and can provide
you with "ice breakers" at parties.

Cancer Prompted Me to Ditch the Worry Habit

I am a worrier by nature. Even as a child I was often ridden with angst. My favorite time to worry is the middle of the night. I call it my "3 AM worry-fest." Some of my best worry topics are:

- my health
- money
- my relationships
- my kids' health and safety
- my job

If I don't have anything legitimate to worry about, I can easily make something up in a pinch. (Such as: "What if there is a tidal wave in the middle of the night and I have to get the kids to high country? How will we survive when we get there? I should really go pack a survival kit right now.")

I just read a book that is making me reconsider my worry habit. *Dying to Be Me* is the story of Anita Moorjani's near-death experience, and subsequent miraculous recovery from cancer. This woman was literally on her deathbed, her skeletal body had open lesions, her organs had begun to shut down, and she was given less than thirty-six hours to live. While in a coma, Anita "crossed over" and came back with such amazing insight and clarity that it cured her of her cancer. It is a true medical miracle that continues to baffle the worldwide medical community.

What interested me in this book is not her description of the afterlife, the feeling of unconditional love and euphoria, or even meeting departed loved ones on the other side. That was a given for me before reading this book. What I wanted to know is this: what gave you cancer in the first place and how did you get rid of it?

When asked what gave her cancer, Anita says, "I can sum up the answer in one word: fear." She believes that all disease starts first on an energetic level, before manifesting as disease in the body. Ironically, one of the things she was most afraid of was getting cancer. According to Anita, because she worried so much and tried so hard to please others, she did not express her true self, and it was literally killing her.

When asked about her miraculous healing, Anita talks about the importance of self-love: "I can't stress enough how important it is to cultivate a deep love affair with yourself." Her near-death experience made her realize the importance of taking care of her own needs and not putting herself last all the time. (Sound familiar?)

So what I have concluded from this riveting book is that the only real thing I have to fear is fear itself. By worrying about my cancer returning, I am actually increasing the likelihood of it happening, since cancer feeds on fear! I don't think that living a fearful life alone guarantees cancer, no more than smoking cigarettes guarantees cancer. But it does put one at greater risk. Therefore, to survive cancer, one of the things I must do is let go of my worries and fears and trust in God's divine plan for my life. Like Anita Moorjani, I must try to live my life fearlessly and love the magnificent being that I am.

Get your priorities straight: Love
yourself and live your life fearlessly!

HEALTH TIP #76
Health Priorities Are (in This Order) Air, Water, Food

You want to get through chemo and radiation with the least amount of side effects.

You want to reduce your risk for further cancer growth.

You want to have a better relationship with your partner.

You want to learn how to fly a plane.

All these things and anything else you might want to ever do in your life, depend on three things: air, water, and food. One person who has perfected teaching this idea is Master Chef Dave Choi.

Chef Dave Choi has been helping people get back to these three basic fundamentals of life for decades. First, as the owner of six successful vegan restaurants in Chicago, and, more recently, as a teacher and dietary guide for those who are going through an illness like heart disease, diabetes, or obesity. Many of the people that Chef Dave helps have cancer, including many children. To treat any illness or disease, Dave says to start with the three primary basics of life: air, water, and food. Without sincere gratitude and respect for these things, everything else is impossible.

First, we all breathe and we all are getting air into our lungs, but we don't always do it in a healthful way. Your lungs and every cell of your body need deep, cleansing breaths throughout the day. This awakens your mind and gets oxygen deep into your body so that every cell has what it needs to live. It also relaxes the body and the mind. Buddhist monks train themselves to breathe deeply, stimulating their diaphragm at all times, keeping them in a constant state of relaxation. (And they live to be a hundred!)

Chef Dave explains, "Your body knows how to heal itself, but it needs the right tools to do it. Cancer patients, especially, have to pay attention to this because the chemotherapy and radiation wipes out their immune system. Their body is like a burnt-down house with just some windows left. In order to rebuild the house, you need the right tools."

Next, we need clean water to help flush out toxins and keeps things flowing. Chef Dave suggests drinking room-temperature water. This prevents a waste of your body's energy to warm the water up to body temperature after you drink it. That's precious energy that could be used on healing.

Lastly, Chef Dave believes that eating alkaline foods as opposed to acidic foods creates an unpleasant environment for cancer growth, as cancer loves acid. While most foods are in the midrange of acidic vs. alkaline, the highly acidic foods include tomatoes, citrus (excluding lemon), dairy, meat, coffee, and alcohol. Most chemicals and preservatives make your body acidic as well.

Alkaline foods like broccoli, pine nuts, black sesame seeds, kale, asparagus, and avocado defend your body from cancer growth. It is always a good idea to include plenty of alkaline foods every day to counter the acids that accumulate in your system. In the decades that Chef Dave has been cooking for the sick, he has seen that a more alkaline diet helps with healing and inflammation, so he prepares meals for those he helps using as many highly alkaline foods as possible.

"Cancer also loves dairy, meat, yeast, and sugar," he says. So Dave doesn't use any of those when he cooks for cancer patients. He suggests eliminating these foods as well to assist your body in the healing process and achieve optimum health. But Chef Dave suggests that instead of thinking of the food as "vegan," you think of it as "earthy grounded food": Things that don't run, fly, or swim and come from the earth. He tells those who aren't sure about making the dietary change, to try it for one week and then see what your body is telling you. Your body knows what it needs. This isn't a "diet" that you follow for a few weeks to lose weight or "detox," this is a lifestyle that will not only help you to lose weight but will also help with your mental well-being, attitude, and energy level.

> Air, water, food. Make these your top three priorities when setting healthy lifestyle goals.

Chef Dave works with many who are so sick they've lost hope. For those who doubt themselves and have feelings of hopelessness because of their illness, Dave asks them to draw a little silly bumblebee and put it in a place where they can easily see it. When they feel this way, he tells them to look at the bee for two reasons. Aerodynamically, the bumblebee's size and shape should make it impossible for it to fly. "This fat bee with these tiny wings shouldn't be able to fly, but it just does. Just looking at that bee in flight should tell you that anything is possible." He also tells people to look at the bee to remind them to "just be." Let your life happen. "Bee" in the moment.

Good air, clean water, and healthy plant-based food give your body the tools it needs to achieve health. When you have achieved good health, everything else becomes possible.

You can find "Chef Dave Choi" on Facebook at: www.facebook.com/chefdave.choi

Cancer Redefined My Relationship with Food

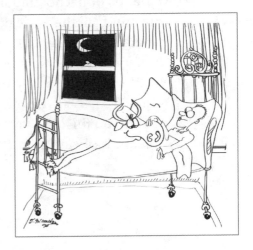

If there is one thing I have learned about surviving cancer, it is that I need to be very aware of what I put into my body. When I first started my cancer-fighting diet, I took it to the extreme. I bought Kriss Carr's book, *Crazy Sexy Diet*, brushed the cobwebs off my juicer, and decided that I would subsist on vegetable juice alone. What's the obsession with chewing anyway? I reasoned that it was high time I gave my teeth a break. While the book suggested that I start out slowly, using only one type of vegetable, I am not one to ease into things. I threw every veggie I could find in the juicer and drank it down as quickly as I could. Not a good idea. (In retrospect, I really should have listened to Kriss.) Let's just say that I had pains in my stomach akin to the early stages of labor. It just did not sit well, and, eventually, despite my best efforts to keep it down, I puked. So ended my crazy, not-so-sexy diet.

I recently met a cancer survivor from Prince Edward Island who told me that not only does she grow her own vegetables, but she also raises her own livestock so that she can be sure her food is completely organic. I briefly considered doing that. But, hey, I am the type of person who picks worms up off the sidewalk with my bare hands and puts them back in the dirt. I am pretty sure that, come slaughter time, I would have bonded with Ole Bessie. In fact, she would probably be sleeping at the foot of my bed. No, that diet would not work for me.

So I have taken the middle road. I have nearly eliminated meat-based foods and sugar from my diet and increased the fruits, veggies, beans, and lentils. This is a diet I can live with. The only issue arises when I go out to a restaurant.

On one such occasion, my teens, Kaitlyn and Donovan, and I decided to eat out, nothing fancy, but a treat all the same. The menu wasn't exactly vegetarian-friendly, but they did offer a nice spinach salad, which would fit well with my healthy diet. I practiced my order in my mind, "A spinach salad with raspberry vinaigrette on the side and a glass of water, please." Service was slow, and all around me I could see other people with their mounds of nachos, mountains of fries, and baskets of wings. I tut-tutted in my mind, all the while practicing my order, "A spinach salad with raspberry vinaigrette on the side and a glass of water, please," getting hungrier and hungrier as time went by. Finally, the waitress came to take our order. "I'll have a large fish and chips and a glass of red wine," I heard a voice blurt out. *Oh My God!* That was my voice. Kaitlyn said, "Mom, are you sure you want to do this? You know how finicky your stomach is." I gave her my most solemn look and said, "Kaitlyn, I'm willing to risk it."

Eat healthy, but don't beat yourself up
if you have a treat from time to time.

HEALTH TIP #77
If Bill Clinton (aka I'll-Have-a-Shake-with-That-Burger) Can Eat Healthy, Anyone Can!

Yes, *that* Bill Clinton. The one who could be seen taking a break in the middle of his morning jog to inhale two egg sandwiches with extra cheese.

All it took was some chest pain and a couple of heart procedures to make him realize that his fast-food diet was killing him—fast. With the help and guidance of some experts, Bill has learned to follow a 100 percent plant-based diet and exercises regularly. Since becoming a vegan, he has dropped 20 pounds and said his cholesterol is perfect and he feels great. He may also be on his way to *reversing* his heart disease.

I have been eating vegetarian-like for the past six years and 99 percent vegan-like for the past two (I am a sucker for a nice piece of wild salmon on occasion). I can honestly say that, not only do I feel great, I feel great without sacrificing wonderfully delicious food. The #1 question people ask is, "Where do you get your protein?"—as if meat and dairy were the only sources of protein on the planet. Stealing a line from several vegans, I say, "I get my protein the same place a 400-pound gorilla gets his: plants." There is plenty of protein in all foods: in vegetables, fruits, seeds, grains, nuts, and legumes. And I have hundreds of plant-based foods to combine to make thousands of satisfying recipes! (And tofu does not have to be in a single one!)

Of course, once Oprah found out that Bill and I had gone vegan, she decided to jump on the bandwagon as well. Recently, an episode of the Oprah show aired in which she challenged her entire staff to "go vegan" for one week.

Three hundred and seventy-eight members of her staff accepted the challenge to eliminate animal products from their diet: no meat, fish, dairy, eggs, or honey for seven days. Also avoided was anything artificial, including sweeteners, flavors, color, preservatives, MSG, and chemicals.

For some, it was a real challenge. There was one staffer who had basically lived on junk food and fast food her whole life. She said that about three days into the vegan diet, she "went into fast-food withdrawal" where she felt physically sick, but after that day, and after staying with the diet, she just kept feeling better and better and actually has committed to "going vegan" from that point on. She reports that she has more energy, is sleeping better, and (not to gross anyone out) she poops every day now, instead of once every eight days! (Sounds to me like she was full of sh*t!)

Oprah brought up some startling statistics:

- 75% of all healthcare dollars are spent on diet-related illnesses.

- 10 billion animals are slaughtered each year in the United States alone (10 billion seconds ago it was the year 1559 . . . just to give you some perspective).

- Our diets have changed more in the last 100 years than in the last 10,000 years because of all the processed food, additives, preservatives, and chemical components.

The biggest thing people thought they would have a problem with was giving up their favorite foods like tacos, burgers, and pizza. But with the help of Oprah's guest, Kathy Freston, they learned that they can have their favorite things transformed into healthy vegan items, and they would actually taste great!

Kathy Freston, bestselling author and wellness expert, showed that any animal product you eat has a plant-based substitute. But the philosophy of eating vegan is not to make "vegan chicken nuggets," but to make you aware of what you are putting into your body and really fuel your body with quality wholesome foods that will enhance your life and prevent illness. Technically, potato chips and soda are vegan, but you don't have to be a health expert to know that they are not exactly healthy.

In one part of the show, the camera crew went into the house of an Oprah staff member. She took all the products that contained animal substances out of her fridge. She was left with a bottle of mustard and a jar of olives. That really made her realize that most of what she ate contained animal products. It was this realization that made her want to change—even if it was just a small change.

> Does the term *vegan* scare you? Then just use the friendlier term: *plant-based*. It offers some "dietary wiggle room" and usually doesn't invoke an "Oh, one of THOSE" response.

So . . . what's my beef with beef?

One of the problems with animal products is the quality. Cattle, milk cows, and other farm animals are naturally designed to graze on grass, get fresh air, and move freely. Once upon a time, farms had pastures and green meadows for cattle grazing. Today, industrialized farms operate on quantity, not quality. Factory farms—or the correct term, Confined Animal Feeding Operations (CAFOs)—are not conducive to healthy animal life. CAFOs use low-dose antibiotics to control the infection risk that overcrowding produces. Instead of grazing on green pastures, the feed consists of animal byproducts, GMOs (genetically modified organisms), pesticide-laden corn, and arsenic-laced chicken feathers. (Chickens are fed arsenic poison to affect growth rates. The arsenic-laced feathers can be fed to cattle as fillers in feed.)

Besides the quality, there is evidence that red meat protein and saturated fat (meat fat) increase the risk of cancers. The American Cancer Society's most current recommendation for nutrition to reduce risk of cancer encourages "limiting red meat." Here's how my brain works: if less is better, none is better-er.

At the end of the show, some of the staff were interviewed. Out of the three hundred and seventy-eight staffers that ate vegan for one week, a collective four hundred and forty-four pounds were lost. One guy lost eleven pounds in just that one week! He said he was really skeptical at first and really thought he was going to hate the food, but said he was surprised at how good it tasted and now he is feeling better than he has felt in his entire life. He remained vegan after the show's experiment.

Some said they couldn't give up all of their favorite animal-product foods, but eating that way for the week really made them realize just how much animal product they were ingesting, and most said they are going to cut down on their intake and would definitely start paying attention to what was in their food.

> Making small changes in your diet and moving toward plant-based foods has many health benefits including reducing your risk of cancer.

Here's a suggestion, for starters: Take one or two days in the week and try to eat plant-based for those days. Then you could add days in the week if you choose, as you get more used to the idea.

As for Oprah, she said she still needs to eat her eggs (but she gets them from a farm across the street so she can see how the chickens live and what they eat). She did say, however, that the show made her think about what she is putting into her body, and she challenged the viewers to adopt a "vegan-ish" attitude about their diets. (Vegan-ish equals Plant-based.)

"If we can't all be vegans, let's at least try to be vegan-ish," she said.

Oprah, how did you get so smart? Maybe her plant-based eating is boosting her brainpower.

We all want to feel good and live better. Eating a plant-based diet is one way to accomplish that goal. Pay attention to what you eat today. Read the labels. How much of it is animal product?

For some help with getting started on a plant-based diet, and information into the benefits, check out the following books and website:

- *The Complete Idiot's Guide to Plant-Based Nutrition*, by Julieanna Hever, MS, RD, CPT

- *The China Study*, by T. Colin Campbell, PhD

- www.KathyFreston.com

An Excuse to Buy New Clothes

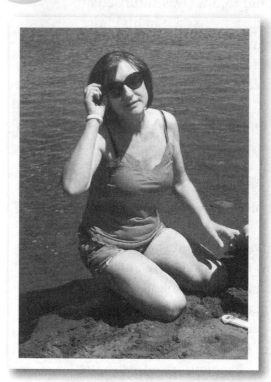

Flo, six months before mastectomy

I figured that by six to eight weeks post-mastectomy, I would have been fitted with a breast prosthesis. Unfortunately, due to swelling in the incision area and burns from my radiation, it would be many months before I got my fake boobie. Being the resourceful person that I am, I managed to improvise (let's just say Ben's teddy bear lost a little weight). However the teddy-inspired boob didn't always stay in place. Given that I had few options, it was up to me to make peace with my new lopsided physique. As far as I was concerned, there was no better way to make peace with my bod than by adorning it with new clothes!

Although my closet was bursting at the seams with clothing, I could honestly say, "I have nothing to wear." You see, all of *those* clothes were bought to fit the body of a woman with two matching breasts (what was the fashion world thinking?). Take for example the little number I am wearing at the beach in the photo above. I am pretty sure that if I wore that with my teddy-boob, it would only be a matter of time before someone noticed. Ya think?

So what did I do? I dusted off the ole VISA and hit the mall in search of a new style. My old motto, "If you've got if, flaunt it," was just not cutting it. I therefore adopted a new motto: "If you've got it, flaunt it. If you ain't got it, hide it." Hence the assortment of black, flowing tops. So there I am, decked out in my new threads. Whadda ya think? (Stay posted for the Victoria's Secret spread after my reconstruction.)

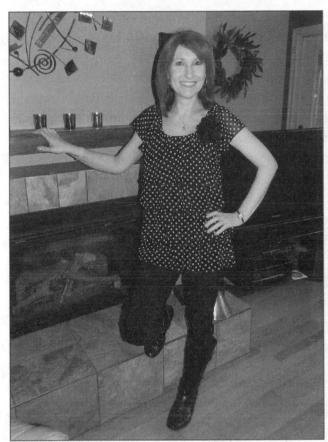

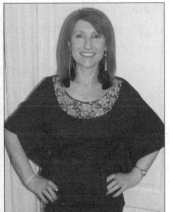

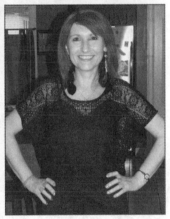

Cancer will likely change your body. You may lose or gain weight, lose your hair, or even lose a breast or two. Make peace with your new body and dress it in a way that makes you feel both beautiful and comfortable.

HEALTH TIP #78
When Dressing for Comfort, Don't Forget Your Feet

In case you haven't noticed, Flo and I want you to include exercise in your daily routine because we believe it brings benefits to so many areas of your healthy life. The easiest way to get started is simply by using your feet.

Walking or running doesn't require special equipment or a fancy gym. But it does require that you fit your feet properly to maximize your workout and prevent injuries. (Injuries equal excuse to sit on the couch.)

Your foot is a wondrous example of perfect construction. The collection of small bones, muscles, tendons, and ligaments are able to withstand constant battering and daily pressure from the entire weight of your body. You owe it to those metatarsals to provide them with some proper support, especially when you exercise! If you can, I would suggest visiting a specialty shoe store that will fit your foot with the right shoe for your needs. This may seem silly or "over the top," but even just walking a few miles a day in poorly fitted shoes can damage not only your feet but your knees, hips, and back as well. (Remember? The foot bone's connected to the leg bone . . . the leg bone's connected to the hip bone . . . the hip bone . . . okay, you get the picture.)

Last year I made the decision to get professionally fitted for running shoes. Part of my decision came from the fact that several years earlier I fit myself for walking shoes to walk in the 60-mile, three-day cancer walk and ended up losing my big toenail from poorly fitting walking shoes. (No laughing, please!) Several years later, I started training for my first half-marathon . . . in my five-year-old cross trainers with the ripped soles that also doubled as my gardening shoes. Wanting to keep all toenails intact for this race, I knew I needed help, so I went looking for some. I feel like the "running fairies" guided me to Joe. Joe owned three Fleet Feet stores. (Fleet Feet is a nationwide chain of independently owned stores that specialize in running and walking apparel and always gives one-on-one service to meet your needs. I swear I didn't get paid to write that.) Joe had been fitting people with the proper athletic shoes for over twelve years. Joe had a degree in Exercise Physiology. Joe was nice and patient. I liked Joe.

My professional fitting for running shoes went something like this and would be the same for someone looking for proper walking shoes as well:

- I had a conversation with Joe about what my goals were and about any injuries, past or current.

- Then Joe watched me walk barefoot so he could see my "foot strike," or how my foot moved through my footstep. This was important, I was told, because different shoes are made for different foot strikes, so some brands work with my own personal stride, and some do not.

- My foot was measured while I was seated (unweighted) to determine my correct arch height when my foot was aligned correctly.

- Then my foot was measured standing, or weighted, to see if the measurement changed. Based on the difference of the two readings (unweighted and weighted), a determination was made on the flexibility of my foot. Joe explained that flexibility is great to have in a relationship but is NOT a good thing to have with your feet. Feet were meant to act like a rigid level, so your shoes should be designed to assist in achieving that. Sometimes inserts are used to help shore up your sole.

- Several recommendations were made for shoes and I tried a few on. I was able to walk around the store, but because I was going to use them for running, I was also able to take a "test drive" in the parking lot.

- Then Joe and I had the "socks talk." Just like shoes, the proper socks can make or break you. Joe said socks should wick moisture away and keep your feet dry during workouts. They should also be seam-free and tight fitting to avoid blisters.

After my extensive evaluation, Joe determined I was a pronator (I wasn't insulted, that just means my foot turned out when I ran), and I needed extra rigidity inside the shoe. Corrections were made, and compared to my gardening shoes, I felt like I was running on a cloud. Using these running shoes, I was able to successfully complete training, injury-free, and rocked my first half marathon. During my training, my running shoes fast became my best friends. While shoes usually last for about 400 to 500 miles of use, I'll know that my shoes are "getting old" when my legs start to feel tired and sore. Joe also explained that you should wear your walking or running shoes only for the activity for which they were designed. Wearing walking shoes for tennis playing, for example, is not only dangerous, and might put you at risk for injury, but it will also wear your shoes out much faster.

Joe also stressed the importance of proper nutrition and hydration. While important for overall health, Joe explained that running on an empty tank or when you're dehydrated causes you to become easily fatigued and that causes your stride to change, putting you at risk for injuries even if you have the perfect shoes. (Smart guy, eh?)

> To prevent injuries and maximize your exercise experience, put your right foot forward . . . in the right shoe!

While you may not be as lucky as I was to find a "Joe," the salesperson that helps you should be knowledgeable and experienced. (Compare Joe with the nineteen-year-old part-timer that helped my daughter find running shoes. She came home with a shoe too small that had a price tag too big and ended up cluttering the bottom of her closet instead of helping her with her fitness.)

If you are unable to be fitted, or would rather fit yourself, that's fine. Just make sure you follow the guidelines for proper fit. You'll know the right shoe when you put it on and try it out. You should never have to "work in" an exercise shoe. It should be comfortable from day one.

When you've found the right shoe, start exercising and never stop!

For more information on buying a running shoe, check out www.the runningadvisor.com/running_shoes.html. For more information on buying walking shoes, visit www.mayoclinic/health/walking/HQ00885_D.

Eat Pray Love

Elizabeth Gilbert was on to something when she wrote the bestselling book *Eat, Pray, Love*. After my diagnosis, I more fully and consciously embraced these three things, and, ironically, despite having cancer, I'd never experienced a stronger feeling of well-being in all of my life! I have since made it my commitment to eat, pray, and love my way to a healthier and happier me.

Eat: Since I got serious about my cancer-fighting diet, not even a piece of gum will sneak past my lips unless it is sugar-free. Apparently, cancer LOVES sugar, and I have no intention of feeding the enemy. My diet is now mainly plant based, with lots of "living foods" like sprouts and fresh spinach. I am amazed at the connection between what I eat and how I feel. Even my old companion, irritable bowel syndrome, has completely disappeared.

Pray: Since my diagnosis, I continue to make prayer and meditation a focus of each day. This is not just based on "blind faith" but also on scientific evidence that proves the power of prayer and meditation in promoting good health and overall well-being. In *Love, Medicine and Miracles*, bestselling author Dr. Bernie Siegel strongly advocates meditation for cancer patients, saying, "I know of no other single activity that by itself can produce such great improvement in the quality of life." Works for me!

Love: Ah, love. The first thing that probably comes to mind is the butterflies and rainbows feeling of falling in love. I was very fortunate to experience that type of love at about the same time that I was diagnosed with cancer. What a wonderful gift! I believe that the feeling of love creates a healing vibration in the body. However, through my cancer journey, I have come to discover that the true gift of love is only possible if you first love yourself. If you are harboring any resentment or ill feeling, especially toward yourself, forgive and let it go. Realize that you ARE love, and allow yourself to experience the healing vibration of this wonderful feeling.

Eat, Pray, and Love your way
to a healthy and happy life.

HEALTH TIP #79
Eat, Pray, Love . . . but First Wash Your Hands

The average person washes their hands more than eight times a day. That said, it would behoove you (yes, I said *behoove*) to make sure your hand soap does not contain unhealthy chemicals. And you can't go by the labels, unfortunately, because the word *natural* is being overused and abused more than the word *awesome* these days.

Case in point: A "well-known" brand of hand soap sold in a major chain store across the United States and Canada labels this hand soap on the front of its packaging as "naturally derived." Here is a list of the ingredients. You be the judge.

- water (so far, so good)

- sodium laurel sulphate (not exactly from nature, but okay)

- cocomide DEA (while it starts out as coconuts, it is mixed with chemicals and ends up as a possible carcinogen and irritant)

- cocamidopropyl betane (known skin irritant)

- glycerine (fine)

- aloe vera gel (hey! Something naturally derived!)

- vitamin E (fine)

- citric acid (from citrus fruits, fine)

- sodium chloride (salt, okay)

- benzophenone 4 (a chemical that causes a high degree of dermatitis when tested)

- sodium citrate (fine)

- methylisothiazolinone/methylchoroisothiazolinone (*hmm* . . . the EPA lists this as a registered pesticide for industrial use. Listed under the heading "Prevention, pesticides, and toxic substances," it is used to prevent mold and bacteria on heavy equipment, cooling systems, paints, dip tanks, and sprayers. The safety recommendations state "users should wash hands before eating, drinking, chewing gum, using tobacco, or using the toilet."

Let me get this straight: You have to wash this stuff OFF your hands *before* using the toilet?

And are they using this hand soap containing this very chemical to wash said chemical off their hands? *That's* not gonna work.

I'm confused. And we've still got three more ingredients to go.

- parfum (fragrance that can hide up to fifty different chemicals including cancer-causing 1,4 dioxane)

- yellow #5 (this artificial color also known as tatrazine, was associated with hyperactivity in children and removed from the UK safe list)

- green #5 cl 61570 (not exactly from green plants, now, is it?)

Well, at least the bottle is made from 100 percent recycled plastic.

No, you're not *eating* this stuff, but remember: Your skin is a carrier, not a barrier, and if you're using it (or something worse) up to eight times a day washing your hands, it's likely these chemicals are being absorbed into your system.

Don't be fooled by words like *naturally derived* or *contains natural ingredients*, as in this case, only five out of the sixteen ingredients could (with imagination) be considered "natural."

Better, safer, healthier choices are out there. One is castile soap. Made from plant oils instead of beef fat, lye, or a colorful collection of chemicals, castile soap is safe, natural, and very effective in cleaning. Found in most supermarkets and pharmacies, it is available in bar and liquid form. Essential oils (from plants, as opposed to synthetic fragrance oils) are sometimes added for a wonderfully aromatic experience. One brand of castile hand soap that I love is Dr. Bronners (www.drbronner.com). A family-owned company that practices fair trade and good energy, the Bronners have been making castile soap for over 150 years. The story of the founder, Emil (Dr.) Bronner, is fascinating as he really was way ahead of his time and overcame great adversity to make a product he believed in. If good energy and pure values have anything to do with good soap, this is the best soap in the history of soap. Their hand soaps and body washes are wonderful, and they also sell large refill containers, so you can save on the packaging.

Clean up your act and make the switch to a healthier soap. It's probably the easiest and least painful thing you can do to reduce your chemical exposure.

Cancer Taught Me the Importance of Living in the Present

A rabbit who narrowly escapes capture from a fox shows many of the signs of the "fight-or-flight response": quick and shallow breathing, shakiness, and a pounding heart. The fight-or-flight response is a natural bodily response built into animals (including humans) to help them confront or escape danger. When we sense danger, whether it be seeing a bear walk toward us in the woods, or being told that we have cancer, our fight or flight response gets activated. Chemicals like adrenaline, noradrenaline, and cortisol are released into our bloodstream, which causes our body to undergo some very dramatic changes. Our respiratory rate increases. Blood is shunted away from our digestive tract and directed into our muscles and limbs to allow us extra energy and fuel for running and fighting. Our heart rate quickens, our pupils dilate, and our awareness intensifies. We become physically and psychologically prepared for fight or flight in the face of the danger. However, people differ from animals in that we often have our fight or flight response kicked into full gear long after the real threat of danger has passed.

Soon after the rabbit escapes capture by the fox, it calms down and goes back to the business of being a rabbit. It does not go to sleep at night thinking, *Jeez, I almost had it today! I could have died. What if that fox had caught me?* Nor does the rabbit wake up thinking, *I don't think I'm going to leave this hole today, that fox could be lurking anywhere.*

For those of us who have experienced cancer, the cancer can be likened to the fox and we to the rabbit. However, unlike a rabbit, many people fail to live in the present moment. We may continue to live in the past by replaying scenes of our diagnosis and treatments over and over in our minds. Or we may worry obsessively about the future. (*What if the cancer comes back?*

or *How long do I have left?*) If we are to experience peace, we must strive to be like the rabbit, and just BE in the present moment. The fact that you are reading this means that you have been given the "gift" of this moment; that is why it is called the "present."

Don't lament the past; don't worry about the future.
Strive to live in the present moment.

HEALTH TIP #80
Sometimes a Little Worry Can Be a Good Thing

There is no doubt that excessive worry will decrease your quality of life and may be associated with aggravating certain illnesses. According to the Mayo Clinic, episodes of anxiety can cause dramatic, temporary spikes in your blood pressure. If those temporary episodes occur frequently, they can cause damage to your blood vessels, heart, and kidneys.

The thought of living a worry-free life is appealing. But what if I told you that some degree of worrying can actually make you live longer?

In 1921 a Stanford University psychologist, Lewis Terman, began studying the lives of 1,500 of the brightest boys and girls he could find. Detailed information was archived about their lives, families, and daily activities as well as their moods in the hopes of shedding some light on how intelligence shapes one's life.

Terman died in 1956, but others were committed to continuing his study. Published in 2011, a book entitled *The Longevity Project,* by Howard S. Friedman and Leslie R. Martin, looks at the 1,500 study participants that were followed over eighty years to determine a broad scope of things. Among them were the personality factors that led to a long life.

One surprising fact was that cheerful, optimistic children were less likely to live longer than those who worry a bit. It was explained that the children who were inherently optimistic and cheerful ended up taking more risks in their lives. It was theorized that these individuals never thought anything bad would happen, and so they ended up engaging in more risky behaviors like smoking and drinking. Their activities were also more risky. I imagine their favorite thing to yell was "Hey guys, watch this!" I'm also thinking they were a lot of fun at parties.

The individual personality traits that were the strongest indicators for longevity were prudence, persistence, and being well organized. Conscientious, responsible people developed better social relationships and achieved more. Because of these qualities, they were given more opportunities in life, which led to being more fulfilled. They also had more stressful jobs, but finding meaning in their work changed the stress from being a negative factor to being a positive factor in their lives, and it ended up having a beneficial effect on their health.

> A little bit of worry can be a good motivator for making healthy changes to your life.

While we are all looking for the fountain of youth, much of it, unfortunately, is out of our control. According to this study, genetics accounts for 30 percent of the longevity puzzle. For just under one-third of us, we really *will* become our parents. (*Gasp!*)

The bottom line is this: needless worry over things that are out of your control can do no good. However, if a little worry forces you to act positively, especially in taking steps to improve your health, it's a good thing! So don't worry . . . or . . . do worry . . . a little.

A Good Reason to Spend More Time in My Garden

Gardening is a way of showing that you believe in tomorrow.
—Author Unknown

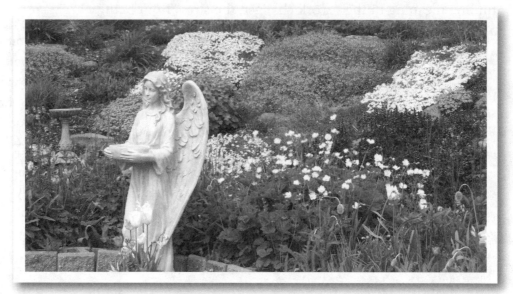

Flo's garden in May

Afew years ago, on a sunny day in June, my friend Sherry dropped by for an unexpected visit and found me in my favorite place: my garden. As I glowed with pride, she commented on my perfectly manicured flowerbeds, neat rows of veggies, and profusion of healthy shrubs and trees. "I don't know how you manage it all!" she exclaimed. "It's a mystery to me how you can take care of three kids, run that big house, and still have a garden that looks this good."

All of the praise must have caused a momentary lapse in my concentration, and I inadvertently invited her inside for a cup of coffee. Hence the mystery was solved. While my flowerbeds were perfectly made, my beds inside were not. I couldn't help but notice the look of shock on her face as a dust bunny the size of a tumbleweed rolled across the hardwood floor in front of her. As I surveyed the dusty landscape, I could have sworn I heard the strains of Old West music. I would not have been the least bit surprised had a cowboy popped out of the closet and challenged us to a shootout. (I had seen stranger things fall out of that closet!)

In my state of embarrassment, I made a vow to myself that never again would I be caught in that situation. I would ration my gardening hours to be used only as a reward for completing housework. For a while, that worked out pretty good. I could walk across my floor without sticking to it (most days), the kids had clean clothes to wear, and I rarely ran out of bread or milk. But then I got cancer.

Cancer gave me a great reason to once again ignore the housework and hang out in my garden. This time, however, it was totally legitimate. You see, I no longer gardened for my own selfish pleasure, or even as a means of housework avoidance. Instead, gardening became therapeutic, and Horticultural Therapy became a critical component of my survival plan.

Gardening is known to increase endurance, flexibility, and strength, providing me with gentle exercise that I could pursue at my own pace. It also gave me an enjoyable way to get some fresh air and increase my poor appetite. Gardening also brought me peace of mind. It is a known stress reliever, providing me with a great distraction from thinking about the "Big C." In addition to being good for my body and mind, gardening also addressed healing at the level of my spirit. Gardening is an act of faith. When I set my tulip bulbs in the fall while undergoing chemo, it was with faith that I would see them bloom in the spring. First, I set the intent with my spirit, and then my body followed suit.

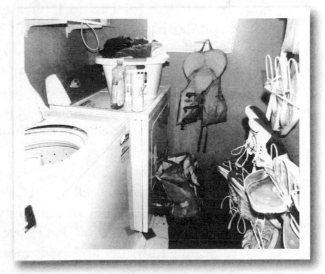

Flo's laundry room in May

So anytime you happen to drop by and find my house in a mess while I am happily puttering around in my garden, feel free to throw in a load of laundry. Hey, I'm not just "gardening," I'm getting my therapy!

Housework can wait!

HEALTH TIP #81
No Dirt? No Space? No Problem!

Would you like to grow your own vegetables but don't have adequate space or soil? You'll be happy to know that there are many ways to grow your own food without a traditional garden.

Home gardening is not only fun, but it also makes sense in a world where you don't know how safe your food is. I just read an article on "fraudulent economically motivated adulteration" in our food sources. Loosely translated, this means "putting crap and fake or synthetic fillers in your food without telling you and passing it off as something else in order to make more money off you." This goes on all the time (I had never heard of it before). The Food Fraud Database (www.usp.org/food-ingredients/food-fraud-database) is a not-for-profit organization listing all the infractions from illegal fraudulent food and the specifics of what was found. The site and the searches are free. (You can sign up with your e-mail for free to get access to other areas of the site if you want.) When I typed in "olive oil" and hit "search," I got ten pages of infractions! Products labeled "100% pure olive oil" were mixed with hazelnut, corn, soybean, sunflower, and other oils, and some of them were colored with beta-carotene to get an authentic olive oil color.

I'm not trying to tell you to avoid olive oil or suggest that you make your own olive oil, but the point is, large mega producers will feed you crap to make a buck. But you don't have to put up with it!

Eating truly "healthy" foods means you should always eat as close to the source as possible, which means eating whole foods with little or no processing. You should also choose organic produce when you can. Organics haven't been exposed to chemical sprays and synthetic preservative coatings. Cancer causing DDT is still found in foods in the United States from imports and from the long life that DDT lives in the soil. What better way to ensure that you are eating healthy, safe, organic food than to grow it yourself!

Gardens are also great to show children that food actually comes from the earth, not from the produce department or the bottom drawer of your fridge. Gardening is an educational activity, which gives kids hands-on science lessons as they participate in the life cycle of a plant from "seed to feed." Growing and nurturing a living plant also boosts their self-esteem and gives them a sense of pride and accomplishment. Best of all, studies show that kids who are involved in the gardening process are more likely to eat their veggies. (Wouldn't *that* be a neat trick?!)

If you are turned off by the thought of how much WORK is involved in gardening, here are some easy ways to produce your own organic veggies. No dirt involved. (But hey, if you want to get dirty, go for it!)

Hydroponics

Hydroponics is an innovative way to grow your own food without using a shovel.

Hydroponics involves using a growing medium (usually ceramic beads or gravel) and flowing water to produce and sustain the growth of plants or vegetables. Growing veggies without dirt has the obvious advantage of keeping you clean, but when there is no dirt, there are virtually no bugs and no weeds! There are many home hydroponics systems that you can place on your deck or patio. General Hydroponics (www.generalhydroponics.com) is one company that offers many options for grow-ing your own food without soil. These systems

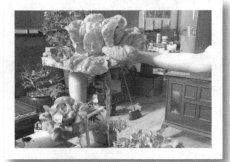

This lettuce was grown with no dirt. Nice head!

look very easy to set up and maintain, and it would be a good option for city dwellers with limited space that would allow for expansion when you want your garden to grow!

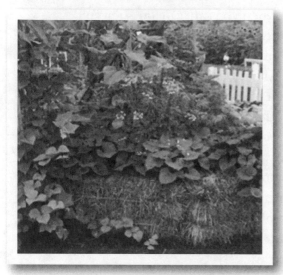

This is what an ideal straw bale garden looks like.

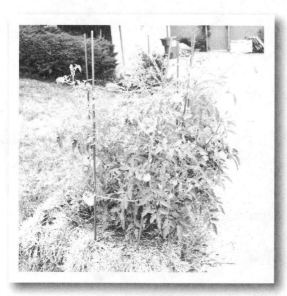

This is what MY straw bale garden looks like. If I cared about neatness more, this would be nice and square, but it serves the purpose and is giving me the most delicious tomatoes I ever grew!

Straw Bale Gardening

I am conducting a little gardening experiment myself. It's called "straw bale gardening," using a bale of wheat straw as the planting medium. You don't need any dirt as you plant directly into the straw. The bale has to be "conditioned" first by either watering for three weeks (the organic way) or by pouring fertilizer on the bale (the fast way). The straw starts to break down to form compost, thereby enriching the plants as they grow. You can use the bale for two years, and then it becomes compost for other areas of your garden. This site—www.strawbalegardens.com—explains it all step by step.

This technique works well in very limited spaces and you can place the bale on a lawn or on concrete and still get great results. I heard of this idea from my husband's coworker, and I knew I wanted to try it when I saw the big delicious homegrown tomatoes he produced from just one tomato plant!

Container Gardening

Another convenient way to grow your veggies is in containers. You can recycle old wood into garden boxes (but make sure the wood has NOT been chemically treated!), or reuse pots, buckets, or other containers. Make sure the containers have plenty of drainage holes, as root systems need air as well as water. Fill with a lightweight potting mix (garden soil is usually too heavy), add in lots of compost, set in your seeds or young plants, and keep them well watered. It's so nice to need no tilling and grow no weeds! Containers do tend to dry out quickly, however, so be sure to keep them well watered. Here is a great site to get you started: http://ohioline.osu.edu/hyg-fact/1000/1647.html.

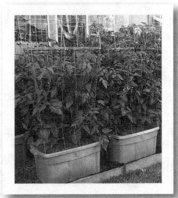

If you feel particularly ambitious, you can build an EarthTainer from simple plastic storage totes. These ingenious portable gardens contain a simple watering mechanism that allows the plant root system to draw water from the bottom of the container supplied though a watering tube from the top. Watering through the tube not only brings the water directly to the root system, but it saves water as nothing is wasted. Visit http://earthtainer.tomatofest.com for instructions and more information.

Community Gardens

If you want the feel of being a real farmer, but just don't have the space, then sign up for a plot or allotment at a community garden. A community garden consists of any group of people that use a common shared gardening area to grow their plants. Usually the land is provided by the city and there is a small fee involved, but much of the work of preparing the soil has already been done for you. Despite their names, they don't really have to be "communal," where everyone shares the work and the harvest, but some are. Gardeners can have their own individual plot within the community garden and, if they choose, can also join with others to grow some crops communally. Contact your local municipality to get started.

> With just a little effort, and almost no dirt, you can grow healthy food right at home!

Take it from a city girl who, at one time, couldn't grow her own hair: there's nothing like the satisfaction of eating fresh, homegrown, pesticide-free veggies!

Cancer Helped Me to Grow as a Psychologist

In my practice as a psychologist, I use a form of counseling known as cognitive-behavioral therapy (CBT). CBT was popularized in the 1980s by Dr. David Burns, bestselling author of *Feeling Good—The New Mood Therapy* and *The Feeling Good Handbook*. The basic premise behind CBT is that your thoughts are directly responsible for how you feel. Therefore, you can improve your moods by choosing more positive thoughts. While the situation itself does not change (the divorce, the illness, the bankruptcy), by changing how you *think* about it, you can change how you *feel* about it. It is all about attitude.

Nineteenth-century philosopher and psychologist William James wrote, "The greatest discovery of my generation is that a human being can alter his life by altering his attitudes of mind." This is a philosophy that I strive to live my life by. I believe that my quality of life is not so much determined by the events of my life, but rather by the attitude that I bring to it and, more specifically, the thoughts I choose to think about it.

I made it my mission in life to always seek out the positive and try to find the silver lining behind every cloud. At times this was difficult, especially with broken relationships and my son Ben's diagnosis of autism, but no matter what the challenge, I strived to stay positive. Then came the ultimate test: I was diagnosed with cancer. Sure, I could talk the talk about the benefits of a positive attitude, but could I walk the walk when I most needed to do so? Would I be able to use the power of my thoughts to feel good through my cancer journey? I believe this book demonstrates that I passed the test!

Attitude is a choice. I did not have a choice in getting cancer, but I did have a choice in how I was going to face it. Choosing to face cancer with a survivor's attitude not only made the experience more bearable, but it also reinforced my belief in cognitive-behavioral therapy and helped me to be a better counselor.

Getting cancer is not a choice,
but the attitude you bring to it is a choice.

HEALTH TIP #82
Choosing the Diet That's Right for You

Anyway you slice it, *diet* is a four-letter word. It evokes feelings of sacrifice and pain. Diets can also come with personal agendas that are defended from attack with sharp knives and forks. Discussing one's diet can become as personal and heated a subject as "boxers or briefs."

My question is: In order to eat healthy, do you have to limit yourself to one type of "diet"? My answer is: Would you limit yourself to just one pair of shoes? Absurd.

Understand first, that you don't just eat food; you have a relationship with food. Eating is not just satisfying your hunger, it is pleasuring your senses of smell, feel, taste, and sight. So when your task is "eat healthier," you have to fulfill and satisfy all these senses, not just replace new foods for old. This can be tricky. That fast-food burger that you associate with immense "pleasure" is going to be hard to replace. Hard . . . but not impossible.

A lot has been learned over the years about how food can be used to prevent and treat illnesses. We know that there is immense power that lies in the food choices you make every day. Foods can have beneficial or detrimental effects at your very basic cellular level, but it seems that food, when eaten whole, as close to its original form (for example, an apple vs. apple sauce), has the most healing power. It was noted that those who ate more foods high in beta-carotene (vitamin A) for example had a lower incidence of lung cancer. So it might make sense that, if high doses of vitamin A were given to subjects, they would have an even lower incidence of lung cancer than those that ate high vitamin A–foods. To researchers' surprise, the lung cancer rates were actually higher in the vitamin A–supplement group than in the vitamin A–food group, suggesting that the magic lies in the whole, pure, unprocessed food, not the broken piece of nutrition in pill form. (Analogy: Take Mona Lisa's smile and put it on Marge Simpson. Somehow, it's just doesn't have the same effect.)

The updated 2012 recommendations for nutrition and exercise by the American Cancer Society are based on a review of the most current and well-documented studies from around the world. The heading for the nutrition part of the recommendations states "Consume a healthy diet with an emphasis on plant foods." Here are their recommendations for a "healthy diet."

- **Choose foods that help maintain a healthy weight.** First, that's a bit vague. Secondly, I detest the term *healthy weight*. Weight tells us nothing about the health of a person. Charts are somewhat helpful in determining your "goal" weight, but many fit, healthy bodies weigh the same as fast-food-eating, out-of-shape bodies. A more accurate measure of health is body fat. Anything over 32 percent body fat is obese. There are special "step-on" scales that measure body fat along with your actual weight. You can also have your 'fat folds" measured by a fitness expert, or you can be immersed in a body-fat tank, which is the most interesting and accurate way of measuring body fat but also may be the most humiliating. Like a giant "dunk tank," your whole body is immersed in water. The weight of the water displaced is calculated with your actual weight and from that, an accurate body fat measurement is obtained. Body mass index (BMI) is another good (and less embarrassing) way of determining if you need to lose weight. The BMI is calculated this way:

$$BMI = \left(\frac{\text{Weight in Pounds}}{(\text{Height in inches}) \times (\text{Height in inches})} \right) \times 703$$

or

$$BMI = \frac{\text{Weight in Kilograms}}{(\text{Height in meters}) \times (\text{Height in meters})}$$

Take your height in inches and multiply it by itself. Then take your weight in pounds and divide it by the "height times height" number. Multiply that number by 703 and that is your BMI. (Or you can just do it the easy way and search "BMI converter" on the computer.)

A BMI between 18.6 and 24.9 is healthy, between 25 and 30 is overweight, and over 30 is obese. Simply put, the food choices that help you maintain a "healthy weight" are plant-based, unprocessed, low sugar, high fiber, and whole. Simple as that. Try this: Examine your next meal and the food that crosses your lips. How much of that meal meets those requirements?

- **Limit consumption of processed meats and red meat.** Limit? Like having one double cheeseburger rather than two? Recommendations are to limit meat intake to two times a week or reduce portion sizes by one half. A serving of red meat is as big as a deck of cards. Now think of the last steak that you ordered from a restaurant. How many decks of cards did you eat?

  The reason limiting meat is listed is because time and time again, studies show that diets high in red meats cause illness. Red meat (beef, lamb, pork) and processed meats (luncheon meats, bacon, sausage, hot dogs) are not only linked to heart disease but also to cancer. One recent study involving over 38,000 men who were followed for over twenty years confirmed this. Processed meats like hot dogs and luncheon meats contain sodium nitrites. It's the nitrosamines that are formed when the nitrites and meat are combined that are the problem. Now that you know this, it's up to you to make the choice at the market and at restaurants. Limit consumption, yes, but it is *you* who will set those limits based on the information you have. Make your guidelines now.

- **Eat at least 2.5 cups of fruits and vegetables/day.** *At least* . . . which means more is better. It doesn't say "eat *up to* 2.5 servings . . . it says AT LEAST! (Sorry to yell, but this is important.) Suffice it to say, fresh fruits and veggies should be the main part of your meals. Change your mind-set and replace the image of your food plate showing neat little piles of veggies with your big slab of meat as the main star. Those veggies and fruits need to take center stage. There are wonderful and delicious choices for vegetables at your market or farmers market. Why are you still choosing white potatoes and iceberg lettuce? Switch it up tonight and reach for sweet potatoes and mixed baby greens of spinach, arugula, and red tip. The highest nutrition comes from the most colorful foods. Gorgeous green avocado, bright red raspberries, and bright orange butternut squash are a few. Try to eat at least three different-colored foods with every meal. (Sorry, ketchup and blue sports drinks don't count!)

- **Choose whole grain instead of refined grain products.** Grains are important for fiber, protein, B vitamins, and iron. A "grain" is a seed. A whole grain is made up of the three parts of the seed: the endosperm, the bran, and the germ, which are not split or processed. The following are examples of whole grains:

- **Barley** has been shown to reduce cholesterol and has more protein than most other grains.

- **Buckwheat** is not in the grain family, but the texture and nutrients are very much the same as other grains.

- **Corn.** Look for non-GMO (genetically modified organism) corn and avoid the word *degerminated*, which means "processed."

- **Millet** is not really a commonly eaten grain, but it is gaining popularity.

- **Oats,** which are rolled, are still whole grains, just flattened. Steel-cut oats are whole oats that have been cut (probably with steel) so they form more of a creamier texture when cooked. Both are whole grains.

- **Quinoa** is technically a seed, but it acts like a grain and is high in "complete" protein, which makes it a great choice for those eating a plant-based diet.

- **Brown and wild rice** are whole grains. White rice has had the outer coating removed and is just not as healthy as brown or wild, sorry folks.

- **Rye.** When buying rye breads or products look for "whole rye" in the ingredient list. The term *rye bread* doesn't mean it's whole-grain rye.

- **Milo or sorghum** is gluten-free and very versatile.

- **Teff** has very small grains and has twice the iron and three times the calcium as other grains. It is slowly gaining popularity.

- **Triticale** is a combo grain of wheat and rye, and it has only been grown for the past thirty-five years. Usually found as a whole grain, even if the ingredients just say "triticale."

- **Wheat** is the most popular grain because of its versatility and high-gluten content, making it perfect for yeast breads and pasta. There are different forms of wheat: berries, cracked, bulgur . . . they are all whole-grain wheats.

If you're one of the many who are sensitive to gluten (a protein in wheat and other grains) you should stay away from wheat, barley, rye, triticale, and oats. (Oats are often grown with wheat, so unless the oats specifically say "gluten-free" you should be suspicious.) For more on whole grains visit the Whole Grains Council at www.wholegrainscouncil.org.

> Look at your diet and try to eat plant-based when and where you can every day.

Now that you have the "main rules" for following a healthy diet, don't be caught up in joining a diet "group" if that's not what makes you happy. Many people say, "I'm going to be a vegetarian" and then feel horribly guilty for wanting grilled chicken in their salad. Do the best that you can do for your health, but be happy with your choices.

I like the term *plant-based*. Plant-based encompasses all the healthy eating groups: vegan, vegetarian, raw foodie, heart-healthy, low calorie, low-fat, diabetic, immune boosting, cancer-fighting, and the list goes on and on. Plant foods should make up most (80% or more) of what you eat every day with very little use of animal products (meat, dairy, fish, chicken, eggs). If you choose to eat "only plants," that's great, but it should be your choice and you should be happy with it and not feel miserable and trapped. The great thing about plant-based eating is that you will notice such a difference in the way you look and feel, that you will be encouraged by your own body to not only continue for yourself, but to get others to hop on board!

For every animal product, know that there is a healthier plant-based choice. Substitute almond or rice milk for unhealthy cow's milk and plant-based butter spreads for butter. These butterlike spreads are NOT margarine and should contain NO hydrogenated oils and nothing artificial. The brand I use and adore is Earth Balance, but there are several others. (Visit www.EarthBalanceNatural.com.)

Here are some great cookbooks to keep you going, and you can always go online or look in the vegan cookbook section of your local bookstore.

- *Everyday Happy Herbivore* by Lindsay S. Nixon

- *The Engine 2 Diet: The Texas Firefighter's 28 Day Save-Your-Life Plan That Lowers Cholesterol and Burns Away the Pounds* by Rip Esselstyn

A Great Save on the Heating Bill

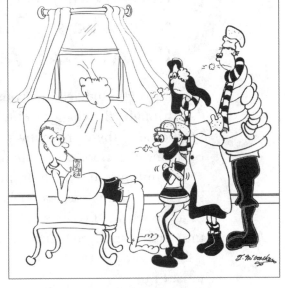

In the winter of 2012, I was pleasantly surprised by a sudden decrease in my heating bill. As I pondered the reason for this stroke of good fortune, my daughter said, "It's no wonder, Mom, this house is like an ice box since you started taking that new pill." Ah, Tamoxifen. While chemopause causes "tropical moments," Tamoxifen can bring on what I can only describe as "oven hours"; prolonged periods of intense body heat. I will kid you not, this can cause discomfort at times, but just consider the money I am saving in heating bills! (So kids, go put on a sweater.)

When my doctor told me I tested positive for estrogen, I said, "Oh darn, more bad news!" Up to that point, all my "positive" results were pretty negative. I tested positive for cancer of the breast, and several of my lymph nodes were positive. However, this was one time when testing positive was just as the label promised—POSITIVE! Having estrogen-positive cancer meant that I could be prescribed an estrogen-blocking drug for five years following my treatments to help prevent a cancer reoccurrence.

Estrogen-positive cancers require estrogen to grow. Tamoxifen does not stop my body from producing estrogen (so I still have a healthy libido), but it does prevent estrogen from binding to cancer cells. So, if there are any cancer cells lingering around in my body, this wonderful drug will latch on to them and help to keep them from reproducing. I am sure you will agree, that is well worth the cost of a few hot flashes.

Don't try to resist your hot flashes.
Recognize when they are coming, and
focus on deep breathing until they pass.

HEALTH TIP #83
Natural Ways to Deal with Menopausal Symptoms
(Without Freezing Your Kids)

And you thought getting your *period* was "the curse"? When you are going through "the change of life" (better known as the "Dr. Jekyll/Mr. Hyde syndrome"), there are many symptoms you might be experiencing. Some of them, like moodiness, will also be "experienced" by those around you.

Symptoms may include hot flashes, moodiness, heart racing, night sweats, insomnia, decreased libido, headaches, forgetfulness, and dryness . . . everywhere. If you are at "the age" or you were lucky enough to be thrust into chemo-induced menopause, you know all this and could probably add a few symptoms to the list. Pharmaceutical remedies are not an option for most of us.

There are many things you can do to improve your menopausal symptoms without taking hormones. They are:

Exercise: Research keeps confirming it (sorry): Regular physical activity reduces your risk of dozens of illnesses as well as the side effects of menopause. And the good news is, you don't even have to sweat. Just being "active," whether by gardening, housework, taking the stairs instead of the elevator, or walking the dog, can have the same benefits for menopause as higher levels of exertion. Regular exercise takes care of many of the symptoms of menopause such as insomnia, improving your mood, and maintaining your weight. Exercise is the number-one thing you can do to improve sleep. And by improving your sleep, you also improve your mood. And it's not just the good night's sleep that will help to put you in your happy place. Exercise helps to produce endorphins, which are your body's own personal "happy pills."

After menopause, you will still be shapely, but the shape may turn out to be a beach ball instead of an hourglass because of the hormonal shift. Exercise will help keep the excess weight from taking over and increase metabolism by regulating cortisol, the hormone that controls fat stores.

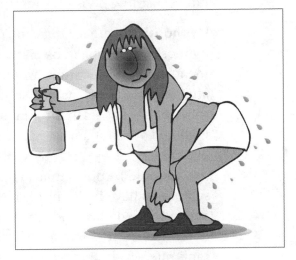

Acupuncture or Chinese herbs: A 2011 study found that acupuncture can help some women with symptoms of hot flashes and mood swings by causing measurable beneficial chemical changes in the body. Usually there is also a trained herbalist in the acupuncturist's office who might suggest Maca, ginseng, or kelp capsules, which are supplements known to reduce hot flashes and help with dryness. There are few risks to acupuncture, and, although it's not free, there is nothing to lose by trying this therapy.

Check your thyroid function: Women around the age of menopause (forty-five to fifty-five) can also develop thyroid abnormalities, which can mimic some of the symptoms of menopause such as dryness and heart palpitations. A simple blood test can tell if your thyroid is healthy.

Increase omega-3 intake: omega-3 fatty acids are important for supple skin, hair, and nails. Increasing omega-3 not only helps with the dryness of menopause, but it also reduces your risk of inflammatory-dependent illnesses like heart disease, arthritis, and cancer. The recommended dose is 1,000 mg twice a day with a meal. *Always check with your healthcare provider before starting supplements.*

Keep having regular sex (a regular orgasm would also certainly suffice): You know the saying "if you don't use it, you'll lose it." This rings true for sex as well. Your kitty will forget how to purr if you don't scratch her neck once in a while. You may need a lubricant to help things along, as vaginal dryness can be an issue. (Read Health Tip #2 about estrogen for more help there.) Always choose a lubricant with natural ingredients and without paraben preservatives. The brand I use is Astroglide Natural; free from alcohol, fragrance, parabens, and artificial color, and it contains aloe (which kitties just love). Visit www.astroglide.com.

Hypnosis: You are feeling cooler . . . cooler . . . COOLER. All kidding aside, hypnosis is proving to be a very useful tool in controlling the symptoms of menopause. In one study, women saw a 70 percent reduction in symptoms after only four sessions, and some women were able to completely rid themselves of hot flashes in three months. These finding were confirmed for those with and without a history of breast cancer.

It should be noted that all tips mentioned here to help with menopausal symptoms have no harmful side effects. Everyone's symptoms are different and every body responds to changing hormones in a unique way. But that doesn't mean you have to suffer and be a permanent "hot mess." If you still can't quench the fire, you may want to look into seeing a naturopath for additional advice.

Again, always check with your healthcare provider if you plan to start any herbal therapy as some can interfere with certain medications.

Don't think you have to suffer through the symptoms of menopause. There's plenty you can do to help yourself, without visiting the pharmacy.

Cancer Can Trump Pretty Much Anything

As predicted, I continued to get a break from dish duty long after my cancer treatments ended. One Sunday, about six months into my recovery, there was a large family gathering at Mom's for turkey and all the fixin's. At the end of the meal, I noticed my sisters' eyes dart nervously around the table. I knew exactly what they were thinking: *Who is going to wash all of these dishes?* It was touch and go there for a while, as both of these sisters had also experienced health issues that year. However, as we all know, cancer can trump a hysterectomy any old day! So once again, I was ushered off to the couch while the job of cleanup fell to my sisters.

I am happy to report that I got a lot of mileage from that particular perk. There were times, however, when the trump value of cancer was not so good. Many times for example, friends and acquaintances would abruptly clam up amid a legitimate complaint, because they seemed to feel that my cancer made their problems seem insignificant. Example: "My husband just left me/I am going bankrupt/All of my friends blocked me on Facebook . . . **BUT I shouldn't complain after all that you have been through.**" Did anybody ever stop to think that maybe I liked to hear about their problems? That came out wrong. What I mean is, I am a counselor. Lending a listening ear makes me feel useful. So, I think the rule of thumb is this: cancer does trump other issues when it comes to washing dishes, but NOT when it comes to being a supportive friend.

It is unethical to use one's cancer to make other people's problems seem insignificant. However, it is totally acceptable to use your cancer as an excuse to avoid household chores. (I feel confident that the entire cancer community will back me up on that.)

HEALTH TIP #84
Friends Can Truly Be Lifesavers

When I was going through chemo, friends I didn't even know came out of the woodwork to help. I remember one particular night my energy tank was on empty and my two young daughters, ages ten and twelve, had just gotten home from school. Not wanting to give them spaghetti for dinner *again*, I searched for something quick and easy to make. I was just unscrewing the jar of peanut butter, when there was a knock at the door and my friend was standing there with a casserole.

"You're a lifesaver!" I said. She came in, and, while the kids ate we talked, laughed, and shared.

I didn't realize that this friendship was *literally* saving my life.

Socialization is the fancy term scientists use for friendships, family, and people you talk to, whether it's face to face, on the phone, or online. That interpersonal connection and human interaction has physical benefits that go far beyond telling you if "those pants make you look fat." Sharing feelings, hearing others' feelings, and helping one another with life's triumphs and tribulations can alter certain chemicals in your body that have to do with stress and immunity.

Stanford University School of Medicine has an entire section devoted to these topics. The Stanford Center on Stress and Health is a research center devoted to studying the effects of stress and support on the mind and body. Directed by Dr. David Spiegel, the center has conducted pages of research on the effect of "socialization" as it relates to immunity in general, and cancer specifically.

It is widely accepted that mental stress has a negative effect on health and immunity. Stress can increase the risk of many illnesses like heart disease and cancer. When conducting experiments to measure stress, sometimes the hormone cortisol is measured. Cortisol is a hormone that is secreted when our mind perceives stress. It readies us for that "fight-or-flight" thing. But chronic stress keeps those levels high and increases the risk of chronic illness.

Dr. Spiegel and his team compared the cortisol levels of women with breast cancer and measured that against their quality and quantity of social supports. Those with better social support (aka friends) had lower cortisol levels. Another study's conclusion states:

> It is reasonable to hypothesize that supportive social relationships may buffer the effects of cancer-related stress on immunity, and thereby facilitate the recovery of immune mechanisms that may be important for cancer resistance.

In other words, it's not a stretch to think that the relationship you have with your friends, and just being with others, is changing your body's chemistry. This helps increase your immunity, which in turn may keep cancer away.

While hugs have their own benefits, a physical body need not be present. It has been shown that Internet support chat groups and interactive blogging sites have the same positive effects on immunity as sitting down and having tea with your buddies face to face. (Just make sure you're getting up every two hours from the computer to do some walking and stretching, as sitting poses it's own health risks even if you exercise regularly.)

> You really can get by with a little help from your friends.

Consider this a prescription to "socialize." Go out with friends, visit with neighbors, and spend time with family. You may want to think about joining a volunteer organization or club to meet new people. Listed below are some great socialization networking sites and forums:

- Imerman Angels (www.ImermanAngels.org). They will match you with a cancer survivor that has the same cancer as you; any cancer, any age. Sometimes it helps to have a friend that knows what you're going through.

- Cancer Survivors Network and chat room (http://csn.cancer.org).

- Cancer Chat Canada (http://cancerchatcanada.ca).

Cancer Made Me Feel Like the Six Million Dollar Man

If you are old enough to remember the TV program *The Six Million Dollar Man,* you will probably recall the line: "Better than he was before: Better, Stronger, Faster." When I consider some of the changes that cancer brought into my life, I sometimes feel like the Six Million Dollar Man.

Better: I am definitely better than I was before cancer, in many ways. I take much better care of my body. I have learned to better cope with stress. I have also come to realize what is really important in life, and I no longer sweat the small stuff. Most important, I have learned to love and approve of myself just as I am. While I would never want to relive my cancer experience (and I would never wish it on anyone!), I can honestly say that it made a better person of me.

Stronger: Friedrich Nietzsche said, "That which does not kill you makes you stronger." There is nothing like a spar with cancer to prove to yourself how strong you really are. Years ago, if someone had told me that at age forty-four I would be divorced, have a child with autism, and be facing cancer, I would have doubted my ability to survive. Not only did I survive my battle, but I experienced some of the most joyful moments of my life while doing so. Cancer may have weakened my body, but my spirit has never been stronger.

Faster: Who am I trying to kid? I'm not actually faster than I was before, but I am more committed to my running practice. My goal is not to win any races, but to make exercise an important part of my survival plan. As long as I am consistent with my plan, slow and steady will win the race!

So here I am, fresh from the battle with cancer and still bearing my battle scars, but feeling like six million bucks (well, at least six hundred bucks). After my breast reconstruction I will also be sporting better boobs than I've had in a long time. Better, stronger, faster AND *bionic* boobs; now that is one of the "perkiest" perks of having cancer.

> Take time to consider the ways that cancer
> may have made a better person out of you.

HEALTH TIP #85
Better, Stronger Bones

Bones are important. Without them we'd all be jellyfish. Age, chemo, and other cancer treatments can deplete the estrogen in our bodies, which turns off the bone-making factory and puts us at risk for osteoporosis. Osteoporosis is the thinning and weakening of bone tissue.

Your body's ability to build and maintain strong bones is a very complex, involved process and one that can be affected by a number of things. For women, chemo induced–menopause is one. Estrogen is a key component in making and maintaining bone. Without estrogen, your "bone-making mechanism" slows down and you end up with "low-density" or "porous" bones. How "porous" your bones are, along with other factors like family history of fractures, smoking history, steroid use, and others, determines your risk of a bone fracture in the future.

We all have to do something to prevent bone loss. Even if you don't have hormone-induced menopause, you're not getting any younger, honey.

During teenaged years, your diet and lifestyle determine how much bone mass you build. By the time you reach your late teens, 90 percent of your bone mass is established. In adulthood, the trick is to keep what you've got and strengthen it. (If you have teenagers, make sure they're getting their recommended daily allowance, 1,300 mg, of calcium and 600 mg of vitamin D to prevent problems for them in their later years.)

Calcium is important in maintaining bone health as it is one of the main components of bone, but we also need it in our blood. If there is not enough calcium in the blood, it might "borrow" some calcium from the bones, thus weakening them. If you have a sufficient amount of calcium in your blood, there won't be as much bone loss, so it's important to eat calcium-rich foods to ensure your serum calcium level is sufficient. There has been some conflicting data recently about calcium supplements and risks, but the majority of healthcare professionals still recommend 1,200 mg of calcium per day to keep bones healthy if you're postmenopausal and 1,000 mg if you're pre-. Your body absorbs calcium most efficiently when taken in amounts of no more than 500 mg at a time. If you're taking supplements, the trick is to take them spaced out, three or four times a day, instead of a mega dose once or twice a day as sudden spikes in blood calcium might cause it to end up in places you don't want, like your heart arteries or your kidneys. Taking calcium three or four times a day also more closely resembles how your body would process it if the calcium came from meals. Obviously, getting your nutrients from whole foods is the best way for your body to absorb it and would also provide the necessary minerals and elements that are needed for proper absorption. Vitamin D, phosphates, magnesium, and vitamin K all play a role in calcium absorption and bone health.

If you take supplements, you should look at the type of calcium you take. Most supplements at the drugstore are calcium carbonate or calcium citrate. These calcium sources come from limestone and oyster shell. We would not ordinarily include these things in our diets.

Another form of calcium comes from algae. I know, you don't eat algae either, but it is edible and it is a plant, which your body is more likely to process than a rock. Algae-derived calcium has been shown to be far superior in absorption and availability than calcium carbonate or calcium citrate, and usually supplies the other elements that help with absorption as well. A 2010 study showed that algae-based calcium was a "superior calcium supplement compared to the other calcium salts tested" (calcium carbonate and citrate). Plant-based calcium supplements are available online and at health food stores. I take Bone Strength by New Chapter, but there are others as well. (I don't get a kick back from them. I just like them.)

Your bones also want you to:

- Limit alcohol to one drink per day.

- Quit smoking.

- Engage in weight-bearing exercise (walking, jumping rope, dancing, yoga, running, weight training; there's that word again: *exercise*).

- Consider taking strontium, a mineral much like calcium that is available in prescription form in the UK and in an over-the counter-form in the United States and is very effective at building bone mass.

Note: When considering any new supplement or a change in your current supplement, please check with your healthcare provider to make sure, in your specific case, that you are helping and not hurting your health.

Remember, it's decisions you make today that will affect your life five, ten, and twenty years from now. Make sure your future includes strong bones.

No bones about it: 1,000 to 1,200 mg of calcium taken properly is the recommended daily allowance for bone health.

My First
Breast Cancer Retreat

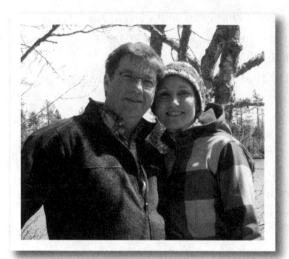

Flo and Shawn

When the last of my radiation treatments ended in April 2012, my boyfriend Shawn and I traveled to Nova Scotia to attend the Skills for Healing breast cancer weekend retreat. I was rather quiet on the drive, which prompted Shawn to ask, "Is everything okay?" Suddenly an image came to mind of a plane landing, and a voice in my head said, *Ladies and gentlemen, we are making our final descent into the land of breast cancer.* It was sort of like the feeling I got the first time I went to the cancer clinic. Although I had been diagnosed for many months, there was a surreal quality about actually being there. A little voice in my head was telling me, *You know, Flo, you must really have cancer if you are sitting in a cancer clinic.* But this time the voice said, *You know, Flo, you must really be a cancer survivor if you are going to one of those retreats.* The word *survivor* is one that I had been struggling with and attending this retreat brought me a little further along in convincing me that I was deserving of the title.

Attending the Skills for Healing retreat was one of the most therapeutic parts of my cancer journey (and since it was free, it was also one of the perks of having cancer!). The facilitators, Dr. Rob Rutledge and Dr. Timothy Walker, simply exuded compassion as they taught skills such as meditation, yoga, how to reframe our thoughts, and how to honor our bodies. For me, these concepts were not new, and, while it was a good opportunity for me to brush up on my existing skills, the real healing came from being part of the group: *the healing circle.*

While I have many "cyber-friends" who share my diagnosis, this was the first time I was actually in a room full of women at various stages of their breast cancer journey. It felt so liberating to take off my wig in a room full of people and not worry about how I looked. For the first time, having breast cancer did not make me different. I was among kindred spirits. Not only was I able to take off my hair, but I also took off my "Super Cancer Hero" cape and spilled my guts about my deepest fears and anxieties. I cried. Not one of those movie star cries, where a few tears creep down the cheek without ever disturbing the makeup. No, this was more of a wounded animal howl accompanied by lots of snot and mascara-stained tears. Oh, but it felt so good to open that floodgate!

I realized that I had been so intent on maintaining a positive attitude, that I sometimes suppressed my "negative" emotions, such as sadness and fear. On this retreat I discovered that when it comes to feelings, it does not have to be one or the other. In other words, allowing myself to feel anger, sadness, and fear does not diminish my positive attitude. Just as it is possible to experience joy amid suffering, so too it is possible to experience "negative" emotions, but maintain an overall positive attitude. In fact, I would say that allowing myself to experience these emotions, without getting stuck in them, has been a critical part of my healing.

Allowing yourself to feel anger, sadness, fear, and
other healing feelings does not diminish your
positive attitude. (Just don't get stuck in them.)

HEALTH TIP #86
It's My Cancer and I'll Cry if I Want To

How often have we been witness to a friend or family member who is upset and crying, and we say to them "It's okay. Don't cry." Or we feel the tears welling up in our throats and we struggle to hold them back and "keep it together."

For crying out loud! Cry already!

Tears aren't just drops of saltwater that drip down your face when you're sad or making onion soup. They are tiny little transporters of stress hormones and other toxins that change the very chemical composition of our body to allow us the ability to "deal with it all."

Not all tears are the same. The tears that come out of your eyes from chopping onions or getting that annoying eyelash in your eye are mainly for lubrication and protection and contain mild antibacterial agents to prevent infection.

Crying is a healthy way to release stress and no one will call you a baby for doing it.

But the tears that are brought on by emotions are very different. They contain high levels of proteins, minerals, and prolactin, a hormone associated with stress and immunity. After the release of these substances through tears, there is a rise in endorphin levels. Endorphins are the body's own natural "happy pills," which is probably why a proven 88.8 percent of people feel better after a good cry.

"Because unalleviated stress can increase our risk for heart attack and damage certain areas of our brain, the human ability to cry has survival value." So says Dr. William Frey, a professor at the University of Minnesota who actually wrote an entire book on the subject entitled *Crying: The Mystery of Tears.* "I have suggested that we may feel better after crying because we are literally crying it out," he writes.

Other animals have tears that only lubricate the eye, but humans are the only mammals on the planet to shed these "emotional tears."

Why are you holding back?

Many people fight tears because they think that crying makes them appear weak, especially men or women that hate stereotypes of crying women like myself. Others don't want to cry in front of their kids or loved ones so as not to make them "feel bad" or worry. But crying brings on empathy and support from loved ones and actually brings people closer to each other, and it also teaches kids the important lesson that it's really okay to cry.

Science says you will feel better after a good cry. Between 6 and 8 PM is the most common time for emotional crying. But you can do it anytime you want. If you've been holding back your tears for the right time . . . how about now?

Cancer Gave Me a Cause

It's not like I didn't have plenty of "causes" to choose from before getting cancer. Between grappling with anxiety for much of my life, being a single parent, and having a child with autism, I have enough causes to write my own *Chicken Soup for the Soul* book (I will call it *Chicken Soup for the Chicken's Soul*). I am not the type to take things lying down, and each challenge in life has kicked me into action. For example, to help me be a better autism mom, I have become a self-made expert in the area of autism (really, ask me anything). I have also read hundreds of self-help books to help me better cope with my anxiety issues.

However, cancer is the one thing in my life that motivated me to action to help *other people*, and therefore I consider it to be my cause. Before you block me from Facebook or change your phone number, I assure you I will not come to you looking for money to support my cause (well, hardly ever). You see, my cause is not to raise money or even to help find a cure for cancer, but rather to help others affected by this disease to realize the benefits of adopting a survivor's attitude (which combines a positive attitude with positive action).

My cancer journey has not been an easy one. Over the course of about a year, I endured countless tests and procedures, three surgeries resulting in the loss of my left breast and associated lymph nodes, six rounds of chemotherapy, and twenty-five radiation treatments. However, in that same year, I met my soul mate and fell in love, I started blogging, I fulfilled a life-long dream of being published, and I started a new business venture. The moral of the story is this: just because you have cancer does not mean that you have to lie down and die.

In the book *Full Catastrophe Living*, bestselling author Jon Kabat-Zinn says, "As long as you are breathing there is more right with you than there is wrong, no matter how ill or how hopeless you may feel."

That is so true! Think of all the things your body has to do to allow you to just sit there and read this book: Your heart is beating, your organs are functioning, your cells are reproducing, your toenails are growing, and you are breathing. That's not even to mention the complex mental processes that are happening to allow you to read and understand these words. Even if you do have cancer, there is a lot more right with your body at this moment than there is wrong. So as long as there is breath left in you, why not make the most of every moment!

Don't let cancer put your dreams on hold.
Live every day to its fullest.

HEALTH TIP #87
The Importance of Dreaming . . . and Sleeping

"I'll sleep when I'm dead."

Well, that may be sooner than you think if you don't get enough quality sleep according to the latest research.

A 2011 study involving 50,000 adults followed over eleven years showed a 45 percent increase in heart attacks among those who reported they suffer from insomnia. That's huge. But not surprising considering other research that has come before it.

Poor sleeping habits are linked to:

- **High blood pressure:** A 2011 study out of Harvard linked poor sleep with an 83 percent increased risk of developing high blood pressure in older adults. One possible factor is that when you sleep, your blood pressure drops, but in poor sleepers that never happens. Over time, it takes a toll on your system.

- **Obesity:** Lack of sleep causes hormone changes, which lead to a slowed metabolism, which leaves you burning less calories and making poor food choices when you're awake. Poor sleep habits were also linked to making poor diet choices when you're awake.

- **Depression/anxiety/mood changes:** During sleep the brain releases chemicals that regulate mood. Insomnia is often a precurser to depression and it has been found that if the insomnia is cured, the depression will be too.

- **Poor memory:** During sleep, our memories are "consolidated." You take what you have learned and seen that day, and convert it to a "hard copy" in your brain to retrieve later if you need it. Disrupted sleep does not allow for this conversion.

- **Diabetes:** Sleep apnea, a condition where sleep is disrupted by an inability to breathe properly, causes a lower sensitivity to insulin, the hormone responsible for regulating blood sugar. A University of Chicago study showed a "robust association" between (obstructive) sleep apnea and insulin resistance, glucose intolerance and the risk of type 2 diabetes, *independent* of obesity.

- **Impaired immunity:** (Hint: Your red flag should be flying with this one since your immune function is related to your risk of cancer.) During sleep your body releases cytokines that aid in fighting infection. Poor sleep habits reduce the production of these proteins so they are not available when your body needs them. This leads to increased susceptibility to bugs and more sickness. This was actually measured in adults receiving the flu vaccine. Those with insomnia did not produce the level of antibodies (flu fighters) from the vaccine that the good sleepers did.

- **Cancer:** Here's a kicker: A 2012 study looking at 412 postmenopausal breast cancer patients showed a definitive link between lack of sleep and more aggressive tumors and recurrence. The study demonstrated that those who reported getting an average of six hours of sleep/night or less developed more aggressive tumors with a greater rate of cancer recurrence. There was no risk difference in premenopausal women, suggesting there is a different underlying process to breast cancer when estrogen is involved. This was the first study of its kind, so more research is needed.

It is obvious from the list that "poor sleep habits" go hand in hand with an "unhealthy body." Insomnia has become more common today because of the "so-much-to-do-and-so-little-time" lifestyle many of us have adopted. And it is often overlooked when people ask the question, "Why do I feel like crap all the time?"

Contrary to what some think, sleeping isn't a form of your body and brain "turning off" or "resting." Your brain remains quite active during this time, with chemical reactions and processes occurring during sleep that allow the brain to "reorganize" and "repair." Growth hormone is manufactured and secreted during sleep, and the amount gradually decreases as we age, which is one of the reasons why infants and children sleep more than adults. (Human growth hormone [HGH] is what the "beautiful people" are injecting to stay younger looking. Maybe there is something to the term *beauty sleep*.)

Your brain undergoes a series of cycles during sleep. You must reach all stages of these cycles 4 to 5 times during the night to get "healthful" sleep.

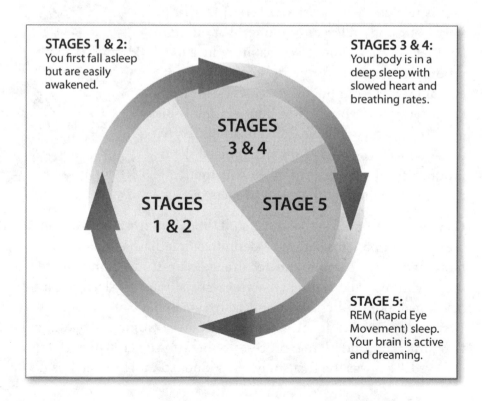

STAGES 1 & 2:
You first fall asleep but are easily awakened.

STAGES 3 & 4:
Your body is in a deep sleep with slowed heart and breathing rates.

STAGES 3 & 4

STAGES 1 & 2

STAGE 5

STAGE 5:
REM (Rapid Eye Movement) sleep. Your brain is active and dreaming.

Disturbed or interrupted sleep does not seem to count. You may be in the bed for eight hours with your eyes closed, but if you don't reach the proper cycles, it's as if you didn't sleep at all.

Poor sleep, or dozing, is just as bad for you as no sleep.

When does it get to the point of "insomnia"?

There are two different kinds of insomnia or sleeplessness. If you have trouble falling asleep (it takes more than thirty minutes to fall asleep) or have trouble staying asleep more than three nights a week for over a month, it's labeled "chronic insomnia." Sometimes there is a specific problem associated with the sleeplessness that causes insomnia for just a short period of time, for example your dog died or you lost your job. That's called "acute" or "secondary insomnia."

> Sleeping isn't a waste of time. It's vital to your overall health.

In more than 80 percent of people there is an identifiable cause for their lack of sleep (secondary insomnia). Whether it's drinking or eating too close to bedtime, too much caffeine, or too much worry, once the problem is identified and corrected, the restful nights return.

For the other near 20 percent of those suffering from insomnia, the sleeplessness is the primary problem and is its own disorder, which should be treated with establishing lifestyle changes, cognitive behavioral therapy, or medications and/or supplements. If you are among this crowd it's important to get help from your doctor or naturopath to get you on the right road to dreamland. It may be discovered that you have sleep apnea or restless leg syndrome (involuntary movements and feelings in your legs that don't allow you to rest). You might not even know you have these two conditions, but they can severely affect sleep patterns and have a negative impact on your health.

It's so annoying when you can't fall asleep, isn't it? Here are some tips that may help:

- **Set a routine:** Try to go to bed around the same time each night. Have a bedtime routine that consists of getting dressed, bathroom stuff (peeing, washing, brushing teeth, flossing), and some form of relaxing activity for ten to fifteen minutes before you try to sleep like reading, listening to music (preferably not heavy metal), or taking a warm bath. Put a few drops of lavender essential oil (*Lavendula angustifolia*, a natural oil, not fragrance oil) in the bathwater to help relieve stress.

- **Avoid alcohol, caffeine, and full meals** at least three hours before bed-time. All these things block the ability of your brain to successfully cycle through the REM stages.

- **No naps** after 3 PM.

- **Regular exercise is key.** Sorry, folks, but it's true; at the very least, twenty minutes, four times a week, but not within two hours of bedtime. (Please note that twenty minutes a day four times a week is far less than you need to build your immunity and lower your risk of cancer and other illnesses.)

- **Dark and cool should be the décor** for your bedroom. Think "cave." This includes turning off computers, TVs, and tablets, as the light in your eyes suppresses the production of melatonin, which is your body's own natural sleeping pill.

- **Earplugs, a mask, or white noise machines** can help eliminate annoying sounds, like your partner's snoring or that neighbor's damn dog.

- **Make a "to-do" list** before you go to bed so you're not thinking about what you need to remember for the next day.

- **Use your bed only for sleep** (and sex . . . but you can have sex in places other than your bed . . . just to be clear). Don't use your bed to hang out and watch TV or catch up on work.

- **Get enough Vitamin B$_6$** as you need this vitamin for the production of melatonin. Some good sources of B$_6$ are bell peppers, sunflower seeds, spinach, shiitake mushrooms, and summer squash. Eat fresh because can-ning reduces vitamin B$_6$ by as much as 60 percent.

- **Meditation** can slow your thoughts down and prepare you for a restful night. Meditation done on a regular basis reduces your overall stress level and can lower your level of cortisol, one of the hormones that causes your body to wake up.

So if you're reading this in bed and it's past your bedtime . . . go to sleep! Your body will thank you for it.

Cancer Gave Me the Courage to Step Outside My Comfort Zone

According to the *Wall Street Journal*, public speaking is the number-one fear of people in North America. Death is number two. In other words, if you were going to a funeral, you would rather be the one in the coffin than the person giving the eulogy. When I was invited to be guest speaker at the Canadian Breast Cancer Foundation's Provincial Annual Retreat, I wasn't sure that I would have the nerve to do it. While I had experience with public speaking, my skills had gotten a little rusty in my time away from work, and the thought of giving a speech to a group of 200 people ranked right up there with bungee cord jumping and running with the bulls for me.

Given that cancer is my new cause, however, I could not pass up this opportunity to spread my message of the benefits of facing cancer with a survivor's attitude. What better place to promote my cause than with a captive audience of women in various stages of their breast cancer journey?

Still, I wasn't sure if I would be able to confront my public speaking fear. When I was a child, my father taught me these words: "Do what you fear and your fear will disappear." There are few things in life scarier than a cancer diagnosis. I reasoned that if I could face cancer head on, then I could certainly take on this challenge. And so I did it! Sure, it was scary to stand before that many people and talk about my cancer experience, but not nearly as scary as hearing those three little words: "You have cancer." If my speech helped even one person, then it was worth it, and, besides, Dad was right. Once I did it, the thought of speaking in public again didn't scare me nearly as much.

Do what you fear and your fear will disappear!

HEALTH TIP #88
Don't Fear the Squash!

Squaaaash! It's fun to say, but as a kid I remember thinking, *I don't think I want to eat something that makes the same sound as a bug when I step on it.*

Thank goodness for adulthood. Now I am mature enough to try new foods and make wonderful recipes from them. The many varieties of squash make for interesting choices.

Summer squash like zucchini, yellow summer "crooked neck" squash, and butterstick (the sweetest damn summer variety there is) all have thin skins. They need to be kept refrigerated or they will soften and "go bad" in about a week or so. Don't store them near gas-producing apples or pears in the fridge or it will make the squash "go bad" quicker. Cucumbers are actually a part of the summer squash family.

Winter squash like acorn, butternut, or carnival tend to have thicker skins and much harder flesh. Some varieties practically require a hammer and chisel to cut them open. But once cooked, the flesh is dense, sweet, and fluffy. The hard skin allows you to store a winter squash in any cool, dark place (like your pantry box) for up to three months. When storing squash with stems, leave the stem intact for the best flavor.

When discussing the benefits of squash here, it is assumed that the squash is fresh, not canned, and it is not boiled, as these processes deplete much of the valuable nutrition contained in these sweet beauties.

> Eating seasonal squash supplies you with cancer-fighting vitamins and a delicious colorful addition to your diet.

The summer varieties in general are high in vitamin C, potassium, vitamin B_6, and fiber (if you're eating the organically grown skins like you should) and have no fat. Winter squash varieties are generally high in vitamin A, vitamin C, calcium, thiamine, niacin, B_6, iron, and potassium, and also have no fat. Summer varieties are delicious raw, and I like to slice these for use as "chips" in many dips I make or to throw them into salads.

Winter varieties are *very* high in vitamin A, as are most orange-colored veggies like carrots. Butternut squash, for example, has an incredible 457 percent of the recommended daily allowance for vitamin A—over 22,000 IUs! Vitamin A is one of the antioxidant vitamins that reduce your risk of illness and disease of all kinds by preventing cell damage and death. (The others are vitamin C and vitamin E.)

I have to admit, it's the winter varieties that get me excited (it doesn't take much, obviously). I am simply intrigued by these dense, heavy veggies with such interesting shapes and names like carnival, cheese wheel, eight ball, gold ball, fairy tale, spaghetti, buttercup, and boo-boo.

No complicated recipes here, just my two favorite ways to prepare summer and winter squashes of all types. For me, this is also the most flavorful and healthy way too.

Summer Squash

Wash and then slice any amount of summer squash into half-inch disks (skin on) and place in a mixing bowl. Drizzle enough organic extra virgin olive oil over the sliced pieces to coat and then mix with a spoon to coat all pieces.

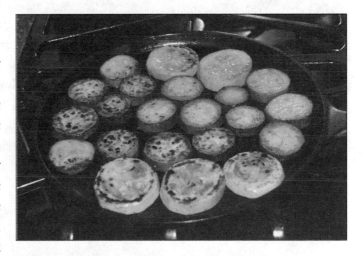

Prepare a cast-iron or similar skillet by heating over medium-high heat. Place slices flat in the skillet and arrange so they are all flat. Season the tops with sea salt and pepper. Cook for about 5 to 7 minutes or until the pieces start to look soft and the underside is speckled with golden brown. Flip over and cook about 4 minutes more. Remove from heat and enjoy! This is the best way of getting the true, sweet, delicious flavor of the squash.

These are crazy good. I love these as a side, but I've also been known to throw them in brown rice or quinoa with other cooked veggies as you can't beat their sweet taste.

Winter Squash

Wash squash and pierce the skin with a fork several times (to make sure it's completely dead). Place on a foil or parchment-lined cookie sheet or baking pan and place in an oven set at 350°F. Place in the center of the oven and cook for 60 to 90 minutes depending on how big the squash is. A 4 to 5 pound squash will take about one hour. Make sure it's done

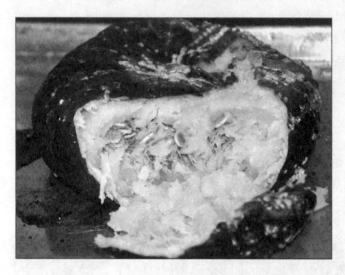

by pushing a long knife straight through in several places. It should be soft all the way through. Avoid overbrowning of the skin, as this will sometimes cause dryness.

Let it cool a bit, then cut open and remove seeds (carefully as it will be very hot). Cut the flesh from the skin. In most cases you can just easily scoop out the flesh from the skin. Place the flesh in a bowl and add a bit of almond or coconut milk, a dash of sea salt, and a drizzle of pure maple syrup. (I mean real maple syrup, not maple-flavored syrup.) Mix well. No exact measurements here, as every squash is a different size. Just experiment . . . it's more fun that way.

With this easy recipe, you'll have a great sub for unhealthy mashed white potatoes.

Did I squelch your fear of squash?

Bonus Reward Points

In my work as an educational psychologist, I would often devise behavior management plans for students, using rewards to improve their behaviors. Many teachers would object to implementing these plans saying, "Why should he be rewarded for doing something he should be doing anyway? That's not how it works in the REAL world." Meanwhile, said teacher has so many reward point collector cards in her purse, she practically needs a crane to lift it to her shoulder.

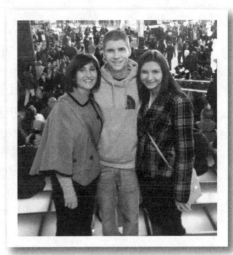

Flo in Times Square
with Kaitlyn and Donovan

So, I would have to say, yes, that is exactly how it works in the REAL world. I buy my groceries at a certain store and I get rewarded with points that can be used toward my next purchase of gas. I buy gas and get rewarded with points that can be redeemed to buy merchandise. I love these points! In fact, the main reason I even drink wine is because of the Air Miles plan (well, maybe not the *main* reason).

I am going to be upfront with you here. Cancer is not a cheap disease to have. If you are one to pinch pennies, you may want to consider getting yourself another, less expensive disease. I would like to recommend one, but that is more Susan's department. While cancer put a dent in my bank account, my reward points skyrocketed! In fact, at the end of my cancer journey, I had collected enough points to take myself on another type of journey. New York, here I come!

Cancer will put a dent in your bank account. However,
the more you spend, the more bonus reward points
you can rack up, so get yourself a collector's card!

HEALTH TIP #89
You Get Points for Buying Food, Too,
but Should You Always Buy Organic?

Food is expensive. And I'm not just talking about lobster and caviar. You could go shopping, spend $100, and come home with nothing but empty calories that satisfy your sweet tooth. (The kid side of you thinks this is just fine, but the adult side of you knows better.)

So you head to the produce aisle of the market (smart) and take a walk along the beautiful rows of shiny colorful apples, plums, cucumbers, and kale (yes, kale!). You reach for a sweet juicy red apple . . . but wait! That apple can contain more poison than the one that nearly killed Snow White!

Pesticides are chemical agents sprayed on growing produce to discourage or destroy anything unwanted from interfering with plant growth; from killing a hungry caterpillar to killing weeds, fungus, mold, mice, or bacteria. Killing all these different living things means using lots of different kinds of chemicals. Chemical pesticide agents have been linked to nervous disorders like ADHD, hormone disorders, and an increased risk of cancer. Ninety-nine percent of Americans tested positive for pesticides in their blood. These chemicals are getting in our bodies because we are letting them in.

"Organic" produce, on the other hand, cannot contain any chemical pesticides by law and are thereby deemed "clean." The Environmental Working Group or EWG (www.ewg.org) does a great job of taking the confusion out of what to buy. The U.S. Environmental Protection Agency (EPA) posts information on pesticide levels every year after testing imported and domestic fruits and vegetables. The EWG takes that information and translates it into two lists of foods called the "Dirty Dozen" and "Clean Fifteen."

The Dirty Dozen lists the foods that have been measured to contain the highest level of pesticides. Some pesticides detected in the produce have been removed from the EPA's "legal use" list, but still find their way into our stores either by way of foreign produce or by omission from the farmer's reports. Either way, you should steer clear of these foods and only buy organic when possible.

The Clean Fifteen is a list containing the foods that measured low for pesticides, so there is no significant benefit from buying these foods as organic. (Unless you just like that the organic versions taste better—and I think they do!)

The lists change every year so check their website for this year's "clean and dirty" foods. Choosing five servings from the "Dirty Dozen" list would result in exposure to fourteen different pesticides, while choosing five servings from the "Clean Fifteen" list would result in exposure to only two. You can reduce your pesticide intake by as much as 80 to 90 percent if you follow the list.

> Limit your pesticide exposure by checking the clean and dirty list.

Washing will help remove bacteria but does little to most pesticides, since many pesticides are "fed" to the plants in their root systems and become one with the plant. (Even those fancy expensive veggie washes won't help with some.) Peeling helps with removing the pesticide layer that gets trapped in the wax applied to most conventional fruits and veggies. (Ever wonder why you can practically see your reflection in a cucumber? It's waxed.)

On a side note: There's a war brewing in the organic world, and it has to do with labeling, federal regulations, and big business. Huge mega corporations have begun the systematic takeover of small organic businesses as they see the profit in the public's awareness of healthy eating. Small independent companies like Izzy, Sweet Leaf, Honest Tea, Ben & Jerry's, and Burt's Bees have been taken over by Pepsi, Coca Cola, Kellogg, and Clorox. Easy-to-read labels with truly natural, healthy ingredients would not be in their best interest. And they spend big money making sure that doesn't happen. Take a moment to find out who owns that "organic" company that makes your organic cereal, and favorite juice. The answer may surprise you.

A great way to avoid pesticides is to buy fresh local produce from either Community Supported Agriculture (CSA) or farmers markets. There, you can actually speak directly to the person responsible for growing the food when you buy it.

Please remember: it's healthier to eat nonorganic fruits and veggies than to omit fruits and veggies because you can't find organic, but in some cases it's worth a look.

Learning Postcancer Etiquette

I have always considered myself to be a polite person. However, after getting cancer, I found myself letting my manners slip a little. For example, I was so caught up in my own health issues that I rarely asked anyone else, "How are you?" Once my treatments ended and I was proclaimed *"cancer-free,"* I realized that I had to brush up on my postcancer etiquette.

When you have cancer, you get used to hearing two things:

1. **"You look great!"** I think that many people equate the word *cancer* with the image of a deathly-pale and emaciated body, and they are genuinely surprised that you can have cancer but still look healthy. So when people told me, "You look great," I realized that they were probably thinking *for someone with cancer*. But I gave the standard cancer patient response anyway: "Thank you!"

   Now that I am no longer in treatment mode, I realize that I can't get away with my standard "Thank you" response. When someone says, "You look great!" they darn well expect that I am going to say, "You too!" possibly followed by, "Have you lost weight?" or "I love that hair color on you."

2. **"How are you?"** When you have cancer and people ask, "How are you?" they are not just being polite. They actually want to know how you are doing. You have a choice of responses to this question: "Doing great, thanks!" OR get into a lengthy discussion of your latest test results and procedures. I usually chose to go with the latter. (Well, hey, they ASKED!)

   Now that there is no evidence of the disease in my body, I have to remind myself that most people don't literally mean it when they ask, "How are you?" "How ya doing?" or "How's it going?" They are just being polite. In this case, the proper postcancer etiquette requires a response such as, "Fine thanks, and yourself?" Or "Good, and you?" The important point is to always remember to ask the person how *they* are doing, and never, ever launch into a detailed explanation of your latest infection scare (well, unless they ask).

There will likely come a time when people
no longer want to hear about your cancer.

HEALTH TIP #90
Hear No Evil, See No Evil, Speak No Evil

"How are you?" This may be the lead-in question to the most often told lie in the history of lies.

If you are an average person, you tell eleven lies per week. (Yeah, you do.) From making excuses for being late to exaggerating the truth, "little white lies" are a part of our lives. What does lying have to with your health? I'm glad you asked, and I'll tell you the truth.

A recent study presented at the 2012 American Psychological Association's meeting tested the theory that lying affects your physical well-being. A group of 110 males and females from eighteen to seventy years old were split into two groups: one group was told not to lie, and the others were given no instructions. (They must assume that the average person is a lying sack of dung, I guess.) Over the ten-week trial period, those that only told the truth had less physical symptoms such as sore throats, headaches, anxiety symptoms, and tension.

"I think lying can cause a lot of stress for people, contributing to anxiety and even depression," said Dr. Bryan Bruno, acting chairman of the department of psychiatry at Lenox Hill Hospital in New York City. "Lying less is not only good for your relationships, but for yourself as an individual. People might recognize the more devastating impact lying can have on relationships, but probably don't recognize the extent to which it can cause a lot of internal stress."

Hmm, I'm going to have think about this one the next time my husband asks how much I spent on those shoes.

The participants in the "truth group" said they invented ways around lying. Some said they had never really tried to tell the truth before (rather than exaggerate) and found it was easier than they thought. Some others found responding to a question with another question was a way out.

> The truth will set you free (of stress).

I don't think answering, "Fine" to the question "How are you?" is a lie, even if you're nauseated, swollen, and your wig is itching you. But I do know people who, when asked that question, say, "I'm making it work," which may be more accurate and a more "healthful" response.

Free T-Shirts

I pulled out my T-shirt drawer one evening and realized that it is practically bursting at the seams. I am not normally a T-shirt gal, so it took me by surprise that I have accumulated so many of these garments. As I rifled through the drawer, I came to realize a perk: Many of these T-shirts came to me FREE for participating in cancer survivor events such as retreats, the Relay for Life and the Run for the Cure. In some cases, I got two T-shirts for the

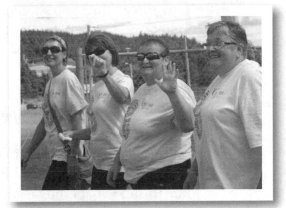

same event: the standard white participant one and the coveted survivors T-shirt (okay, maybe coveted is a bit strong of a word).

Although there is some controversy in the cancer world about the use of the term *survivor* and what it means, there is no denying the special synergy that exists among the group who gets to wear the "coveted" T-shirt. Having shared a similar experience, we feel an automatic kinship with other survivors. (We also get to say, *Cancer . . . been there, done that, got the T-shirt!*)

I am pretty sure that, as I walk or run the track wearing my survivors T-shirt, spectators are looking at me and thinking, *Wow! Look at that cool yellow T-shirt. All I got was a boring old white one. I wonder what I have to do to get to wear the yellow one?* Well, probably they are not thinking that. But I am certain that at least some of the spectators are looking at me and thinking, *Wow! Look at my mom/sister/daughter/friend/girlfriend. She is a survivor!*

Taking part in cancer survivor events can be a joyous experience. Allow yourself to feel the special energy of being part of a survivors' group.

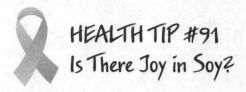

HEALTH TIP #91
Is There Joy in Soy?

The three things you should never discuss at a party are religion, politics, and soy. People have very definite opinions about whether soy is a savior or the devil. Sometimes those opinions are based on misinformation or old information. Let's start with the basics.

The basic whole form of soy, the soybean, is a legume. But the magical thing about this legume is that it's one of the few plants that contain the kinds of proteins our bodies need to survive. The protein profile for soybeans is very similar to that of meat, milk, and egg protein, but it's a plant. It's inexpensive to grow, and there's a lot of it on our planet. Studies continue to show that eating regular servings of soy will help lower cholesterol and reduce the incidence of heart disease.

So what's the problem? One of the big problems with soy is that the soy protein contains phytoestrogens or "plant estrogens." Soy protein doesn't contain the female hormone estrogen, per se, but substances in the soy protein called isoflavones act like estrogens to weakly activate estrogen receptors. In the general population, and in women who have never had cancer, this is actually a good thing because the weak estrogens can block the more potent "natural" estrogens that your body produces from binding with receptors and causing a chemical reaction that may decrease risk of hormone-related cancer. The isoflavones may also help to eliminate trapped estrogens in the fat tissue, which is another way to reduce cancer risk. Soy also contains antioxidants and anti-inflammatory agents that can reduce your risk of cancer in general. So when used in moderation and taken in the right form, it can be a great part of a healthy diet.

But for those with hormone-related cancers like breast and endometrial cancers, it would make sense that the action of the isoflavones activating the receptors would put that population at an increased risk for cancer recurrence. Early animal studies confirmed this. For this reason, most oncologists have told their patients with hormone-related cancers to steer clear of all soy products.

That belief is being challenged by a number of studies, the latest being a 2012 study published in the *American Journal of Clinical Nutrition*, which analyzed data from three separate studies that looked at the diets of over 9,000 women in America and China. They concluded that the data from the studies show that for women who have had ER (estrogen-receptor) positive cancer, those who consumed 10 mg per day or more of soy isoflavones had a 25 percent *lowered risk* of breast cancer recurrence. (Just for comparison, three ounces of soymilk contains 10 mg of isoflavones and three grams of total protein.) This result was not affected by taking the estrogen-blocking drug Tamoxifen. ER negative women showed an even greater benefit with a larger reduction in risk.

So just to recap: Women with a history of breast cancer ate soy and *reduced* their risk of getting cancer again. But before you go "tofu-loco" on me, researchers caution that this study needs to be repeated and verified, as it was a study that gathered its data from three other studies. More questions are always raised with huge claims like this. One of the questions has to do with the diets of the women as children. It is hypothesized that women who grow up eating soy as children react differently to dietary soy than those to whom soy is new. And the minimum amounts of soy protein were noted to be no less than 10 mg per day, but can you eat too much? And what kind of soy protein were they eating? There are many different forms of soy: whole, fermented, and processed.

Processing is a broad term, but it really just means taking something healthy and then grinding it, heating it, separating it by use of chemicals, kicking the crap out of it, and turning it into another substance to be used with other chemicals that will be sold to you as food. Since the main attraction of soy is its protein, this is the part that manufacturers use. The soybean can be put through a process that breaks it into parts and isolates the soy proteins from the carbs and fats. These are called *soy protein isolates* and they are chemically derived—that is, chemicals are used to separate the different parts of the soy. You will find soy isolates in breakfast bars, breads, energy bars, and many frozen foods. They are hard to avoid in most packaged foods, and, if you start reading some of the labels in your pantry right now, I think you'd be surprised where they're hiding. Bodybuilders use soy isolates in powdered form to make "high-protein shakes," and they are widely used in high-calorie supplement drinks. Anywhere manufacturers want to add protein to their product, they add soy isolates.

Manufacturers can also "hydrolyze" the protein to make *hydrolyzed soy protein*, which is very similar to harmful monosodium glutamate (MSG). Again, using chemicals (hydrochloric acid, to be precise) to complete the process, this substance is about as far from the soybean as you can get. Hydrolyzed soy protein and soy isolates both contain glutamates. Glutamates affect brain function and cause other neurological symptoms, and, for this reason, glutamates like MSG, soy isolates, and hydrolyzed soy continue to be studied for safety. Soy can also be processed into pills. Supplements in pill form contain extremely high levels of hormonelike isoflavones and all populations, even those who have never had cancer, are generally discouraged from taking them.

There are other soy foods that are highly processed as well. Soymilk, tofu, and soy cheeses, while not processed to the extent of the soy proteins, still may cause concern. Some state that processed raw soy foods like these contain substances that can block proper vitamin absorption and actually increase your risk for cancer. Only the fermented soy products like soybean miso, tempeh, and natto are beneficial and safe and seemingly have no harmful hormone effects. Fermenting uses the whole soybean and no chemicals for processing. The use of yeasts and fungus alters the protein over time so it becomes healthier for you overall and much easier to digest.

Researchers are always studying the Asian diet because Asians are among those with the lowest incidences of cancer. But when we look at the typical Asian diet, they only eat one serving of soy products per day, which adds up to about 30 mg of isoflavones. The type of soy is usually fermented soy like in soybean miso (miso soup) or tempeh. If they eat tofu, it is a small sliver in soup or small cubes in stir-fry. They don't eat massive "veggie soy burgers," they don't drink soymilk (they don't drink ANY milk actually), and they certainly don't mix up powdered soy isolate megapower shakes!

Aside from the hormone and processing issues, another consideration is that soybeans used in making the soy isolates and proteins are all sprayed to the max with pesticides and are GMOs, or genetically modified organisms. Genetic makeup of crops can be modified to make the plant grow bigger, be more resistant to bacteria or viruses, or be resistant to insects. A full 90 percent of all soy products used in the United States are GMOs. (Soybeans were the first GMO mass-produced crop in the mid-1990s.) GMO crops continue to remain under scrutiny for health concerns related to "gene transfer." When GMO foods are eaten, they are absorbed into the gastrointestinal tract. If the food was genetically modified to be resistant to bacteria, for example, that resistance could be transferred to the cells in your GI tract. This could mean problems in your gut, as the human body relies on certain "good" bacteria to maintain balance in your digestive system. Even when you want to avoid GMO products, labels that say "made with non-GMO soy" can be deceptive, as the product might be made with GMO *and* non-GMO soy and the labeling would still be accurate. To avoid GMO products, look for "organic"

> There's lots of crap flying around about soy. Get informed and make sure none of it sticks to you.

on the label and make sure all ingredients are organic. By law, organic foods cannot be GMOs. This is one time where buying organic might be worth it. But keep in mind that *soy protein isolates* are never organic. GMO crops, and the health concerns they potentially pose, continue to be studied and debated worldwide. There are many things in the past that were deemed "safe" by the powers that be that were reversed later because of overwhelming evidence. Case in point: the pesticide DDT.

Side note: In Europe, GMO foods are required to be labeled as such. Unfortunately, a recent battle in California was lost that would have required companies in the United States to specify on the label if a product contained GMO ingredients. Due to the efforts of major food giants like Kellogg, Coca-Cola, General Mills, Kraft Foods, Heinz, and others, millions of dollars were pumped into ad campaigns that swayed the public to vote the law down. With major corporations owning and running the majority of "organic" businesses these days, you may want to look twice at what they're passing off as "healthy organic food products." For a list of big companies that pose as small organic farms, go to www.OrganicConsumers.org. You can also find out more about GMO food at www.who.int; click on "Health Topics" to navigate to GMO foods.

If you're looking to soy for protein, it's one of the best places to look, as soy is the perfect protein for humans. But you don't need soy to get proper protein intake. Remember, there is protein in everything you eat, and eating "consciously" and including whole plant-based foods will provide you with the perfect amount of protein intake, as eating a plant-based diet will provide 8 to 10 percent protein, which conveniently, is the percentage of protein that should be included in a healthy diet. Here's a list for comparison. I've included tofu, veggie burgers, and soy milk for comparison purposes only.

FOOD	SERVING	PROTEIN (grams)
Tempeh	1 cup	41
Soybeans, cooked	1 cup	29
Lentils, cooked	1 cup	18
Veggie burger	1 patty	13
Chickpeas, cooked	1 cup	12
Tofu, firm	4 oz.	11
Quinoa, cooked	1 cup	8
Peas, cooked	1 cup	9
Peanut butter	2 tbsps.	8
Veggie dog	1 link	8
Spaghetti, cooked	1 cup	8
Almonds	1/4 cup	8
Soy milk, commercial, plain	1 cup	7
Almond butter	2 tbsps.	5
Spinach, cooked	1 cup	5
Broccoli, cooked	1 cup	4

I know, lots of info here. Skimmed through this health tip and just want the nutshell version? Here it is:

- Soy is a great source of protein, providing the kind of protein your body needs for total health, but it also contains hormonal components called isoflavones that can have variable effects depending on the amount and type of soy foods eaten.

- For those who never had cancer or who have a cancer that is not "hormonal," a little bit of soy (1 to 2 servings of healthy soy) in your diet can help prevent further cancer and heart disease. But if you don't normally eat soy, this may not be a reason to start. There are plenty of other things besides eating soy that you can do to reduce your risk.

- A 2012 study shows that women with a history of breast cancer (both ER-positive and ER-negative) who ate soy in their diets reduced their risk of their cancer coming back by 25 percent, but the study needs to be repeated and verified and a lot more questions answered before it is adopted as a rule.

- Organic whole soybeans are the best form of soy with the most beneficial health effects when used in moderation and as part of an overall plant-based diet.

- Fermented forms of soy like soybean miso and tempeh have health benefits that go beyond other forms of soy. They are minimally processed and aged, which makes them easier to digest, and typically very small amounts are used in cooking. These types of soy have been part of Asian cultures for thousands of years. Asian countries have among the lowest cancer incidence rates in the world.

- Soymilk, tofu, and soy cheese are processed forms of soy and are not as healthy as the whole or fermented forms and should not be your first choice when choosing a soy product. If you don't normally eat these types of foods, don't start now.

- Everyone should avoid soy supplements as they contain unnaturally high levels of isoflavones, the "hormone" part of soy.

- Soy protein isolates and hydrolyzed soy protein are highly chemically processed and unhealthy and don't resemble a soybean at all either visually or nutritionally. They may actually be doing some harm. Unfortunately, you are eating these forms of soy every day if you eat processed packaged foods. Check your labels.

- Using soybean oil, since there is no protein in it, does not have any effect on hormonal cancers or heart disease. Soy sauce, as long as it's made the traditional fermented way as opposed to using hydrolyzed soy, and does not contain preservatives or artificial coloring, has no effect, either positive or negative, on cancer either.

- It is important for you to follow the advice of your healthcare professional, but it is also important that your healthcare professional is well informed and up-to-date on the subject of soy.

Skipping the Line at the ER

Subtitle: "How I wound up spending Friday Evening Happy Hour at the Emergency Room."

Well, it all started with a little bird. While visiting my boyfriend Shawn one weekend, I discovered a nest right in one of the flowerpots, surrounded by dahlias and petunias.

I was so honored to have this feathery visitor to our garden that I decided to roll up my sleeves and do a major garden makeover. As I weeded, pruned, and mulched, I felt myself getting more and more tired. Not the normal tiredness that comes with a good honest day's work, but the low energy, chills, and sense of unwellness that could only mean one thing: an infection.

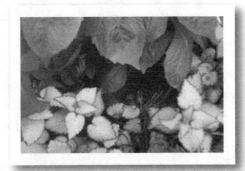

My plans for Friday evening involved sitting on my friend Kathy's patio, having "just-the-one" glass of wine, and enjoying the sunny weather—not sitting in a hospital waiting room! By that point in time, I figured that I had graduated to the status of "cancer survivor" and my trips to the ER were a thing of the past. On a brighter note, however, as soon as I mentioned my history of cancer, I was fast-tracked to the head of the long line! It came as a pleasant surprise to me that I was still getting perks, even though I was no longer technically considered a cancer patient. In no time, I found myself on a stretcher, hooked up to IV antibiotics, and dodging dirty looks from the many patients who had been biding their time waiting to be seen by a doctor. (I spoke to one guy who had been waiting for more than seven hours!)

Surrounded by the familiar hospital smells, the sound of the IV pump, and the feel of the needle in my arm, I found myself experiencing "chemo flashback." I was gripped with fear and a profound sadness, as I felt the hot tears bubble to the surface. *It is just not fair*, I thought. *I am done with cancer, why can't I just move on with my life?* Followed by, *Cancer will always be there, I will never be free of it.* And if that was not enough to really wind me up for a good cry, I added, *Shawn may as well go and find himself a healthy woman.*

I called my cousin Lil, intent on stepping the ole pity party up a notch, but to no avail. Rather than wallowing along with me, Lil said, "Oh, stop your boo-hooing. Forget the chemo flashback and pretend you are shooting up heroin or something!"

So, I ended up spending the entire weekend in the hospital, hooked up to IV antibiotics, and pretending that I was shooting up heroin, so as to avoid another episode of the dreaded chemo flashback. I did learn an important lesson from this experience. Cancer was not just a temporary disruption in my life. Even though my treatments had ended, the road to recovery was a long one. I just had to remind myself to not get discouraged.

Your cancer journey does not necessarily end
when your treatments end. Be prepared for
setbacks along your road to recovery.

HEALTH TIP #92
And as I Always Say, "The Road to Recovery Is Paved with Garlic"

I don't *always* say that, but I do love garlic, and I'm sure a lot of you have started to include more of this odoriferous (that means "smelly") bulb wherever you can in your diet because you've heard of the health benefits. The Greeks knew garlic was special, as they would feed it to their athletes before Olympic games. (I wonder if that's Michael Phelps's secret weapon?) But it's just recently that we are uncovering the science behind just how amazing these beautiful white cloves really are.

Garlic is in the Alliaceae family along with its cousins leeks, shallots, and onions. It is the substance *allicin*, which is contained in great quantities in garlic, that is responsible for its incredible antioxidant properties. In fact, science is discovering that the allicin in garlic is the most potent antioxidant producer there is. Antioxidants prevent oxidation from occurring at a cellular level. Oxidation is the breakdown of cells, causing system disease, aging, and cellular death.

The allicin in garlic breaks down into more than twenty different sulfide compounds (chemicals that contain sulfides) and each has particular benefits.

A recent Canadian study revealed one of the sulfides produced is *sulfunic acid*. Sulfunic acid is an extremely potent antioxidant. The allicin found in garlic decomposes very rapidly, thereby releasing an enormous amount of this acid that acts at an amazing speed in your body.

"The reaction between the sulfunic acid and radicals is as fast as it can get, limited only by the time it takes for the two molecules to come into contact. No one has ever seen compounds, natural or synthetic, react this quickly as antioxidants," stated the lead researcher on the team.

Good news for those of us who want to prevent cancer, heart disease, and getting old. (Okay, you'll still get old, but you'll look good doing it.)

Note: To release the most allicin out of your garlic, let it rest for fifteen minutes to one hour at room temperature after it is peeled or crushed before adding it to recipes—something not many of us do. Garlic used in cooking is very healthy, but eating it raw in recipes gives you the highest level of cancer-fighting benefits.

Along with the production of sulfunic acid, garlic also causes our bodies to produce more of the natural substance *hydrogen sulfide*. Elevated levels of naturally produced (your body actually *makes* this stuff) hydrogen sulfide also act like regulators that relax the blood vessels, promoting healthy blood flow to all areas of your body and promoting healthy blood pressure.

Boosting hydrogen sulfide production has also been shown to reduce the incidence of certain cancers, including breast, prostate, and colon.

It has also shown some promising effects on heart muscle tissue. Researchers at Albert Einstein College of Medicine found that injecting hydrogen sulfide into mice almost completely prevented the damage to heart muscle caused by a heart attack.

Garlic is best used as a fresh bulb. The studies on garlic pills is cloudy as it has not been verified that the amazing benefits of fresh garlic can be harnessed once it is ground into pill form.

To get the health benefits of garlic, you should eat at least two medium-sized raw cloves a day—that's two of the little pieces that come out of a whole bulb. Because the allicin is released as soon as the garlic is peeled, the health benefits of jarred cloves, while still present, are not as potent as fresh. Garlic stored in water at room temperature loses half its allicin in six days, and garlic stored in vegetable oil loses half its allicin in less than one hour.

Garlic is delicious in main dishes like veggies and pasta, but it also works equally well in snacks like hummus. If you've never had hummus, you're really missing out on a wholesome snack that is healthy *and* delicious. Made from chickpeas, it has the consistency of peanut butter and can be used as a spread on sandwiches, as a dip, or in wraps.

> Use garlic to keep evil *and* illness at bay.

Here's my favorite recipe for hummus. Traditional hummus contains tahini, a sesame paste, but tahini is not a normal staple of most kitchens, so I omitted it. If you happen to have some tahini lying around, you can throw in 1 tablespoon and add 15 calories, 1 gram of fat, and 0.5 gram of protein to the nutritional content of a serving size.

GARLIC-Y HUMMUS

YIELD: ABOUT 2 CUPS

1 (15-ounce) can chickpeas, drained and rinsed,
or 2 cups cooked chickpeas

2 tablespoons fresh lemon juice

2 tablespoons chopped fresh parsley
(dried flakes won't work here)

$1^1/_2$ tablespoons extra-virgin organic olive oil

2 cloves garlic, crushed (let it rest for 15 minutes
after it's peeled to get the most allicin!)

Dash of cayenne pepper

Dash of black pepper and sea salt, to taste

Directions:

If your chickpeas are not cooked, soak overnight and simmer in water $1^1/_2$ hours or until tender. (Note: soaked and cooked chickpeas contain no BPA, but canned may.)

Place all ingredients in food processor or blender and combine until creamy and smooth. Add some water if it's too thick. It should spread like peanut butter.

Use cut up celery, baby carrots, red peppers, raw summer squash, pita bread, or crackers to dip. This makes a great spread for sandwiches or in wraps.

Either eat together with your loved ones or use caution (or breath mints) with close contact.

NUTRITION PER $^1/_4$ CUP:

Calories: 65; Fat: 3 grams; Protein: 2.5 grams; Fiber: 2.5 grams

Eavesdropping on the Ward

There I was, months after my cancer treatments had ended, back in the hospital battling off an infection in the area of my incision (FYI, there are no perks of having infections). I'll admit, I am not one to share my living space with strangers. So anytime I had to stay in the hospital, I opted for a private room. Since this particular stay was an emergency, however, there were no private rooms available so I was forced to stay on a ward with the common folk. I know . . . I know . . . Beyoncé would never put up with that, and I seriously considered writing a stern letter to the hospital administration.

The interesting thing about sharing a room with three other people is the false sense of security that they get thinking that the thin curtain surrounding their beds (falling one foot short of the floor) provides any semblance of privacy. So while lying in my bed, staring at the ceiling, I overheard some doozies of conversations! Here is a sampling:

Conversation #1

Woman: I don't want the IV type of chemo; I want the pill. Mavis took the pill, and she didn't even lose her hair. I'll just tell the doctor to give me the pill. I'm sure it's all the same.

Man: Now, Mother, don't be hasty. I've heard that if you eat lots of corn niblets while you are on chemo, your hair will grow back all yellow and curly. Just think, you won't have to get your hair dyed or permed anymore!

(An actual conversation between a woman in her seventies and her son)

Conversation #2

Woman 1: IF SOMEONE DON'T GET ME SOME #@%#% DRUGS SOON, I'M GONNA BLOW THIS PLACE UP!

Woman 2: Calm down, Shelly. It is your own fault. If you hadn't been so drunk last night, you never would have fallen and broken your arm in the first place.

Woman 1: I'VE BEEN HERE FOR NEARLY TWELVE HOURS AND IF I DON'T GET OUTTA HERE SOON I'M GONNA STRANGLE SOMEONE WITH THIS @^%$**^ IV CORD!

(Don't quote me on this, but I believe that conversation happened between two nurses. However, I was a bit loopy from the drugs, so it could have been a patient and her friend.)

Conversation #3

Woman: *PPPPPFFFFFFFFFFFFFFFTTTTTTTTTTTTTTTT-tut-tut-tooooooooot!*

Me: Excuse me, lady, but that curtain does not stop noises from crossing over to my side of the room, nor does it stop smells!

(As an update to the corn conversation, another cancer survivor told me that the only thing she could keep down during her chemo treatments was creamed corn, and her hair NEVER grew back. I think it is safe to conclude from this one isolated case study that while eating corn niblets causes your hair to grow back yellow and curly, eating creamed corn causes permanent baldness. I cannot stress this enough people: eat NIBLETS!)

Even a hospital stay can be fun
if you keep a sense of humor about you.

HEALTH TIP #93
Need Fresh Niblets? Look in Your Neighborhood Markets

Food is one of those three necessities for life (the other two being water and air), and "unhealthy food" is just as bad for you as sucking in a lungful of exhaust fumes. Buying local is one way to ensure that the food you're eating is as healthy as possible. You may think that because you live in an urban area, there aren't any farms. That may be true, but it doesn't mean you can't get fresh local produce all season long.

Farmers Markets

Farmers markets are outdoor "instant" marketplaces that can be held seasonally or all year depending on the rules of the city. Farmers pay a price to set up a stand to sell to the public. These are all the rage, and there's probably a market very close to you no matter where you live. Some things to remember before you buy:

- Check out the website for the market you plan to visit and look at the rules for vendors. This will tell you what you're likely to find there. Some markets only sell food while others sell food and crafty items. Some markets require licensure to sell eggs, dairy products, or canned goods, while others do not. Some markets require all nonproduce foods to be prepared in a "community kitchen," which is an industrial kitchen you rent (rather than using your own kitchen), which ensures cleanliness. It's always nice to know that the strawberry preserves you put on your toast this morning weren't mixed up in Aunt Fannie's bathtub.

- Look for signs that say RESALE and then avoid that vendor. Most farmers markets require a sign be posted if the produce did not come from that specific vendor's farm. There are vendors who will take a trip down to a bigger farmers market or other farm, buy up bulk produce, and then try to sell it at a smaller market at higher prices to make a profit. A reputable market will have a market manager onsite on sales days and will be enforcing these rules.

- Know your produce. If you want figs and you know there's a vendor who has them, first research what the "perfect fig" looks like. If you are just browsing and you see some corn that you might want to buy, ask what variety it is and then make sure it looks like that variety. Check out the color, feel, and appearance. Strip down some of the husk and look for worms or deformed kernels (a sign of fungus). Ask the farmer about the variety of corn and what they use for pest control. Smart phones are great in these cases. If the farmer says it's Silver Queen variety, for example, you can look on a search engine to see if that variety is "in season" in your part of the country and what to look for when buying the perfect ear.

- The produce you buy at a local market is ripened on the vine or in the ground. You don't have to worry about forced ripened veggies. In supermarkets, mass-produced fruits and veggies are "gassed" by using ethylene gas to "force ripen" the produce so it looks better and more colorful. Advocates say it does not effect the taste, but anyone that has ever eaten a vine-ripened tomato versus a supermarket tomato can tell you that not only is the flavor better from a vine-ripened tomato but the consistency is better as well.

- You also don't have to worry about the wax coating applied to supermarket produce so they look pretty for you when you stroll down the aisle. We all know that the sweetest and most nutritious apple is not the prettiest one, but the one with the best personality.

- If you're not picky, go to the market about fifteen minutes before the market closes. Farmers DON'T want to lug all that unsold produce back home, so this would be a good time to stock up on those corn niblets and other great food.

Community Supported Agriculture (CSA)

If you want to support your local farmer and get top-quality produce, try a CSA. When you subscribe to a CSA, you get a weekly supply of produce from the farm you choose for a set price. The farm will give you a certain amount of produce in your weekly box, depending on what is harvested that week. CSAs not only give you fresh and local produce, but they also give you seasonal. Some CSAs require you to come to the farm to pick up your weekly stash, and others will deliver to pickup locations around the area on a certain day for your convenience.

CSAs are a win-win situation for the farmer and the consumer. You pay ahead of time, which helps the farmers prepare for the growing season, and they get to know who they are feeding. It allows the consumer exposure to many fruits and veggies that aren't available at the supermarket. Lots of farms will even include recipes that go along with the produce included with the weekly box.

The best part is, it's all run locally. The food goes from farmer to you with no middleman and no big-government involvement. (Let's see how long THAT lasts.) And the food is not limited to produce. Many CSAs offer milk, eggs, cheese, bread, or other goods that are made on the farm. The city or town usually monitors food safety regulations.

You can increase the quality of your food and help your local economy by shopping at CSAs and farmers markets. (They also have the freshest niblets in town.)

Now if you are a picky eater, CSAs may not be for you because you get what you get and that's what you have to eat. (Man, I sound like my mother.) But it's nice to know that you are supporting the farmer and the farmer is feeding you. There's no comparison as far as freshness and quality goes, and you'll be a part of a healthy community.

If you're thinking of joining a CSA, you may want to ask some questions of the farmers:

- How long have you been farming?

- How many people do you serve?

- Is everything in the box from your farm, and if no, where is it from?

- Did you have any problems last year? How were the crops?

- What do you use for pest control?

- Do I get a set box? Or can I choose my own produce to go in the box?

- Could I get some references from your current CSA customers?

To find a farmers market or a CSA in the United States in your area you can go to www.localharvest.org, or search: "find [your town] farmers market."

Living a Kick-Ass Life

S hortly after being diagnosed, I went to visit my cousin and lifelong friend, Lil. As she cracked open a bottle of Merlot, I proceeded to bawl my eyes out about my dismal future with cancer. Lil, being the no-nonsense person that she is, would have none of it. "Stop your whining," she said. "You will still be hot, even with one boob. You are going to beat this thing, and then you'll go on to live a kick-ass life. Mark my words!"

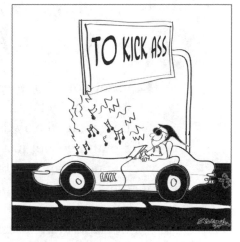

As I slowly transitioned from my cancer-fighting mode into survivor mode, I found myself fulfilling Lil's prophecy. I am living what I con-sider to be a kick-ass life! If you are having visions of me zip-lining, bungee jumping, or running with the bulls, let me stop you right there. I prefer to take my adrenaline rush in smaller doses, thank you very much. Take, for example, the time I put my SUV in the garage for repairs and was delighted to discover that my loaner for the day was a white sports car, complete with a full tank of gas, the new car smell, and a rockin' stereo! The old Flo would have been cautious about using this flashy vehicle, but kick-ass Flo said, "I'm taking this baby for a ride!"

I ignored my chores and spent my afternoon cruising along the coast, visiting garden centers and nurseries along the way (yes, folks, I am really living life on the edge now). I blatantly ignored the speed limits and even burned some rubber taking off from a stop sign. Bear in mind that an entire funeral procession once passed me on the highway, and I have been pulled over by the police for driving too slow. With my favorite tunes blasting on the stereo, I sang at the top of my lungs while playing imaginary drums on the steering wheel. *"Life is a highway, I wanna ride it all night long. . . ."* Drinking in the beauty of the scenic coastline on that perfect sunny day, I was simply buzzed on life!

> Go and live a kick-ass life,
> whatever that may mean to you.

HEALTH TIP #94
You've Kicked Ass, but Have You Kicked the Habit?

I am not going to bore you with the harmful effects of smoking. We all know them by heart.

Instead, let me try using some positive reinforcement to get you to consider quitting—not just for your health, but also for those around you. If you are not a smoker, but you love (or really, really like) someone who is, open the book to this page and leave it in a prominent place (such as next to their pack of cigs). It's not nagging if they just *happen* to see it.

Consider these facts:

- **After twenty minutes without a cigarette:** Heart rate and blood pressure normalize.

- **After twelve hours without a cigarette:** Carbon monoxide level drops to normal.

- **After one day without a cigarette:** Increased damage to skin stops.

- **After two days without a cigarette:** Taste buds start to regenerate. Nose hairs and nerves that effect smell begin to repair.

- **After two weeks without a cigarette:** Circulation begins to improve.

- **After three months without a cigarette:** Lung function improves up to 30 percent.

- **After one year without a cigarette:** Risk of heart disease is cut in half.

- **After five years without a cigarette:** Risk of cancer of the mouth, throat, esophagus, and bladder are cut in half. Risk of stroke is that of a non-smoker.

- **After ten years without a cigarette:** Risk of lung cancer is cut in half.

- **After fifteen years without a cigarette:** Risk of heart disease is the same as a nonsmoker.

Okay, I know I said I would keep this positive, but since you are already reading this . . .

- Cigarette smokers not only have a higher risk of heart and lung disease, but also erectile dysfunction, decreased sperm count, and macular degeneration, which is a leading cause of blindness.

- Secondhand smoke damage causes asthma, cancer, and sudden infant death syndrome. If you are smoking in your car with your child, even if you are holding the cigarette out the window, you are exposing them to the harmful effects of smoking.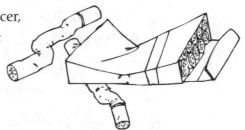

- Just because you don't smoke a pack a day doesn't mean you're fine. Even just two cigarettes a day have harmful effects.

- Cigarette smoking is the leading cause of heart and cardiovascular disease, accounting for more than 2.4 million premature deaths per year.

- When I was a nurse, I watched one of my favorite patients die of cancer. The last thing he did before he died was smoke a cigarette . (He was so weak, his family had to hold it up to his lips so he could take a drag.) He would always say, "How I wish to God I never picked one of these things up."

Good news and bad news . . .

Once you quit, your lungs will continue to heal for many months. Because of that, you may notice that you produce more mucous after you quit than while you were smoking. (This is usually when the quitter says, "To hell with this—I felt better on cigarettes.")

But realize that all the tiny goblet cells (cells that produce helpful mucous that eliminates impurities from your lungs) that were destroyed with smoking are growing back! They will produce mucus to try to clean out your lungs. Don't hate them! Nurture them along so they can do their job for you once again to keep your lungs clear of nasty impurities.

Naturopathic doctor, Negin Misaghi, has some tips to share on some things you can do to help your lungs heal. These tips can also be applied to any lung problems: asthma, bronchitis, or even just a cough from a cold.

- Smoking causes a deficiency in Lung Yin and Lung Qi (energy). Useful foods to nourish lungs include: rice, oats, carrots, mustard greens, sweet potato, yam, spinach, orange, peach, apple, watermelon, tomato, banana, string bean, flaxseed, clam, ginger, garlic, and spirulina and cholorella (types of algae).

- Try to include seaweed and flaxseed in your diet, which help to renew the mucous membranes that line the lungs.

- Mucous is good! The production of mucous is healthy in this case and is your body's way of expelling toxins and impurities. Don't stifle the mucous by taking antihistamines or drugs that "dry you up" unless absolutely necessary.

- Dairy causes the body to produce mucous. Since your lungs will already be producing excess mucous, limit or avoid your intake of milk, cheese, and yogurt.

- Increasing water intake will help to liquefy the mucus and help you to get rid of it. Steam will also help—either in the shower, or by making a tent holding a towel over your head as you lean over a pot of steaming water and breathe deeply. Adding Himalayan pink salt (available online or at health food stores) to the water will help even more.

- Increase your lung intake by taking walks, starting a yoga routine, or practicing mindful breathing or meditative breathing during the day. The air needs to be forced deep down in your lungs to go where air has never gone before.

- Stay away from other smokers for the obvious reason of cravings, but secondhand smoke will damage the lungs you are trying to heal.

- Stay away from air cleaners or automatic air filters that emit ozone into the air as these will compromise your lungs.

- Sadness, grief, and worry deplete Lung Qi and manifest as feelings of tightness in the chest, breathlessness, and sighing. Your meditation and deep breathing exercises will help here. Consider seeing a therapist if you have deeply rooted unresolved issues.

Remember:

- Never quit quitting! It takes most people four tries to quit, so if you've tried before, try again! Maybe this time it will take.

- The best results occur when therapy involves counseling and support groups as well as nicotine withdrawal medication. There are natural methods of quitting; however, because they are natural there is no good data to list success rates. I am not a proponent of unnecessary drugs, but in this case, if other methods, including natural ones, have not worked, the benefits of not smoking far outweigh the risks of taking prescription pharmaceuticals short term while you quit.

- If you need help with quitting you can check out these sites and consult your healthcare provider for more help:

  - ➤ www.smokefree.gov
  - ➤ www.helpguide.org/mental/quit_smoking_cessation.htm
  - ➤ www.cancer.org/Healthy/StayAwayfromTobacco/GuidetoQuitting Smoking/index
  - ➤ www.yourdiseaserisk.wustl.edu

Do I really have to list a healthy living tip here?

Cancer Helped Me to Find My Spirit

For many years, I described myself as a "spiritual seeker." What it was exactly that I was seeking, I am not quite sure. However, I invested thousands of dollars in hundreds of books by the top spiritual gurus of our day, such as Wayne Dyer, Eckhart Tolle, Thich Nhat Hanh, and Deepak Chopra. I also did classes and workshops on topics like Mindfulness Meditation, Reiki, Angel Therapy, and Crystal Therapy. In the back of my mind, I believed that if I only hit on the right book or the right course, I would be an enlightened spirit and my life would be fixed.

I figured there were many benefits to being an enlightened spirit. First of all, it would allow me to master the Law of Attraction, and I would be showered with prosperity and love (by "love" I mean a good man, as I was also seeking that!). Secondly, my intuition would be magnified to the point that, not only would I always make the right decisions based on my gut feelings, but I might even develop psychic skills. Then I would get to impress my friends by saying stuff like, "Jackie, I see you on a plane. Are you planning a trip in the near future?" Most important, I would be able to live my life in a state of blissful peace and not be bothered by worldly problems. Yes, my friends, all of the secrets of the universe would be revealed to me if I could just find that one enlightening book or course.

I developed a ritual of spiritual exercises, which I practiced every day. As the term *exercise* implies, it was hard work. I often did not feel like hauling my butt out of bed at 6 AM to do the spiritual work, but visions of myself as an enlightened spirit kept me going. So each morning I would sit on the cold hard floor, in an uncomfortable position, and try to quiet my mind in meditation.

After my diagnosis, I decided to cut myself some slack. I continued to do my meditations, but instead of sitting in a traditional meditation pose on the floor, I would lie on my bed or just sit on a comfortable chair. Rather than do Mindfulness of Breathing meditation (which often just irritated me because I could never seem to quiet my mind), I decided to listen to guided meditation CDs. This allowed me to combine my deep breathing exercises with visualization. Guess what? Meditation wasn't work anymore; it actually became fun! I started rising at 5:30 each morning to allow me extra time to relax and listen to these guided meditations. This form of meditation instills in me a feeling of love, joy, and peace, which I try to carry into my day.

Reading my many books has been an important part of my spiritual education. However, rather than seek out new books and gurus after my diagnosis, I began to reread my old favorites. I discovered that the words of these great teachers were different when read through the lenses of cancer. I began to discover common themes that ran through many of these books, themes such as the importance of self-love and forgiveness (even the Lord's Prayer talks of forgiveness), living in the present moment, and using the power of positive thinking and affirmations.

When cancer came into my life, I did not really have time to pursue my spiritual seeking by pushing myself to meditate harder, read more books, or do more courses. Ironically, when I stopped seeking, I discovered that what I had been looking for was there all along. I found my spirit!

How do I know when I am connected with my spirit? It is when I experience that feeling of joyful bliss. This feeling did not come from reading a book or doing a course. Rather, it pops up when I am gardening, meditating, hugging my children, or just looking at a beautiful sunset. Becoming an "enlightened spirit" did not suddenly "fix" my life or shower me with wealth (although I DID find a good man!). Becoming an enlightened spirit meant simply realizing that God is within me and all around me. When I am seeking that connection to the divine, I can find it in the eyes of my children or in a single flower.

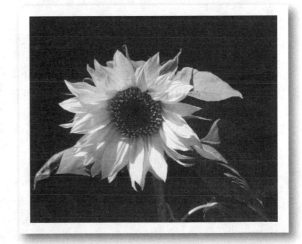

Sunflower grown by Flo's son, Ben

> "If we could see the miracle of a single flower clearly,
> our whole life would change."   —Buddha

HEALTH TIP #95
If You're Going to Breathe, Be Mindful

I can't emphasize breathing enough. Yes, if you are reading this, you are breathing right now and it is automatic, but *mindful* breathing is different. With mindful breathing you can bring your mind (and your body) to a place of peace and, in doing so, reduce stress and improve your health in many ways. Unlike deep breathing or meditative breathing, mindful breathing can be done anywhere at any time.

Peter Doobinin, founder and guiding teacher at Downtown Meditation Community in New York, gives some helpful instruction to improve on what you have been doing all your life. Peter states:

> As human beings, we breathe every moment of our lives. And yet, we pay very little attention to our breathing. If, however, we learn to be mindful of our breath, it will have great impact on the quality of our well-being.
>
> It's helpful to put aside some time every day, to step back from the busyness of our lives, and to meditate, to practice being mindful of the breath. It's also extremely helpful to be mindful of the breath at different times during the day, as we go about our daily tasks. We can be mindful of the breath at almost any time, while we're working, driving a car, talking to our kids. Nobody even has to know!
>
> In being mindful of the breath, you put your attention on the movement of the breath. You feel the breath, at one specific place. It could be the nose, the throat, the chest, the abdomen. You put your mind on the breath and you attempt to keep it there. If your mind drifts off, bring it back to the breath. If it drifts off again, bring it back again. It may wander off, like a young child, again and again. That's okay. Just keep bringing it back.

When practicing mindfulness of breathing, it's important to put your mind on the breath at some point where the breath feels comfortable. If your belly hurts, don't feel the breath there; choose another spot, perhaps the nose.

As you're mindful of your breath, allow it to be easeful, pleasant-feeling. The breath, by its nature, is easeful, pleasurable. So you don't have to try to "make it" that way. Simply allow it to be comfortable. You can tell yourself: "Breathe in the most comfortable way." Then get out of the way. Let your body breathe comfortably. Defer to your body's innate wisdom. It knows what to do; it knows how to breathe comfortably, easefully.

If you make a regular habit of being mindful of the breath, you'll certainly come to know many benefits. You'll experience greater ease, greater well-being. You'll begin the crucial process of learning to let go of your excessive thinking. Thinking is a manifestation of stress. When we're mindful of the breath, we move our awareness from the thinking realm, into the body. We begin to de-stress. We begin to experience tranquility.

Tranquility . . . doesn't that sound nice? And you'll get it just from breathing!

When I first started to practice mindful breathing it was weird. I would try to breathe a certain way and control it and then I would get out of breath! I must have looked like an idiot sitting there . . . very quietly . . . hyperventilating! When I continued to practice, it got a lot easier. Now I can do it anywhere. (I'm doing it right now. . . .)

> Be the most thankful for your breath, because without it, you have nothing.

It wasn't until I could be mindful without trying to control my breathing that it made sense. It really is very calming and brings you back if you're anxious or have a lot on your mind. It's also a great metaphor for life. Be *mindful* but don't try to *control* it. Just let it happen.

Just breathe. . . .

Realizing I Am Worth It

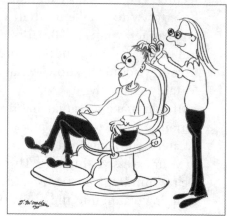

When I lost all of my hair just two weeks after starting chemo, I was not the least bit disturbed. I had heard many stories of women whose pre-chemo hair was replaced by a head of luxurious curls when their chemo ended. I never did really like my hair; it was too thin, too fine, and too mousey brown. I would gladly sacrifice that hair for a big mane of sexy curls!

After chemo ended, I would rush off to a mirror every morning and examine my head under a bright light, eagerly anticipating my chemo curls. But, alas, they never appeared. Instead of the prize-winning locks, I got the consolation prize: even thinner than before, baby-fine hair, with what I can only describe as bald patches on the top and sides. While I was grateful that I had some hair, I couldn't shake the feeling that I had somehow been ripped off!

I promised myself that, as soon as this hair was long enough, I would go some place nice to have it styled by a professional who could at least give the illusion of nice hair. For weeks I agonized over where to go. I finally settled on a place that, from the outside, looked upscale yet affordable.

As soon as I walked in, I knew I had made the right choice. I had never seen so many beautiful people (the staff) gathered in one place. I was lost in a sea of flawless skin, gorgeous hair, and impeccable clothes . . . and that was just the men! Several of the staff approached me at the same time to take my coat and offer me tea, coffee, or a glass of wine from the minibar. A GLASS OF WINE, NO LESS! I had never before been offered a glass of wine at a hair salon—how classy. Oh yes, I had come to the right place all right!

Next, Stephen, my stylist, colored my hair, and I was treated to a complimentary paraffin wax treatment on my hands. I couldn't take my eyes off my beautiful and youthful image in the mirror. Stephen confessed that the salon uses special lighting and mirrors to shave ten years off your reflection. ("If I have to look at myself in a mirror all day, I wanna look good!" said Stephen.) I was feeling pretty pampered by that time, but next came the piece de resistance: the shampoo room.

Folks, I kid you not, the shampoo room exceeded any spa experience that I have ever had. The room was dimly lit with soft music, candles, and aromatherapy. But the best part of all was the leather, heated, massage chair, which gently massaged my back, buttocks, and legs as I had my hair washed. To say, "had my hair washed" is a gross understatement. Actually, a beautiful man gently and expertly massaged my head and neck for a good twenty minutes. I thought I had died and gone to heaven, I could not stop myself from smiling.

Suddenly, a thought occurred to me that completely wiped the smile off my face: *Wine? Complimentary hand treatment? Massage?* I was way out of my league. I could not afford this place! I felt myself panic as I mentally calculated how much wiggle room I had left on my VISA.

Sure enough, when I went to check out it was confirmed: This type of treatment comes at a price. Let's just say, the hundreds I had saved by not having my hair done in over a year? Gone in one fell swoop. What did I do? Well, I smiled, added a generous tip, and walked out of there feeling like a million bucks. Because I am worth it!

Chemo can wreak havoc on your hair and skin. When your treatments end, book yourself a day at the spa. You are worth it!

HEALTH TIP #96
You Are Also Worth Safe Spa Products

Your skin is a sponge. I don't mean a smelly old kitchen sponge. I mean a beautiful soft sea sponge that will deeply absorb anything applied to it.

Most women don't really pay attention to what they apply to their skin, especially if the commercial for the said skin product shows a woman with a flawless face twirling in a flowery field of daisies and promises that you will be twirling in daisies with a flawless face too, if you just use their product. (Never mind that the product contains three different chemical preservatives and four different cancer-causing agents.)

Manufacturers are very tricky when it comes to cosmetics and skin care. They know marketing, and they spend millions of dollars on knowing just the right things to show you or say in the ad that will get you to hand over your money. But what exactly are you paying for? Sometimes it's hard to know. The ingredients for many cosmetics may not be listed on the packaging, or it may be listed so small you can't read them. When you can read them, the ingredients look like they belong on a chemistry teacher's shopping list. You are smarter than that.

> Make sure you know what you're putting on your body, because it ultimately ends up in your body.

It is possible to choose healthy, wholesome products and look equally as flawless (and still twirl in those daisies). You just have to know what to look for.

It is a common misconception that there are government rules and regulations in place to test cosmetics for safety. The fact is, the United States currently has no such regulations in place (for the past several years, legislation has been proposed, but the proposals have yet to make it out of committee). As a result, more than 500 products available in the United States contain ingredients that were banned by other countries. So it is up to you to know what is contained in that lotion that you slather on your face twice a day. Here are some quick general tips to help you choose the right one:

- Look at the list of ingredients. Is the list short? Or does it require a foldout label and a translator? Do you recognize the first four ingredients on the list? Ingredients are listed in the order of highest percentage, so the first four should be recognizable. If you don't know what they are, take the time to look them up on several sites and cross-check for accuracy to see if they pose a health risk (www.safecosmetics.org).

- Watch out for tricky labeling. You may see a label that lists the "active ingredients." Those are the only ingredients that the company wants to reveal to you. Sometimes you have to go to their website or actually call a 1-800 number to get the entire full list of ingredients. And when they play this game, the other ingredients usually are hidden for a reason.

- Since the United States doesn't certify cosmetics to be organic, choose a company that has organic certification in another country.

- Watch out for words like *natural* and *made with organic ingredients*, which has absolutely no meaning in cosmetic labeling. A label that states, "made with organic ingredients" can still contain other, not-organic, cancer-causing ingredients.

- Avoid mineral oil as this might as well be named "motor oil." It literally is derived from the same fossil fuels, and since you don't drink motor oil, neither should your skin. Mineral oil ("baby-type" oil) does nothing to improve the health of your skin. It covers and sometimes smothers your skin, but inside, your body literally rejects it. Many plant-based oils, like coconut oil, are structurally similar to sebum, the oil substance your skin naturally produces for moisture, and are a much healthier and logical choice.

- We are suckers for pretty labels. A green bottle made of bamboo does not mean what's in that bottle is natural. If you're concerned about it coming from nature, just get the 411 on the ingredients.

Clean up your facial beauty products. Then clean your face.

The Opportunity to Help Other People

Sometimes in conversation, I will casually mention something about my psychic, and it generally results in a few raised eyebrows. To me, my annual psychic reading is as normal as my annual dental checkup. I don't think it is weird at all. In fact, I have been going to psychics on a regular basis for fifteen years, not just to get a sneak peek into my future (although that has been very helpful at times), but more important, to help guide me on my life path.

For the past four years, I have been going to Kelliena (www.kelliena .com). The last time I spoke to her in person was in Halifax in July 2011, three months after I had been diagnosed with breast cancer. At that point, my treatments had not yet started, and I was unsure of my prognosis for survival.

When Kelliena started the session by asking if I had any questions, I frantically said, "Do you see any sickness or death around me?!"

She gazed over my shoulder and then looked back to me and said, "No, they are rejoicing!" (By "they" she meant my angels and spirit guides, of course.)

Rejoicing! I thought. *What kind of back-stabbing angels and guides are you anyway to rejoice at my misfortune?*

The thought had barely entered my mind when Kelliena once again gazed over my shoulder and continued, "They are telling me that you are going to help so many people through your journey with cancer."

Well, that meant diddlysquat to me at that time. I was just trying to survive one day at a time and could not understand how *my* cancer was going to help *other* people. I dismissed her prediction and forgot all about it. Fast forward to five months later. My blog was taking off, and I was getting hundreds of comments and e-mails from my readers. One lady, a nurse, commented: "You are going to help so many people through this blog." BINGO! Kelliena's prediction came back to me, and, finally, it made perfect sense.

After more than twenty years of working in the helping profession, being unable to work due to my cancer treatments was a real challenge for me. In total, I was away from my workplace for seventeen months. During that time, however, it gave me a great deal of personal satisfaction to know that I was still helping people through my blog, even if just by bringing a smile to someone's face. And I pray that as you read this book, you will find something in my words to make your journey a little easier.

Just because you have cancer does not
mean you can't be of service to others.

HEALTH TIP #97
Just Because You Are Not a Scientist
Doesn't Mean You Can't Understand the Research

The news media loves big headlines such as "New Study Shows Vitamin D Ineffective." This was actually a headline not long ago. Can you imagine the surprise and the level of interest that was generated among the tens of thousands of people taking vitamin D supplements? But that's exactly what the news media wanted. It forced those with an interest, and that was a lot of people, to tune in for the details. When you hear headlines like these that are alarming, don't jump to conclusions. First, ask yourself these questions: *What kind of study? Where was it done? Who sponsored the study? Who is reporting the study? How many people were involved? Was this a new study or one that was replicated? What were the actual results?*

Once these questions are answered, you can decide if this news is noteworthy or not.

What Kind of Study?

Research studies can be done many different ways. Studies always start with a question, called a hypothesis, and a guess as to how the questions will be answered. Then a method is determined to get the answer. Some studies are done by observing the effects on different groups. There are usually one or two groups that receive the "drug" or "treatment" and a control group that does not, so a comparison can be made as to whether the drug or treatment was effective.

Sometimes the study is a study of other studies. Research results from experiments that have already been done, which all asked the same question, are compiled into one big study of data. One scientist will look at all those studies, use that data, and come up with one conclusion. When listening to results from these types of studies it's important to consider "causal relationships." For example, if a scientist looked at rain and open umbrellas, she might conclude that the open umbrellas caused the rain because when you see one, you see the other, just as a child might conclude that darkness is caused by putting on pajamas. The two events may be related, but one did not cause the other.

Where Was It Done?

Think about what is being studied and where it was done. If a drug is being tested, more credibility would be given to studies done at a university, for example, than the drug company's research lab.

Who Sponsored the Study?

The funding makes a big difference in how much credibility the study has, although it may be good data anyway. For example, I saw a headline that read, "Milk Fights Cancer." After I read the study a bit, I realized it was a study funded 100 percent by one of the big American dairy associations. When I looked more closely at the study, the title was exaggerated at best.

Who Is Reporting the Study?

Studies can be tilted this way and that to get the outcome that is favorable to certain agendas. It may be discovered that vitamin X is just as effective for a certain illness as drug Z. The company that manufactures drug Z might publicize a study showing the negative side effects of vitamin X, for example.

How Many People Were Involved?

Was it a study of 10 people or 10,000 people? The credibility goes hand in hand with the size of the study.

Was This a New Study or One That Was Replicated?

Good science depends on data that can be reproduced over and over to get the same result each time. If this is a brand-new study with new findings, I would want to see if the results could be reproduced by someone else.

What Were the Actual Results?

In the example I gave at the start of this health tip, the headline read, "New Study Shows Vitamin D Ineffective." After reading the entire study from the actual source and not a news-reporting source, the actual facts were that for osteoporosis, vitamin D is ineffective in older populations in doses lower than 800 IUs per day. What they didn't bother to report was that it was shown to be highly effective for preventing osteoporosis in older populations in doses between 800 and 2,000 IUs per day. The news reported only part of the story, and it caused quite a stir. It made me so angry to think that there were older folks who, after hearing that misquoted news report, decided not to take their vitamin D, putting them at greater risk for osteoporosis.

> Research is great when it is credible and unbiased. When you hear news that might affect you, stop and get the real facts before you accept it as true.

Scientific research is how we learn what works and what doesn't. Make sure you find out all the facts and read the study for yourself at the source before making any changes in your routine.

Raising Awareness

When my son, Ben, was three years old, I knew there was something wrong. Having nearly twenty years of experience as an educational psychologist, I analyzed the possible diagnoses: cognitive delay, learning disability, autism, or some other syndrome? Whatever they called it, it would not change the reality of his deficits. He could not talk, his motor skills were delayed, and he had no desire to socialize with other people. When he was finally diagnosed with autism in April 2008, I breathed a sigh of relief. If he was going to wear some label to describe his lack of communication and socialization skills, then the autism label gave him the best chances of getting the support he needed. There is a huge awareness campaign around the autism spectrum disorders these days. Awareness brings lobbying, which brings money, which brings solutions. Since Ben's diagnosis we have had a trained ABA therapist come to our home every day to work with him, paid for by the government. That is what comes of increasing awareness.

Many people question the value of raising awareness, and just what it is that we are raising awareness of. Personally, I think that awareness is a good thing, as resources will go to where awareness is the greatest. One of the perks of having cancer for me is that it puts me in the position to help raise awareness about this disease and, hopefully, be part of the force that helps to finally find a cure.

When Susan and I decided to write this book together, we committed to raising awareness for a cancer charity. With so many good charitable organizations out there, we had a difficult time narrowing down our choice. The obvious choice for us was to support Stand Up To Cancer. What appeals to us most about this organization is its nonpolitical nature.

When I was first diagnosed, I had no idea about the politics of breast cancer. In some ways, the breast cancer community can be likened to a battlefield with two distinct camps: "survivors" (defined by some as those who "beat cancer") versus stage-4 (metastatic breast cancer or MBC) patients. Susan and I were both very lucky in that our cancer was discovered at stage

3, before it had metastasized to distant sites. At the moment, there is no evidence of disease in our bodies. However, we don't view ourselves as being in different camps from those with MBC, or from anyone with any type of cancer for that matter. The way we see it, being a survivor is all about attitude, not about the presence or absence of cancer cells in one's body.

It surprised me to learn about the politics of cancer and how each faction seems to be in competition for their own piece of the "find-a-cure" pie. The bottom line is this: At the moment, there is no cure for any type of cancer. On this battlefield, we are all fighting the same fight. Right now, those with stage 4 are at the front lines of the battle. However, the sad truth is, when one of our comrades falls, there will likely be another of us called to the front lines to take his or her place.

What we like about Stand Up To Cancer is their mission to encourage collaboration instead of competition among the entire cancer community. This is very fitting with our mission, which is to help those with cancer realize that it is possible to live a healthy and a happy lifestyle, regardless of your diagnosis. No matter what the stage of cancer, or what the body part affected, we all want the same thing: a world that is free from cancer. Let not our differences divide us! **This is where the end of cancer begins: when we unite in one unstoppable movement and Stand Up To Cancer.**

Being part of an awareness campaign can be a very rewarding experience. Reward yourself by taking on a cause.

HEALTH TIP #98   The Rewards of Broccoli

Mention broccoli to some and you will get an immediate wrinkled-nose reaction. I honestly think the people that don't like it have never really eaten it without prejudice. When you're a kid and you are "forced" to eat something, it survives in your memory as something horrid and you avoid ever eating it again.

But broccoli and the whole cruciferous family (Brussels sprouts, cabbage, kale, cauliflower, bok choy, cabbage, arugula, watercress, radishes, and turnips) contain the highest levels of cancer-fighting substances found in nature. Two, in particular, have been shown to inhibit the development of cancer. Indole-3-carbinol and sulforaphane are produced from the digestion of cruciferous veggies. Once in your system, they reduce inflammation, protect the body from cell damage, and render carcinogens helpless. Including cruciferous veggies in your diet has been shown to be a factor in lowering your risk of prostate, colorectal, lung, and breast cancer. And the research continues. There are cancer drugs that are currently being developed for use as treatment that are derived from diindolylmethanes commonly found in cruciferous veggies. How's *that* for powerful?

The way most people eat broccoli is by smothering it with cheese or cream sauces. Adding dairy and extra fat to this green goddess is like putting aluminum siding on the Taj Mahal. Yeah, you can do it . . . but why would you?

If we put our heads (of broccoli) together there are more ways to prepare it than just boiling it. Boiling broccoli, or any vegetable for that matter, removes many of the important nutrients and they get dumped down the drain after cooking. If you don't believe me, just check the color of the water after you've boiled some.

Steaming is much healthier and easier, and cooking this way eliminates the risk of burnt food. Steaming broccoli also retains that beautiful dark green color. If you don't have a steamer, simply place a metal colander on top of a large pot filled with about five inches of water. The colander should fit securely on the pot and not be touching the water. Place the washed broccoli in the colander and cover. (It's okay if some of the steam escapes out from the sides. It will still cook properly.) Turn the heat on high and allow the water to boil under the colander for about 15 minutes or until the desired tenderness. Stir-frying or quick frying in a tiny bit of oil is another healthy preparation method. But before you reach for the melted cheddar cheese, try topping this green miracle with melted plant-based butter like Healthy Balance mixed with finely ground nuts like almonds, or just drizzle olive oil and lemon juice over it and finish with pine nuts and a pinch of sea salt.

Another way of eating your veggies is to use them in healthy recipes. This one makes a good side dish or paired with a salad for a main dish. This recipe uses broccoli and has the word *cake* in the name. See? You can have your broccoli and eat your cake, too.

BROCCOLI CAKES

YIELD: 15 CAKES

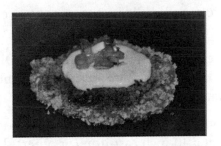

1 large head of broccoli, larger stalks removed (about 6 cups)

$1/2$ cup prepared quinoa

3 tablespoons olive oil, preferably extra-virgin organic,
plus more for cooking

5 to 6 scallion greens, chopped to make 1 cup

1 small onion, chopped

2 cloves of garlic, crushed

$1^1/2$ cups cooked chickpeas (garbanzos)
or 1 (15-ounce) can, rinsed

1 teaspoon sea salt

$1/4$ teaspoon black pepper

$1/2$ teaspoon paprika

1 teaspoon turmeric

$1/4$ teaspoon celery salt

1 cup unbleached all-purpose flour

2 cups panko-style breadcrumbs

$1^1/2$ tablespoons Old Bay or other seafood seasoning

White Sauce (optional)

$1/2$ cup vegan mayonnaise

2 scallions, whites only, finely chopped

1 teaspoon lemon juice

Directions:

1. Wash and cut broccoli, small stems and florets, into chunks. Steam for 20 minutes or until broccoli is tender when pierced with a fork. Meanwhile, cook quinoa according to directions on the package. Set aside.

2. Sauté scallions, onion, and garlic in 2 teaspoons of olive oil over medium heat until onions are translucent (8 to 10 minutes).

3. Add all ingredients except flour, breadcrumbs, and Old Bay to food processor. Add 2 teaspoons of olive oil and pulse until blended. Process on high until very smooth. Transfer to bowl and add the flour. Mix well.

4. In a small bowl, combine Panko crumbs, 1 tablespoon olive oil, and Old Bay, and mix well. Heat a 10-inch cast-iron (or other) skillet and add a tablespoon of oil. Disperse evenly. Using a $1/4$ cup scoop or large spoon, and filling just shy of full, drop batter into breadcrumb mixture and coat evenly. Use a spoon to help coat the batter, as the batter will be sticky. Place coated batter in the pan and press down slightly with the back of the spoon to flatten. Three cakes should fit in a 10-inch skillet. Cook about 8 minutes on each side until sides are golden. Add 2 teaspoons of oil to pan for each additional batch.

Broccoli is the vegetable that loves you back.

5. For white sauce, mix vegan mayo, scallion whites, and lemon juice well. Top broccoli cakes with white sauce if desired and garnish with chopped scallion greens.

NUTRITION:

Serving size: 1 cake

Two cakes provide you with 130% of your daily intake of vitamin C.

Calories: 180; Fat: 7.7 grams; Protein: 4.5 grams; Fiber: 2.8 grams; Vitamin C: 65% of the RDA; Iron: 6.6% of the RDA

White sauce serving size: 1 teaspoon

Calories: 43; Fat: 4 grams

Cancer Introduced Me to a New Way to Get a Buzz

"Hello, my name is Florence and I am a blogger. I knew it was becoming a problem when I started to steal time away from my kids to blog. Eventually, I just let myself go. I found myself checking my blog stats rather than brushing my teeth. Of course, the inevitable happened. I got a cavity. God, I'll never forgive myself for that. But I just couldn't resist the buzz. That's when I decided to join Bloggers Anonymous."

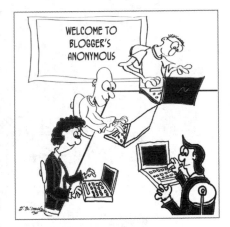

Okay, it didn't actually get to the point of having to join a 12-step program (and the jury is still out on what caused the cavity), but the truth is, I am hooked on blogging! It gives me a buzz that I can only compare to buying new clothes or finding a great deal on potted perennials.

You see, I am the type of person who loves to set concrete, measurable goals for myself, goals like: lose 5 pounds, run 10 kilometers, or find 100 perks of having cancer. The closer I get to my goal, the more excited I get. So you can just imagine my anticipation as I sat on the cusp of one of the greatest victories of my life: finding 100 perks of having cancer!

Hey, I heard that—some of you are questioning how writing a blog can be considered such a victory. Not to toot my own horn, but finding 100 good things about having cancer was no easy task. Being so close to my goal, I felt like I was nearing the end of a marathon, and I was simply HIGH on my sense of accomplishment.

Even though I make jokes about my cancer experience, I would like to make it clear that my goal has never been to make light of this very serious illness. For me, focusing on the perks was my way of staying positive through a very difficult time in my life. I did not write these perks after I was declared "cancer-free" and looking back on the experience through rose-colored glasses. Rather I wrote them while undergoing treatments and surgeries and not knowing what the outcome would be for me. Blogging not only provided a great distraction from my illness, it also gave me a positive and creative outlet for my feelings. Writing my blog, and now this book, has certainly been one of the most therapeutic perks of having cancer.

Don't let cancer stop you from
setting goals for yourself.

HEALTH TIP #99
If Your Goal Is Healthier Eating,
Start with Your Cookware!

Yes, throw away those pots and pans made of Teflon, aluminum, and silicone. They may be making you sick, and there is a healthier, cheaper, and more logical solution: **cast iron**.

Cast-iron pots have been around for thousands of years (yes, thousands!) The material for cast iron comes from iron ore, found in the earth, mixed with oxygen and carbon. A molten mixture is made by superheating, and then the mixture is poured into sand casts and cooled. When the cast is cooled, the sand is blasted off and voilà! A pan is made. No matter who you buy from or where you find your pans, all cast-iron pots and pans have been made the same way for the past 130 years. Beware of cast iron from China, however, as the quality of iron ore is subpar and can give your cookware "hot spots" instead of an even, uniform heat.

What's wrong with Teflon, calphalon, and copper? To begin with, the U.S. government has mandated that all Teflon manufacturers change the chemical composition of Teflon by the year 2015. Until then, the nonstick pots and pans will be emitting toxic gasses when heated, putting us at risk for cancer and causing flulike symptoms and possible birth defects.

Calphalon is a nonstick chemical made with aluminum. The research is not conclusive, but there are indications that cooking in aluminum can increase risks of Alzheimer's disease and multiple sclerosis.

Copper is fine healthwise, but it's crazy expensive. Who wants to spend $90 on an eight-inch fry pan?

Cast Iron Makes Sense in So Many Ways

- Cast iron is very affordable. Not only can you get complete sets of cookware for about $50, but also if you look, you are sure to find cast-iron pots and pans at yard sales and thrift stores for just a few bucks. No matter what the conditions, they can always be reseasoned (the term for getting the surface back to being "cookable").

- Cast iron will never peel, flake, chip, or warp . . . ever!

- The best cast iron is old cast iron. You can use the same pan for hundreds of years and beyond. Pass it down to your kids, grandkids, and great-grandkids! The more you use it, the better it gets.

- Cast iron retains heat better than other pans so your food stays hot even after the stove is off. The heat is distributed more evenly, making it the favorite cookware for shallow or deep-frying and the preferred cookware of master chefs.

- Cooking in cast iron increases the iron content in your food. Iron is an important mineral for overall health.

- A well-seasoned cast-iron pan far surpasses any chemical nonstick surface for supreme "nonstickiness." Food slides out without a spatula.

- You can move food from stove top to oven without concern.

- If you don't like black cookware, you can choose enameled cookware in a variety of colors. The enameled version has all the same properties as the black cast iron, but it can match your kitchen. (The enamel can chip, but that's the only difference.)

- You can use cast iron outdoors over an open fire and indoors on electric or gas heat.

- Cast-iron pans make excellent weapons. One hit over the head and your assailant is stopped in his tracks (or has a face in the shape of a frying pan).

- Cast iron comes in a multitude of shapes and sizes. You can get muffin and cornbread pans in fun shapes like cactus or ears of corn.

Cast-Iron Care Is Easy

- Never use soap! Wash with hot water and a stiff nylon brush. If food is stuck, add some water and place it back on the stove. The heat will boil the stuck residue off. Never put cast iron in the dishwasher.

- Towel-dry immediately. Do not air dry, as water is your pan's enemy.

- Never place a hot pan into cold water as it could cause thermal cracking.

- Use nonmetal utensils to avoid scratching the "seasoned" surface.

- Apply a light coating of oil to the pan while it's still a bit warm before putting it away.

So Why Doesn't It Ever Rust?

The secret is in the seasoning. Oil must be baked in and continually applied to make the surface water resistant. If your pan is not seasoned properly or not cared for, it can rust. But the great thing is, you can always reseason to restore it back to its original cooking condition. You literally cannot destroy it!

Most pans you get new are "preseasoned," which means they are ready for the stove or oven. But if you've found one at a garage sale or left one sitting in water, it can cause the pan to get dull, light gray areas on the surface. When this happens, it needs reseasoning. Here's how:

- Scour off rust or dull areas with a fine steel wool.

- Wash in hot soapy water (yes, this time, you can use soap) using a stiff brush.

- Apply a thin even coating of melted cooking oil of your choice inside and out.

- Place foil or cooking sheet on the bottom rack of the oven to catch any oil drips.

- Set oven to 350 to 400°F.

- Place cookware upside down on the top rack of the oven.

- Bake for 1 hour. When done, turn the oven off, but leave the pan in.

- When cooled, store in a dry place and use as if new.

Another great reason to use cast iron is your goal to get stronger arms. Since cast iron is heavy, the more cooking you do, the stronger you'll get. Cook more . . . get strong and healthy. Watch for my DVD: *The Frying Pan Workout.* (I'm kidding, of course.)

I love my cast-iron pans, and I now have a set that allows me the pleasure of using only cast iron for everything I cook. I have two from my mom and my mother-in-law, and then I bought a set from Lodge. Founded by Joseph Lodge, this family-owned company has been making cast-iron cookware since 1896 and is the number-one company making cast iron in the United States today. You can visit them at www.lodgemfg.com to start or add to your cookware collection. They also have great recipes and cookware tips.

> Cooking with cast iron is not only healthy; it's smart and economical, too.

You might even become such a fan that you will want to join the International Dutch Oven Society. Check out their website (www.idos.com) for tips and recipes. "Come an' git it" indeed.

I Am a Survivor!

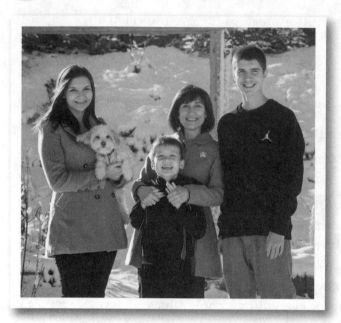

When I began my blog in October 2011, I described myself as: *"A forty-four-year-old breast cancer 'warrior' . . . meaning that I am actively battling the disease, but not yet far enough along to call myself a 'survivor.'"* I believed that the term *survivor* was reserved for those who were declared cancer-free and that I had not yet earned myself that title. I figured that once my treatments were done, and there was no evidence of disease left in my body, only then could I call myself a survivor.

On March 30, I drove myself to the hospital for my last radiation treatment. As I walked back to my car afterward I thought, *So, this is it. It's done. Can I now finally call myself a survivor?* There were no banners or fireworks to mark the occasion. No news camera crews were rushing at me asking, "So, Florence, how does it feel to be a survivor?" In fact, the staff at the Cancer Center hadn't even bothered to get me a cake. It was then that I made an important realization.

Being a survivor is not about killing cancer cells. For all I know, there could still be tiny, living cancer cells lurking in my body, ready to take up residence elsewhere. What if I wait for the much anticipated five-year mark? Then do I call myself a survivor? Well, I know of cases where cancer returned fifteen or even twenty years after the initial diagnosis. So can one really ever say that they SURVIVED cancer? I guess it is only if we die of something else that we truly can say we survived cancer.

That was my *Aha* moment! The moment I realized that being a survivor is not about what cancer does to your body, but about what it does to your spirit, and that I had been a survivor all along. Cancer did not diminish my faith in God or weaken my relationships with my loved ones. It did not steal my hopes and dreams. It did not make me doubt my belief in myself and my ability to face any challenge. Cancer weakened my body, but my spirit has never been stronger.

No matter what your diagnosis, you too can be a survivor, because being a survivor is not about outliving cancer. It is about attitude. You did not have a choice in getting cancer, but you do have a choice in the attitude you bring to it. When you use all of the resources within and around you to give the best fight you possibly can to beat this disease, then you are living your life as a survivor. When you continue to take on new challenges, set new goals for yourself, and attempt to fulfill lifelong dreams to the best of your ability, you are a survivor. Living with a survivor's attitude does not necessarily mean that you will outlive the cancer, but it will give you the best chances of doing so. It will also ensure that you make the most of whatever time you have left on this earth, whether that be four months or forty-four years. The way I see it, cancer may one day take my body, but it will never take my spirit. I AM A SURVIVOR!

Repeat after me: I AM A SURVIVOR!

HEALTH TIP #100
Make a Survival Plan (Hmm . . . Better Use a Pencil)

Plan ahead or find trouble on the doorstep.
—CONFUCIUS

The best laid plans of mice and men often go astray.
—ROBERT BURNS

(Burns said this after he accidentally mowed over a
perfect mouse's nest in a field.)

would love to hear these two great thinkers debate their points. While it may sound like conflicting pieces of wisdom, the fact is, they are both correct. Plans are necessary whether you are building a house or going out to dinner with friends. But trees fall on almost-finished houses, and baby-sitters cancel at the last minute. Therefore, it is necessary to make plans but be prepared to change them.

I feel justified in adding my own quote:

Over time, you will change your plans, but your plans, when followed, will ultimately change you.

—S. GONZALEZ, RN

I found "Susan's Survival Plan," dated 2006, in the documents section of my computer. I wrote it just after I finished chemo. It included:

- Exercise at least 45 minutes, 5 times a week

- Vegetarian diet, no hydrogenated oils.

- Selenium supplement daily (someone in the waiting room told me this).

- Look into beginning osteoporosis prevention medication (was I really looking for MORE medication?).

- Daily breast (chest wall) and lymph node self-exams (paranoid, ya think?).

- Use paraben-free soap.

This plan, which sounded great to me at the time, obviously had its flaws. As I learned and researched and spoke to other experts in the field, I've changed some things. This part of my survival plan now looks something like this:

- Exercise 4 to 5 hours a week (I break it up for convenience).

- 99% plant-based diet (no meat, dairy, eggs, processed, or artificial anything. Organic when possible. . . . I still like wild salmon one or two times a month).

- Take omega-3 in the form of chia seeds or supplements, vitamin D, acidophilus, shiitake, maitake, and reishi mushroom supplements, and curcumin supplements daily.

- Take plant-based calcium and strontium when I can, for bones.

- Monthly chest wall and lymph node self-exams.

- Ultimate goal to eliminate all harmful synthetic chemicals from any personal-care product that I use.

- Eliminate exposure to plastics whenever possible.

- Include meditation and mindful breathing in my daily routine.

There are dozens of other things on "the plan" as I continue to gather information from reliable sources. My survival plan is evolving, and so am I. In fact, even in the course of writing this book, I've made changes.

If you are faced with a health crisis of any kind, making a plan can be very empowering. I called mine a "survival plan," but you might be more comfortable with the term *recovery plan* or *healing plan*. The point is, you are taking charge of your health. There is no "one size fits all" when it comes to "surviving" cancer. While there are general things like healthy diet and exercise that are an important component of any good health plan, how you choose to implement the plan must fit with your lifestyle and philosophy.

No matter where you are in your cancer journey, and no matter what stage, think about these three areas of your life and make a plan that you can follow.

Body

Consider what you are putting in and on your body. How can you make your body stronger and more immune resistant? What healthy physical changes (such as diet, exercise, taking supplements, avoiding toxins, and so on) can you make today without sacrificing your happiness? (And how do you know you *won't* be happy with a change?)

Mind

Are you fully aware of the mind-body connection? What practices, such as positive thinking, visualization, affirmations, and others can you include in your daily life that will enhance its power to help you heal, not only your body, but your mind as well?

Spirit

Are you practicing exercises to build your spiritual muscle? Prayer, meditation, practicing gratitude, being with others, and spending time in nature are all good spiritual exercises. Are you surrounding yourself with those who are positive, loving, and respectful of you? Are you engaging in activities that maximize your joy?

Your survival plan is a reminder that you are working toward an ultimate goal of living a full, rewarding, healthy, and happy life, no matter what your diagnosis or prognosis. So grab yourself a pencil, and make sure it has a big eraser!

You are not helpless in giving your body and mind what they need to be healthy and resist illness. Get your information, make your plan, and start living.

Cancer Plan 4 Life

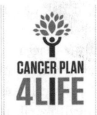

Congratulations on reading this book and empowering yourself with the tools you need to live your life as a survivor! Remember, being a survivor is not about the presence or absence of cancer cells in your body. It is all about attitude. When you use all of the resources within you and around you to give the fight of your life to survive cancer, to prolong your life, or to prevent a reoccurrence, then you ARE a survivor.

We believe that the key to cancer prevention and cancer survivorship lies in making healthy lifestyle choices. In this book, you have been presented with literally hundreds of healthy living tips for body, mind, and spirit. The vast majority of these tips deal with improving the health of the body through proper nutrition, exercise, and taking supplements as needed. However, we believe that true health is only possible when you also address your emotional, mental, and spiritual well-being. Affirmations, prayer, meditation, and forgiveness exercises are some of the tools talked about in this book to help you achieve a state of balance and peace.

If you have not already done so, now is the time to make your Survival Plan. We do not expect that you adopt every practice in this book. Take what resonates with you and leave the rest. As your plan evolves, you will find yourself coming back to this book as you move closer and closer to your goal of achieving optimal health.

Some people are very self-motivated, and they will take their plan and run with it! Others may need a little more guidance and structure on their journey to optimal health. It is for those people that we have created a life transforming four-week program called Cancer Plan 4 Life (www.cancerplan 4life.com).

Cancer Plan 4 Life (CP4L) is essentially "cancer rehab." It is a four-week online cancer survivorship program designed to increase your chances of surviving cancer and reduce your risk of a reoccurrence. While there is no guaranteed cure for cancer, research shows that proper diet, exercise, and lifestyle choices can significantly impact longevity and survival rates.

Our wish for you is optimal health. Optimal health means performing at your personal peak level of physical, mental, emotional, and spiritual functioning. It involves setting health goals that you can realistically achieve to feel your personal best! CP4L empowers you to make positive lifestyle choices that will help you to achieve your optimal level of health, no matter what your diagnosis or prognosis. If you are serious about living the survivor's lifestyle, you owe it to yourself to check out www.cancerplan4life .com!

Recommended Websites

The following is an alphabetical listing of all of the recommended websites mentioned throughout this book. Each entry includes the perk/tip number for easy cross-reference.

American Art Therapy Association: www.arttherapy.org (perk/tip 1)

American Cancer Society: www.cancer.org (perk/tip 12)

American Cancer Society's Guide to Quitting Smoking: www.cancer.org/ acs/groups/cid/documents/webcontent/ 002971-pdf.pdf (perk/tip 94)

Association of Cancer Online Resources: www.acor.org (perk/tip 12; worldwide)

Astroglide: www.astroglide.com (perk/tip 83)

Aubrey Organics: www.aubrey-organics.com (perk/tip 8)

Avalon Organics: www.avalonorganics.com (perk/tip 8)

Badger Products: bug balms and sunscreens www.badgerbalm.com (perk/tip 3, 55)

Breast Cancer Yoga: www.breastcanceryoga.com (perk/tip 54)

Brita Water Filters: www.brita.com (perk/tip 41)

Burt's Bees: www.burtsbees.com (perk/tip 3)

Canadian Cancer Advocacy Network: www.ccanacc.ca/ (perk/tip 12)

Canadian Cancer Society: www.cancer.ca (perk/tip 12)

Cancer Advocacy Coalition of Canada: www.canceradvocacy.ca/ (perk/tip 12; Canada)

Cancer Hope Network: www.cancerhopenetwork.org (perk/tip 12; United States)

Cancer Index: www.cancerindex.org (perk/tip 12; worldwide)

Cancer Support Community: cancersupportcommunity.org (perk/tip 12; worldwide)

Centers for Disease Control and Prevention—Physical Activity: www.cdc.gov/physicalactivity (perk/tip 7)

Centers for Science in the Public Interest: www.cspinet.org (perk/tip 47)

International Dutch Oven Society:
www.idos.com (perk/tip 99)

Jason Natural products:
www.jason-personalcare.com (perk/tip 8)

John Masters Organics:
www.johnmasters.com (perk/tip 8)

Lavera Cosmetics (sunless tanner):
www.lavera.com (perk/tip 8) (perk/tip 55)

Lodge Cast Iron: www.logdemfg.com
(perk/tip 99)

Lung Cancer blood test:
www.hellohaveyouheard.com (perk/tip 38)

Maple Medicinals Wild Branch Mushrooms:
www.maplemedicinals.com (perk/tip 22)

Mayo Clinic walking shoe information:
www.mayoclinic?health/walking/HQ00885
_D (perk/tip 78)

Memorial Sloan Kettering Cancer Center:
www.mskcc.org/cancer-care/
integrative-medicine (perk/tip 22)

Metal Detecting: www.gometaldetecting.com
(perk/tip 37)

Mountain House: www.mountainhouse.com
(perk/tip 70)

Mountain Rose Herbs:
www.mountainroseherbs.com (perk/tip 3)

Mrs Dash: www.mrsdash.com (perk/tip 58)

National Cancer Institute: www.cancer.gov
(perk/tip 12)

National Geographic's Smart Plastics
Guide: www.pbs.org/strangedays/
pdf/StrangeDaysSmartPlasticsGuide.pdf
(perk/tip 45)

Nitro-pak: www.nitro-pak.com/products/
freeze-dried-foods (perk/tip 70)

Nutrition Data omega calculator:
www.nutritiondata.com (perk/tip 10)

Ohio State University Extension:
http://ohioline.osu.edu/hyg-fact/1000/1647
.html (perk/tip 81)

Oncochat: www.oncochat.org (perk/tip 12;
worldwide)

100% Pure Cosmetics:
www.100percentpure.com (perk/tip 8)

Organic Consumers:
www.organicconsumers.org (perk/tip 91)

President's Council on Fitness Sports &
Nutrition: www.fitness.gov (perk/tip 7)

Quitting smoking:
www.cancer.org/Healthy/StayAwayfrom
Tobacco/guidetoquittingsmoking/index
(perk/tip 94)

Quitting smoking:
www.helpguide.org/mental/quit_smoking_
cessation.htm (perk/tip 94)

Quitting smoking: www.smokefree.gov
(perk/tip 94)

Radiation Risk Calculator: www.xrayrisk.com
(perk/tip 56)

Radon info: www.epa.gov/radon and www.hc-sc.gc.ca (enter "radon" in the search bar) (perk/tip 17)

Ready Store: www.thereadystore.com (perk/tip 70)

Running Advisor: www.therunningadvisor .com/running_ shoes.html (perk/tip 78)

Safe Cosmetics: www.safecosmetics.org (perk/tip 96)

Scotch Naturals nontoxic nail polish: www.ScotchNaturals.com (perk/tip 4)

Self-Breast Exam Instruction: www.breastcancer.org (perk/tip 38)

Siteman Cancer Center Disease Risk calculator: www.yourdiseaserisk.wustl.edu (perk/tip 94)

Sleep Foundation: www.sleepfoundation.org (perk/tip 33)

Stand Up To Cancer: www.standup2cancer .org (perk/tip 60)

Stanford Hospital & Clinics Workshop: http://stanfordhospital.org/clinicsmed Services/clinics/complementaryMedicine/ scimForegiveness.html (perk/tip 63)

Stanford University School of Medicine's Stanford Center on Stress and Health: http://stresshealthcenter.stanford.edu (perk/tip 84)

Straw Bale Gardens: www.strawbalegardens .com (perk/tip 81)

U.S. Department of Health and Human Services Product Database: www.householdproducts.nlm.nih.gov/ index.htm (perk/tip 47)

Water Quality: www.water.epa.gov (perk/tip 72)

Whole Grains Council: www.wholegrainscouncil.org (perk/tip 82)

Wholemega: www.newchapter.com/fish-oil/ wholemega (perk/tip 10)

World Health Organization on GMO foods: www.who.int (click on "health topics" to find GMO information) (perk/tip 91)

Suggested Reading & Viewing

The China Study by T. Colin Campbell and Thomas M. Campbell II

One of the largest studies ever conducted, Dr. Campbell and his international associates studied the diets of 6,500 Chinese residents and found striking differences in the incidence of all kinds of diseases (including cancer) among the plant-based eating Chinese population and animal-based eating population of the United States. The subject of the book is science but is written in a way that is easy to understand.

The Complete Idiot's Guide to Plant-Based Eating by Julianna Hever

This is a great book for someone just starting out on a plant-based journey. Easy to read pages with special side notes take the guesswork out of planning your menus. There are also great recipes and resources listed.

The Engine 2 Diet: The Texas Firefighter's 28-Day Save-Your-Life Plan That Lowers Cholesterol and Burns Away the Pounds by Rip Esselstyn

Rip is a firefighter and triathlete (don't you love him already?) whose dad, Dr. Caldwell Esselstyn, helped former president Bill Clinton go vegan and improve his health. His book is laid out as a four-week program and focuses on different aspects of a vegan diet each week. The recipes at the back of the book are easy to make and follow the diet plan in the front.

Everyday Happy Herbivore by Lindsay S. Nixon

This cookbook is easy to follow and read with quick-look indications about how long a recipe will take to make, how expensive the ingredients are, and more. I love the pictures and variations she provides if I'm out of an item.

Feng Shui for Dummies by David Daniel

This book follows the other "for Dummies" varieties, making it easy for even the most simpleminded of us to follow.

Gorgeously Green: 8 Simple Steps to an Earth-Friendly Life by Sophie Uliano

Even though this book seems like an environmentally focused book, it actually gives hundreds of resources for healthy products that you use everyday. I find myself constantly consulting it.

The Healing Power of Doing Good by Allen Luks with Peggy Payne

Packed with actual stories and scientific support, this book goes into great detail to explain why helping others will also help our own health.

How to Pray: Tapping into the Power of Divine Communication by Helene Ciaravino

A friendly little book that does not lend itself to one religion, the author makes it very easy to start praying even if you don't know where to start.

Left to Tell by Immaculee Ilibagiza

This book shows the power of forgiveness to create a beautiful life. Immaculee was the victim of the Rwandan genocide where her whole family was massacred. She found a way to forgive those who murdered her family and, in doing so, reclaimed her life.

The Link Between Religion and Health: Psychoneuroimmunology and the Faith Factor by Harold Koenig and Harvey Jay Cohen

This is one of the few books citing scientific research on the connection between religion and health. They look at all religions and the common factors that lead to healthier followers.

The Longevity Project by Howard S. Friedman and Leslie R. Martin

A study spanning over eighty years, this book reports on its findings looking at health trends and long lives and gives us some surprising guidelines for both.

Love, Medicine & Miracles: Lessons Learned About Self-Healing from a Surgeon's Experience with Exceptional Patients by Bernie S. Siegel

As a surgeon, Dr. Siegel has witnessed medical miracles. He explores the reasons for these miracles and helps you to understand what you can do to help heal yourself.

Loretta J. Standley at www.drstandley.com

An extremely interesting, diverse, and knowledgeable woman who is an expert in affirmations and other healing practices. Her website is full of various ways to help healing and achieve happiness.

Miss Diagnosed: Unraveling Chronic Stress by Erin Bell

A quick-read, Erin takes you on her own personal journey to find the answers to her health problems. In an easy-to-follow anecdotal format, she explains chronic stress using her own experience and also gives good scientific resources for her solutions.

Patch Adams

A film released in 1998 starring Robin Williams, based on the book *Gesundheit: Good Health Is a Laughing Matter* by Patch Adams and Maureen Mylander.

Silent Spring by Rachel Carson

Now in its fortieth year of print, *Silent Spring* was the book that launched the environmentalist movement in this country. Rachel Carson saw that the systematic poisoning of land, water, and air would someday destroy the environment and make us sick. She was right, of course, and explains her position in this book, which would later be used in Congressional hearings to fight chemical companies and change laws.

When a Parent Has Cancer: A Guide to Caring for Your Children by Wendy Haprham

Written by a doctor, mother, and cancer survivor to give you specific ways to deal with situations that arise with children when a parent has cancer. It also comes with a children's book, *Becky and the Worry Cup*, that helps kids face their fears.

When the Body Says No: Exploring the Stress-Disease Connection by Gabor Maté

This book is an impressive argument for the mind-body connection citing Dr. Maté's work over his decades of research. He uses science as well as anecdotal stories to convey the message that the mind and body are connected and one can be used to influence the other.

Why Millions Survive Cancer: The Success of Science by Lauren Pecorino

The author of this up-to-date (2011) book traces every cancer through the breakthroughs and illustrates how far we've come, but also how far we have to go. She gives great insight into what we know now about prevention through lifestyle changes and points out that there is a lot of "good news" when dealing with cancer research.

The Year My Mother Was Bald by Ann Speltz

This adorable, kid-friendly book uses humor and accurate facts to explain what goes on when your mom has cancer. Written in a diary format, it's easy for kids ages nine and older to read.

References

PERK/TIP #1

Breslow, D. M. 1993. "Creative Arts for Hospitals: The UCLA Experiment." *Patient Education & Counseling* 21:101–110.

Malchiodi, C. A. 2002. *The Soul's Palette: Drawing on Art's Transformative Powers for Health and Well-Being.* Boston: Shambhala, xi.

Nainis, N. 2009. "Art Therapy." *Journal of the American Art Therapy Association* 25(3):115–121.

PERK/TIP #2

Dew, J. E., Wren, B. G., and Eden, J. A. 2003. "A Cohort Study of Topical Vaginal Estrogen Therapy in Women Previously Treated for Breast Cancer." *Climacteric* 6:45–52.

Oprah.com. January 29, 2009. "HRT Q & A with Dr. Christiane Northrup." Oprah webcast transcript. Accessed July 2011. www.oprah.com/ health.

Ponzone, R., Jacomuzzi, M. E., Maggiorotto, F., Mariana, L., and Sismondi, P. 2005. "Vaginal Oestrogen Therapy After Breast Cancer: Is It Safe?" *European Journal of Cancer* 41:2673–2681.

PERK/TIP #3

Agency for Toxic Substances and Disease Registry (ATSDR). "Public Health Statement for DDT, DDE, DDD." Accessed March 2013. www .atsdr.cdc.gov/ phs/phs.asp?id=79& tid=20.

Extension Toxicology Network: DEET. "Pesticide Information Project." Accessed September 2012.

http://pmep.cce.cornell.edu/profiles/extoxnet/car baryl-dicrotophos/deet-ext.html.

www.scjohnson.ca/msds/OFF! Clip-on Mosquito Repellent.pdf.

National Pesticide Information Center. "DEET Technical Fact Sheet." Accessed July 2012. http:// npic.orst.edu.

SC Johnson. "MSDS OFF! Clip-On Mosquito repellent." Accessed September 2011.

U.S. Environmental Protection Agency. "EPA R.E.D. facts DEET." Accessed August 2012. www .epa.gov/ oppsrrd1/REDs/factsheets/0002fact.pdf.

PERK/TIP #5

Cancercare. "Helping Children Understand Cancer." Accessed August 2012. www.cancercare.org/ publications/49-helping_children_understand _cancer_talking_to_your_kids_about_your _diagnosis.

Fox Chase Cancer Center. "Talking To Your Children About Cancer." Accessed August 2012. www.fccc.edu/patients/support/children.html.

PERK/TIP #7

Kumanyika, S. 2009. "Trial of Family and Friend Support for Weight Loss in African American Adults." *Archives of Internal Medicine* 169:1795–1804.

McCullough, L. E., Eng, S. M., Bradshaw, P. T., Cleveland, R. J., Teitelbaum, S. L., Neugut, A. I., and Gammon, M. D. 2009. "Fat or Fit: The Joint Effects of Physical Activity, Weight Gain, and Body Size on Breast Cancer Risk." *Cancer* 118:4860–4868.

Moore, S. C., Patel, A. V., Matthews, C. E., Berrington de Gonzalez, A., Park, Y., Katki, H. A., and Lee, I-M. 2009. "Leisure Time Physical Activity of Moderate to Vigorous Intensity and Mortality: A Large Pooled Cohort Analysis." *PLoS Medicine* 9. Accessed December 2012. doi:10.1371/journal.pmed.1001335.

Oncology Nurse Advisor. "Exercise May Fortify Immune System of Cancer Survivors Against Future Cancers." Accessed November 2012. www.oncologynurseadvisor.com/exercise-may-fortify-immune-system-of-cancer-survivors-against-future-cancers/article/263851/#.

World Health Organization. "World Health Organization: Physical Activity and Adults." Accessed August 2012. www.who.int/dietphysicalactivity/factsheet_adults/en/index.html.

PERK/TIP #9

Ovadje, P., Hamm, C., and Pandey, S. 2012. "Efficient Induction of Extrinsic Cell Death by Dandelion Root Extract in Human Chronic Myelomonocytic Leukemia (CMML) Cells." *PLoS Medicine* 7(2): e30604. doi:10.1371/journal.pone.0030604.

Rodriguez-Fragoso, L., Reyes-Esparza, J., Burchiel, S. W., Herrera-Ruiz, D., and Torres, E. 2008. "Risks and Benefits of Commonly Used Herbal Medicines in Mexico." *Toxicological Applied Pharmacology* 227:125–135. doi:10.1016/j.taap.2007.10.005.

PERK/TIP #10

Kiecolt-Glaser, J. K., Belury, M. A., Andridge, R., Malarkey, W. B., Hwang, B. S., and Glaser, R. 2012. "Omega-3 Supplementation Lowers Inflammation in Healthy Middle-Aged and Older Adults: A Randomized Controlled Trial." *Brain, Behavior, and Immunity* 26:988–885.

Le, T. T., Huff, T. B., and Cheng, J. 2009. "Coherent Anti-Stokes Raman Scattering Imaging of Lipids in Cancer Metastasis." *BMC Cancer* 9:42. doi:10.1186/1471-2407-9-42.

Stulnig, T. M., Berger, M., Sigmund, T., Raederstorff, D., Stockinger, H., and Waldhäusl, W. 1998. "Polyunsaturated Fatty Acids Inhibit T-Cell Signal Transduction by Modification of Detergent-Insoluble Membrane Domains." *Journal of Cell Biology* 142:637–644.

University of Maryland Medical Center. "Omega-3 Fatty Acids." Accessed November 2011. www.umm.edu/altmed/articles/omega-3-000316.htm.

PERK/TIP #12

Berkman, L. F., and Syme, S. L. 1979. "Social Networks, Host Resistance, and Mortality: A Nine-Year Follow Up of Alameda County Residents." *American Journal of Epidemiology* 109(2):186–204.

Glanz, K., Rimer, B. K., and Wiswanath, K. 2008. *Health Behavior and Health Education: Theory, Research, and Practice.* California: John Wiley & Sons, 190–206.

Kroenke, C. H., Kubzansky, L. D., Schernhammer, E. S., Holmes, M. D., and Kawachi, I. 2006. "Social Networks, Social Support, and Survival After Breast Cancer Diagnosis." *Journal of Clinical Oncology* 24:1105–1111.

Spiegel, D., Sephton, S. E., Terr, A. I., and Stites, D. P. 1998. "Effects of Psychosocial Treatment in Prolonging Cancer Survival May Be Mediated by Neuroimmune Pathways." *Annals of New York Academy of Science* 840:674–83.

Turner-Cobb, J. M., Sephton, S. E., Koopman, C., Blake-Mortimer, J., and Spiegel, D. 2000. "Social Support and Salivary Cortisol in Women with Metastatic Breast Cancer." *Psychosomatic Medicine* 62:337–345.

Winzelberg, A. J., Classen, C., Alpers, G. W., Roberts, H., Koopman, C., Adams, R. E., and Taylor, C. B. 2003. "Evaluation of an Internet Support Group for Women with Primary Breast Cancer." *Cancer* 97:1164–1173.

PERK/TIP #13

Mowrey, D., and Clayson, D. 1982. "Motion Sickness, Ginger, and Psychotropics." *The Lancet* 319:655–657.

PERK/TIP #15

Centers for Disease Control (CDC). "Recommendations to Prevent and Control Iron Deficiency in the United States." Accessed July 2012. www.cdc.gov/mmwr/preview/mmwrhtml/00051880.htm.

Mainous III, A. G., Wells, B. J., Koopman, R. J., Everett, C. J., and Gill, J. 2005. "Iron, Lipids, and the Risk of Cancer in the Framingham Offspring Cohort." *American Journal of Epidemiology* 161:1115–1122.

McKinley Health Center. "Dietary Sources of Iron." Accessed July 2012. www.mckinley.illinois.edu/handouts/dietary_sources_iron.html.

Yee, Y. S., and Khadijah, S. 2011. "Iron and Cancer." *E-Journal of Traditional & Complementary Medicine*. Accessed November 2012. http://ejtcm.com/2011/03/18/iron-and-cancer-2/.

PERK/TIP #18

Calafat, A. M., Ye, X., Wong, L. Y., Reidy, J. A., and Needham, L. L. 2008. "Urinary Concentrations of Triclosan in the U.S. Population 2003–2004." *Environmental Health Perspectives* 116:303–307.

Cooney, C. "Personal Care Products: Triclosan Comes Under Scrutiny." *Environmental Health Perspectives* 118:A242.

eNews Park Forest. March 6, 2013 (press release). "Minnesota State Agencies Will No Longer Purchase Products Containing Triclosan." Accessed March 27, 2013. www.enewspf.com/latest-news/science/science-a-environmental/40958-minnesota-state-agencies-will-no-longer-purchase-products-containing-triclosan.html.

Luks, A., and Payne, P. 2001. *The Healing Power of Doing Good*. Nebraska: iUniverse.com, Inc., 64.

Odabasi, M. 2008. "Halogenated Volatile Organic Compounds from the Use of Chlorine-Bleach-Containing Household Products." *Environmental Science & Technology* 42:1445–1451.

Stoker, T. E. 2009. "The Effects of Triclosan on Puberty and Thyroid Hormones in Male Wistar Rats." *Toxicological Science* 107:56–64.

UC Davis Health Systems. "Anti-Bacterial Personal Hygiene Products May Not Be Worth Potential Risks." Accessed September 2012. www.ucdmc.ucdavis.edu/welcome/features/20080903_anti-bacterial/index.html.

Zorrilla, L. M., Gibson, E. K., Jeffay, S. C., Crofton, K. M., Setzer, W. R., Cooper, R. L., and Stoker, T. E. 2009. "The Effects of Triclosan on Puberty and Thyroid Hormones in Male Wistar Rats." *Toxicological Science* 107:56–64.

PERK/TIP #20

Ohio State University Medical Center. April 25, 2006 (press release). "Black Raspberries: Fruitraceuticals of the Future." Accessed September 2012. http://fst.osu.edu/caffre/news/Black%20raspberries,%20'fruitaceuticals'%20of%20the%20future.pdf.

PERK/TIP #21

Rose, L. F., Mealey, B., Minski, L., and Cohen, D. W. 2002. "Oral Care for Patients with Cardiovascular Disease and Stroke." *Journal of the American Dental Association* 133:375–445.

Allin, K. H., Nordestgaard, B. G., Flyger, H., and Bojesen, S. E. 2011. "Elevated Pre-Treatment Levels of Plasma C-Reactive Protein Are Associated with Poor Prognosis After Breast Cancer: A Cohort Study." *Breast Cancer Research* 13:R55. doi:10.1186/bcr2891.

Michaud, D. S., Joshipura, K., Giovannucci, E., and Fuchs, C. S. 2006. "A Prospective Study of Periodontal Disease and Pancreatic Cancer in U.S. Male Health Professionals." *Journal of the National Cancer Institute* 99:171–175.

National Public Radio (NPR). February 11, 2005 (podcast). "Gum Disease and Heart Disease." www.npr.org/templates/story/story.php?storyId=4 495598.

PERK/TIP #22

Torkelso ., C. J., Sweet, E., Martzen, M. R., Sasagawa, M., Wenner, C. A., Gay, J., and Standish, L. J. 2012. "Phase 1 Clinical Trial of Trametes Versicolor in Women with Breast Cancer." *ISRN Oncology.* Article ID 251632. doi:10.5402/2012/ 251632.

PERK/TIP #24

Grandjean, P., Andersen, E. W., Budtz-Jørgensen, E., Nielsen, F., Mølbak, K., Weihe, P., and Heilmann, C. 2012. "Serum accine Antibody Concentrations in Children Exposed to Perfluorinated Compounds." *Journal of the American Medical Association* 307:391–397. doi:10.1001/jama.2011.2034.

Hubbs, A. F., Cumpston, A. M., Goldsmith, W. T., Battelli, L. A., Jackson, M. C., Frazer, D. G., and Sriram, K. 2012. "Respiratory and Olfactory Cytotoxicity of Inhaled 2,3-Pentanedione in Sprague-Dawley Rats." *The American Journal of Pathology.* doi:10.1016/j.ajpath.2012.05.021.

Kropp, T., and Houlihan, J. 2005. "Evaluating Human Health Risks from Exposure to Perfluorooctanoic Acid (PFOA): Recommendations to the Science Advisory Board's PFOA Review Panel." www.epa.gov/sab/pdf/kropp-ewg.pdf.

U.S. Environmental Protection Agency. "Exposure Assessments Methods for Perfluorinated Compounds." Accessed February 2012. www.epa.gov/heasd/regulatory/projects/d1b_right_to_know.html.

PERK/TIP #26

Mora-Ripoll, R. 2011. "Potential Health Benefits of Simulated Laughter: A Narrative Review of the Literature and Recommendations for Future Research." *Complementary Therapeutic Medicine* 19:170–177.

PERK/TIP #30

Emmons, R., and McCullough, M. 2003. "Counting Blessings Versus Burdens: An Experimental Investigation of Gratitude and Subjective Well-Being in Daily Life." *Journal of Personality and Social Psychology* 84:377–389. doi:10.1037/0022-3514.84.2.377.

PERK/TIP #31

Ciaravino, H. 2001. *How to Pray: Tapping into the Power of Divine Communication,* New York: Square One Publishing, 19–27.

Koenig, H. G., and Cohen, H. J. 2002. *The Link Between Religion and Health: Psychoneuroimmunology and the Faith Factor.* New York: Oxford University Press, 93–96.

Meisenhelder, J. B., and Chandler, E. N. 2000. "Prayer and Health Outcomes in Church Members." *Alternative Therapeutic Health Medicine* 6:56–60.

PERK/TIP #32

Headey, B. 1999. "Health Benefits and Health Cost Savings Due to Pets: Preliminary Estimates from an Australian National Survey." *Social Indicators Research* 47:233–243.

Siegel, J. 1990. "Stressful Life Events and Use of Physician Services Among the Elderly: The Moderating Role of Pet Ownership." *Journal of Personality and Social Psychology* 58:1081–1086.

PERK/TIP #33

Perks of Having Cancer (blog). April 11, 2012. "Guest Blogger: Dr. Bernie Siegel." www.perksof cancer.com/2012/04/11/900/.

Stewart, M. "Effective Physician-Patient Communication and Health Outcomes: A Review." *Canadian Medical Association Journal* 152:1423–1433.

PERK/TIP #34

Harvard Health Publications. 2009. "Napping May Not Be Such a No-No." Accessed October 2012. www.health.harvard.edu/newsletters/Harvard _Health_Letter/2009/November/napping-may -not-be-such-a-no-no.

Purnell, M. T., Feyer, A. M., and Herbison, G. P. 2002. "The Impact of a Nap Opportunity During the Night Shift on the Performance and Alertness of 12-H Shift Workers." *Journal of Sleep Research* 11:219–227.

Signal, T. L., Gander, P. H., Anderson, H., and Brash, S. 2009. "Scheduled Napping as a Countermeasure to Sleepiness in Air Traffic Controllers." *Journal of Sleep Research* 18:11–19.

PERK/TIP #35

Campbell, T. C., and Campbell, T. M. 2006. *The China Study*. Dallas: BenBella Books, 65.

PERK/TIP #37

National Institutes of Health (NIH). "Participating in Activities You Enjoy—More Than Just Fun and Games." Accessed September 2012. www .nia.nih.gov/health/publication/participating -activities-you-enjoy-more-just-fun-and-games.

Tinsley, H. E. 1995. "Psychological Benefits of Leisure Participation: A Taxonomy of Leisure Activities." *Journal of Counseling Psychology* 42:123–132.

PERK/TIP #39

Hong, H., Kim, C. S., and Maeng, S. 2009. "Effects of Pumpkin Seed Oil and Saw Palmetto Oil in Korean Men with Symptomatic Benign Prostatic Hyperplasia." *Nutrition Research and Practice* 3:323–327.

Hudson, C., Hudson, S., and MacKenzie, J. 2007. "Protein-Source Tryptophan as an Efficacious Treatment for Social Anxiety Disorder: A Pilot Study." *Canadian Journal of Physiology and Pharmacology* 85:928–932.

Hyun, T. H., Barrett-Connor, E., and Milne, D. B. 2004. "Zinc Intakes and Plasma Concentrations in Men with Osteoporosis: The Rancho Bernardo Study." *American Journal of Clinical Nutrition* 80:715–21.

Suphakarn, V. S., Yarnnon, C., and Ngunboonsri, P. 1987. "The Effect of Pumpkin Seeds on Oxalcrystalluria and Urinary Compositions of Children in Hyperendemic Area." *American Journal of Clinical Nutrition* 45:115–121.

PERK/TIP #41

New Hampshire Department of Environmental Services. "Environmental Fact Sheet/ARD-EHP-13 Trihalomethanes: Health Information Summary." Accessed September 2011. http://des.nh.gov/ organization/commissioner/pip/factsheets/ard/ documents/ard-ehp-13.pdf.

University of Minnesota/Extension. "Treatment Systems for Household Water Supplies: Activated Charcoal Filters." Accessed November 2011. www .extension.umn.edu/distribution/natural resources/dd5939.html.

Wilmot, E. G., Edwardson, C. L., Achana, F. A., Davies, M. J., Gorely, T., Gray, L. J., and Biddle, S. J. 2012. "Sedentary Time in Adults and the Association with Diabetes, Cardiovascular Disease and Death: Systematic Review and Meta-Analysis." *Diabetologia* 55:2895–2905.

PERK/TIP #43

Kuo, F. 2010. "Parks and Other Green Environments: Essential Components of a Healthy Human Habitat." *National Recreation and Parks Association.* Accessed July 2012. www.nrpa.org/uploadedFiles/nrpa.org/Publications_and_Research/Research/Papers/MingKuo-Summary.PDF.

Maas, J., Verheij, R. A., Groenewegen, P. P., de Vries, S., and Spreeuwenberg, P. 2006. "Green Space, Urbanity, and Health: How Strong Is the Relation?" *Journal of Epidemiology and Community Health* 60:587–592.

Takano, T., Nakamura, K., and Wantanabe, M. 2002. "Urban Residential Environments and Senior Citizens' Longevity in Megacity Areas: The Importance of Walkable Green Spaces." *Journal of Epidemiology and Community Health* 56: 913–918.

Ulrich, R. 1984. "View Through a Window May Influence Recovery from Surgery." *Science* 224: 420–421.

PERK/TIP #45

American Fertility Association (in blog posted by Jackie Lombardo). May 17, 2011. "Chemicals in Umbilical Cord Blood." www.theafa.org/blog/chemicals-in-umbilical-cord-blood/.

Ayyanan, A., Laribi, O., Schuepbach-Mallepell, S., Schrick, C., Gutierrez, M., Tanos, T., and Brisken, C. 2011. "Perinatal Exposure to Bisphenol A Increases Adult Mammary Gland Progesterone Response and Cell Number." *Molecular Endocrinology* 25:1915.

Baker, M., and Chandsawangbhuwana, C. 2012. "3D Models of MBP, a Biologically Active Metabolite of Bisphenol A in Human Estrogen Receptor A and Estrogen Receptor B." *PLos ONE* 7: e46078. doi:10.1371/journal.pone.0046078.

Harvard School of Public Health. November 2011 (press release). "Consuming Canned Soup Linked to Greatly Elevated Levels of the Chemical BPA." Accessed November 2011. www.hsph.harvard.edu/news/press-releases/2011-releases/canned-soup-bpa.html.

Kendziorski, J. A., Kendig, E. L., Gear, R. B., and Belcher, S. M. 2012. "Strain Specific Induction of Pyometra and Differences in Immune Responsiveness in Mice Exposed to 17a-Ethinyl Estradiol or the Endocrine Disrupting Chemical Bisphenol A." *Reproductive Toxicology* 34:22–30.

Liao, C., Liu, F., and Kanna, K. 2012. "Bisphenol S, a New Bisphenol Analogue in Paper Products, Currency Bills, and Its Association with Bisphenol A Residues." *Environmental Science and Technology* 46:6515–6522. doi:10.1021/es300876n.

National Geographic's Strange Days on Planet Earth (PBS). "Smart Plastics Guide." Accessed March 28, 2012. www.pbs.org/strangedays/pdf/StrangeDaysSmartPlasticsGuide.pdf.

PERK/TIP #46

American Cancer Society. "Cancer Facts and Figures: 2013." Accessed March 2012. www.cancer.org/acs/groups/content/@epidemiologysurveilance/documents/document/acspc-036845.pdf.

National Cancer Institute. "Surveillance Epidemiology and End Results." Accessed June 2012. http://seer.cancer.gov/statfacts/html/all.html.

World Health Organization International Agency for Research on Cancer. "World Cancer Factsheet." Accessed June 2011. http://gicr.iarc.fr/files/resources/20120906-WorldCancerFactSheet.pdf.

PERK/TIP #47

Center for Science in the Public Interest. March 5, 2012. "Lab Tests Find Carcinogen in Regular and Diet Coke and Pepsi. Accessed July 2012. http://cspinet.org/new/201203051.html.

Darbre, P. D., and Fernandez, M. F. 2013. "Environmental Oestrogens and Breast Cancer: Long-

Term Low-Dose Effects of Mixtures of Various Chemical Combinations." *Journal of Epidemiology and Community Health* 67(3):203–205. doi: 10.1136/jech-2012-201362.

Department of Health and Human Services Food and Drug Administration. February 2011. Citizen Petition submitted by the Center for Science in the Public Interest to revoke regulations authorizing the use of caramel coloring in foods. Accessed November 2012. http://cspinet.org/new/pdf/caramel_coloring_petition.pdf.

Environmental Working Group Skin Deep Database. "Sodium Lauerth Sulfate." Accessed October 2012. www.ewg.org/skindeep/ingredient/706089/SODIUM_LAURETH_SULFATE/.

Environmental Working Group Skin Deep Database. "Sodium Lauryl Sulfate." Accessed October 2012. www.ewg.org/skindeep/ingredient/706110/SODIUM_LAURYL_SULFATE/.

Good Guide. "Coco Glucoside Guide." Accessed August 2012. www.goodguide.com/ingredients/166258-coco-glucoside.

State of California Environmental Protection Agency (EPA) Office of Environmental Hazards Assessment. November 2, 2012. "Chemicals Known to the State to Cause Cancer or Reproductive Toxicity." Accessed November 2012. http://oehha.ca.gov/prop65/prop65_list/files/filesp65single110112.pdf.

PERK/TIP #48

American Cancer Society. "Antiperspirants and Breast Cancer Risk." Accessed September 2011. www.cancer.org/cancer/cancercauses/othercarcinogens/athome/antiperspirants-and-breast-cancer-risk.

Darbre, P. D. 2005. "Aluminum, Antiperspirants and Breast Cancer." *Journal of Inorganic Biochemistry* 99:1912–1919.

PERK/TIP #50

Davenport, L. 1996. "Guided Imagery Gets Respect." *HealthCare Forum Journal* 39:28–32.

PERK/TIP #54

Black, D. S., Cole, S. W., Irwin, M. R., Breen, E., St. Cyr, N. M., Nazarian, N., and Lavretsky, H. 2012. "Yogic Meditation Reverses NF-[kappa]B and IRF-Related Transcriptome Dynamics in Leukocytes of Family Dementia Caregivers in a Randomized Controlled Trial." *Psychoneuroendocrinology* 38(3):348–355. doi:10.1016/j.psyneuen.2012.06.011.

DeStasio, S. A. 2008. "Integrating Yoga into Cancer Care." *Clinical Journal of Oncology Nursing* 12:125–130.

MindBodyGreen. "How Yoga Can Help Cancer Patients." Accessed August 2012. www.chicagomanualofstyle.org/tools_citationguide.html.

Streeter, C. C., Gerbarg, P. L., Saper, R. B., Ciraulo, D. A., and Brown, R. P. 2012. "Effects of Yoga on the Autonomic Nervous System, Gamma-Aminobutyric-Acid, and Allostasis in Epilepsy, Depression, and Post-Traumatic Stress Disorder." *Medical Hypotheses* 78(5):571–579. doi:10.1016/j.mehy.2012.01.021.

Streeter, C. C., Whitfield, T. H., Owen, L., Rein, T., Karri, S. K., Yakhkind, A., and Jensen, J. E. 2010. "Effects of Yoga Versus Walking on Mood, Anxiety, and Brain GABA Levels: A Randomized Controlled MRS Study." *Journal of Alternative & Complementary Medicine* 16:1145–1153.

PERK/TIP #55

Butler, S., and Fosko, S. 2010. "Increased Prevalence of Left-Sided Skin Cancers." *Journal of the American Academy of Dermatology* 63:1006–1010.

EWG's Skin Deep (Environmental Working Group). "Health Agencies Question Sunscreen Efficacy." Accessed October 2011. http://breaking

news.ewg.org/2012sunscreen/sunscreens-exposed/health-agencies-question-sunscreen-efficacy.

EWG's Skin Deep (Environmental Working Group). April 4, 2011. "The Claim: You Cannot Get Sunburned Through a Car Window." As reported in the *New York Times*. Accessed November 2012. http://breakingnews.ewg.org/2012sunscreen/sunscreens-exposed/health-agencies-question-sunscreen-efficacy/.

Trouiller, B., Reliene, R., Westbrook, A., Solaimani, P., and Schiest, R. H. 2009. "Titanium Dioxide Nanoparticles Induce DNA Damage and Genetic Instability in Vivo in Mice." *Cancer Research* 69:8784–8789.

PERK/TIP #56

Idaho State University. "Radiation and Risk." Accessed June 2011. www.physics.isu.edu/radinf/risk.htm.

International Atomic Energy Agency. "Factsheets and FAQs." Accessed June 2011 www.iaea.org/Publications/Factsheets/English/radlife.html.

MIT News. "Radiation: How Much Is Considered Safe for Humans?" Accessed June 2011. http://web.mit.edu/newsoffice/1994/safe-0105.html.

U.S. Food and Drug Administration (FDA). "Radiation Emitting Products." Accessed June 2011. www.fda.gov/radiation-emittingproducts/radiationemittingproductsandprocedures/medicalimaging/medicalx-rays/ucm115329.htm.

PERK/TIP #58

Franco, V., and Oparil, S. 2006. "Salt Sensitivity: A Determinant of Blood Pressure, Cardiovascular Disease and Survival." *Journal of the American College of Nutrition* 25:247s–255s.

PERK/TIP #59

Gaziano, J. M., Sesso, H. D., Christen, W. G., Bubes, V., Smith, J. P., MacFadyen, J., and Buring, J. E. 2012. "Multivitamins in the Prevention of Cancer in Men: The Physicians' Health Study II Randomized Controlled Trial." *JAMA* 308(18): 1871–1880. doi:10.1001/jama.2012.14641.

Help Guide. "Vitamins and Minerals: Understanding Their Role." Accessed August 2012. www.helpguide.org/harvard/vitamins_and_minerals.htm.

PERK/TIP #60

Bliss, R. M. 2004. "Insulin Imitators: Polyphenols Found in Cinnamon Mimic Job of Hormone." *Agricultural Research* 52. Accessed October 2012 .www.ars.usda.gov/is/AR/archive/apr04/cinnam0404.htm.

Christofk, H. R., Vander Heiden, M. G., Harris, M. H., Ramanathan, A., Gerszten, R. E., Wei, R., and Stuart, L. 2008. "The M2 Splice Isoform of Pyruvate Kinase Is Important for Cancer Metabolism and Tumor Growth." *Nature* 452:230–233. doi:10.1038/nature06734.

Michaud, D. S., Liu, S., Giovannucci, E., Willett, W. C., Colditz, G. A., and Fuchs, C. S. 2002. "Dietary Sugar, Glycemic Load, and Pancreatic Cancer Risk in a Prospective Study." *Journal of the National Cancer Institute* 94:1293–1300.

Taubes, G. April 13, 2011. "Is Sugar Toxic?" *New York Times Magazine*. Accessed September 2012. www.nytimes.com/2011/04/17/magazine/mag-17Sugar-t.html?pagewanted=all.

PERK/TIP #62

American Cancer Society. "Turmeric." Accessed September 2012. www.cancer.org/treatment/treatmentsandsideeffects/complementaryandalternativemedicine/herbsvitaminsandminerals/turmeric.

Chainani-Wu, N. 2003. "Safety and Anti-Inflammatory Activity of Curcumin: A Component of Turmeric (Curcuma Longa)." *The Journal of Alternative and Complementary Medicine* 9:161–168. doi:10.1089/107555303321223035.

Maheshwari, R. K., Singh, A. K., Gaddipati, J., and Srimal, R. C. 2006. "Multiple Biological Activities of Curcumin: A Short Review." *Life Sciences* 78:2081–2087.

PERK/TIP #63

Greer, S., and Morris, T. 1975. "Psychological Attributes of Women Who Develop Breast Cancer: A Controlled Study." *Journal of Psychosomatic Research* 19(2):147–153.

Johnson, L. January 1, 2012. "Holding Grudges? Forgiveness Key to Healthy Body." *CBN News.* www.cbn.com/cbnnews/healthscience/2011/june/holding-grudges-forgiveness-key-to-healthy-body/.

Maté, G. 2003. *When the Body Says No: Exploring the Stress-Disease Connection.* Hoboken: John Wiley & Sons, 88–89, 99.

Siegel, B. S. 1986. *Love, Medicine & Miracles: Lessons Learned About Self-Healing from a Surgeon's Experience with Exceptional Patients.* New York: HarperCollins, 202.

Stanford Hospital & Clinics. "Forgive for Good Workshop." Accessed October 2012. http://stanfordhospital.org/clinicsmedServices/clinics/complementaryMedicine/scimForegiveness.html.

University of Miami. "Stress Management Improves Breast Cancer Outcomes." Accessed September 2012. www.miami.edu/index.php/news/releases/stress_management_improves_breast_cancer_outcomes/.

Watson, M., Haviland, J. S., Greer, S., Davidsone, J., and Bliss, J. M. 1999. "Influence of Psychological Response on Survival in Breast Cancer: A Population-Based Cohort Study." *The Lancet* 354:1331–1336.

PERK/TIP #64

American Cancer Society. "Alcohol Use and Cancer." Accessed November 2012. www.cancer.org/cancer/ cancercauses/dietandphysicalactivity/alcohol-use-and-cancer.

Federation of American Societies for Experimental Biology (FASEB). April 23, 2012. "Why Drinking Alcohol Is Linked to Breast Cancer." Accessed November 2012. www.sciencedaily.com/releases/2012/04/120423162245.htm.

PERK/TIP #66

American Institute for Cancer Research. "Diet: What We Eat." Accessed September 2012. www.aicr.org/reduce-your-cancer-risk/diet/.

McDonalds. September 2012. "McDonald's USA Adding Calorie Counts to Menu Boards, Innovating with Recommended Food Groups, Publishes Nutrition Progress Report" (press release). Accessed September 2012. www.aboutmcdonalds.com/content/dam/AboutMcDonalds/Newsroom/Electronic Press Kits/NutritionEPK/McDonalds USA Adding Calorie Counts to Menu Boards.pdf.

Schlosser, E. *Fast Food Nation: The Dark Side of the All-American Meal.* 2001. New York: Houghton Mifflin, 3.

PERK/TIP #67

Aloia, J. F., Patel, M., Dimaano, R., Li-Ng, M., Talwar, S. A., Mikhail, M., and Yeh, J. K. 2008. "Vitamin D Intake to Attain a Desired Serum 25-Hydroxyvitamin D Concentration." *The American Journal of Clinical Nutrition* 87:1952–1958.

Clarke, S. "In Tests, Vitamin D Shrinks Breast Cancer Cells." *Good Morning America.* Accessed April 2011. http://abcnews.go.com/GMA/OnCall/study-vitamin-d-kills-cancer-cells/story?id=9904415#.UMoABY7U4VR.

Harvard School of Public Health. "The Nutrition Source/Vitamin D and Health." Accessed September 2010. www.hsph.harvard.edu/nutritionsource/what-should-you-eat/vitamin-d/index.html.

Masterjohn, C. 2007. "Vitamin D Toxicity Redefined: Vitamin K and the Molecular Mechanism." *Medical Hypotheses* 68:1026–1034.

National Institutes of Health, Office of Dietary Supplements. "Dietary Supplemental Fact Sheet: Vitamin D." Accessed November 2011. www.ods .od.nih.gov/factsheets/VitaminD-HealthProfessional/.

PERK/TIP #68

Del Toro-Arreola, S., Flores-Torales, E., Torres-Lozano, C., Del Toro-Arreola, A., Tostado-Pelayo, K., Guadalupe Ramirez-Dueñas, M., and Daneri-Navarro, A. 2005. "Effect of D-Limonene on Immune Response in BALB/c Mice with Lymphoma." *International Journal of Immunopharmacology* 5:829–838.

Hyman, M. "Glutathione: The Mother of All Antioxidants." *Huffington Post/Healthy Living.* Accessed November 2011. www.huffingtonpost .com/dr-mark-hyman/glutathione-the-mother -of_b_530494.html.

Kim, B. "The Truth About Alkalizing Your Blood." Accessed November 2011. http://drbenkim.com/ ph-body-blood-foods-acid-alkaline.htm.

Mori, A., Lehmann, S., O'Kelly, J., Kumagai, T., Desmond, J. C., Pervan, M., and Koeffler, H. P. 2006. "Capsaicin, a Component of Red Peppers, Inhibits the Growth of Androgen-Independent, p53 Mutant Prostate Cancer Cells." *Cancer Research* 66:3222–3229. doi:10.1158/0008-5472 .CAN-05-0087. PMID 16540674.

Novick, J. "The Incredible Edible Avocado." National Health Association. Accessed November 2012. www.healthscience.org/Articles/avocado _article.htm.

Yang, Y., Paik, J. H., Cho, D., Cho, J. A., and Kim, C. W. 2008. "Resveratrol Induces the Suppression of Tumor-Derived CD4+CD25+ Regulatory T Cells." *International Immunopharmacology* 8:542–547.

PERK/TIP #69

Self-Nutrition Data. "Know What You Eat." Accessed June 2011. http://nutritiondata.self.com/

PERK/TIP #71

Maskarinec, G. 2009. "Cancer Protective Properties of Cocoa: A Review of the Epidemiologic Evidence." *Nutrition and Cancer* 61:573–579. doi:10.1080/01635580902825662.

PERK/TIP #72

Environmental Protection Agency (EPA). January 7, 2011 (news release). "EPA and HHS Announce New Scientific Assessments and Actions on Fluoride: Agencies Working Together to Maintain Benefits of Preventing Tooth Decay While Preventing Excessive Exposure." Accessed September 2011. http://yosemite.epa.gov/opa/admpress.nsf/d0cf6 618525a9efb85257359003fb69d/86964af577c37 ab285257811005a8417!OpenDocument.

Environmental Protection Agency (EPA). "Questions and Answers on Fluoride." Accessed June 2011. http://water.epa.gov/lawsregs/rulesregs/ regulatingcontaminants/sixyearreview/upload/ 2011_Fluoride_QuestionsAnswers.pdf.

Gorman, R. March 2012. "Is Your Tap Water Safe?" *Good Housekeeping Magazine.* Accessed July 2012. www.goodhousekeeping.com/health/womens -health/water-safety.

National Academies Press. 2006. "Fluoride in Drinking Water: A Scientific Review of EPA's Standards." Accessed September 2011. www.nap.edu/ openbook.php?record_id=11571&page=R2.

PERK/TIP #75

Bassett, D., Wyatt, H., Thompson, H., Peters, J., and Hill, J. 2010. "Pedometer-Measured Physical Activity and Health Behaviors in US Adults." *Medicine and Science in Sports and Exercise* 42:1819–1825. doi:10.1249/MSS.0b013e3181dc2e54.

Berkley Wellness Letter. "Preventing Heart Disease." Accessed September 2011. www.wellnesslet ter.com/ucberkeley/foundations/preventing -heart-disease/#.

Kravdal, H., and Syse, A. 2011. Changes Over Time in the Effect of Marital Status on Cancer Survival. *BMC Public Health* 11:804. doi:10.1186/1471-2458-11-804.

Leproult, R., Copinschi, G., Buxton, O., and Van, C. 1997. "Sleep Loss Results in an Elevation of Cortisol Levels the Next Evening." *Journal of Sleep Research & Sleep Medicine* 20:865–870.

Medical Research Council. "Does a Strong Handshake Predict a Longer Life?" Accessed December 2011. www.mrc.ac.uk/Newspublications/News/MRC007212.

Mostofsky, E., Levitan, E. B., Wolk, A., and Mittleman, M. A. 2010. "Chocolate Intake and Incidence of Heart Failure." *American Heart Association—Circulation: Heart Failure* 3:612–616. doi:10.1161/CIRCHEARTFAILURE.110.944025.

Pecorino, L. 2011. *Why Millions Survive Cancer: The Successes of Science.* New York: Oxford University Press, 89.

U.S. Geological Survey (USGS). "The Water in You." Accessed October 2012. http://ga.water.usgs .gov/edu/propertyyou.html.

van den Berg, L. December 18, 2009. "Monash University Public Health Expert Dr. Nathan Grills Says Santa Claus Promotes Obesity, Speeding, Drink-Driving." *Herald Sun* (Australia). Accessed December 2011. www.heraldsun.com.au/news/the-other-side/santa-a-health-hazard/story -e6frfhk6-1225811511670.

PERK/TIP #77

Oprah.com. "Oprah and 378 Staffers Go Vegan: The One Week Challenge." Accessed March 20, 2011. www.oprah.com/showinfo/Oprah-and-378 -Staffers-Go-Vegan-The-One-Week-Challenge.

PERK/TIP #82

Albanes, D., Heinonen, O. P., Taylor, P. R., Virtamo, J., Edwards, B. K., Rautalahti, M., and Huttunen, J. K. 1996. "Alpha-Tocopherol and Beta-Carotene Supplement and Lung Cancer Incidence in the Alpha-Tocopherol, Beta-Carotene Cancer Prevention Study: Effects of Baseline Characteristics and Study Compliance." *Journal of the National Cancer Institute* 88:1560–1570.

American Cancer Society. "Vitamin A, Retinoids, and Provitamin A Carotenoids." Accessed October 2012. www.cancer.org/treatment/treatments andsideeffects/complementaryandalternative medicine/herbsvitaminsandminerals/vitamin-a -and-beta-carotene.

Kushi, L. H., Doyle, C., McCullough, M., Rock, C. L., Demark-Wahnefried, W., Bandera, E. V., . . . and Gansler, T. 2012. "American Cancer Society Guidelines on Nutrition and Physical Activity for Cancer Prevention." *CA: A Cancer Journal for Clinicians* 62:30–67.

Meadows, G. G. 2012."Diet, Nutrients, Phytochemicals, and Cancer Metastasis Suppressor Genes." *Cancer and Metastasis Review.* doi:10.1007/s10555-012-9369-5.

National Cancer Institute. "Cruciferous Vegetables and Cancer Prevention." Accessed September 2011. www.cancer.gov/cancertopics/factsheet/diet/cruciferous-vegetables.

PERK/TIP #83

Elkins, G. R., Fisher, W. I., Johnson, A. K., Carpenter, J. S., and Keith, T. Z. 2012. "Clinical Hypnosis in the Treatment of Postmenopausal Hot Flashes." *Menopause: The Journal of the North American Menopause Society,* doi:10.1097/gme.0b013e31826ce3ed.

Harvard Health Publications. "When Sex Gives More Pain Than Pleasure." Accessed August 2012. www.health.harvard.edu/newsletters/Harvard_Wo mens_Health_Watch/2012/May/when-sex-gives

-more-pain-than-pleasure?utm_source=womens &utm_medium=pressrelease&utm_campaign =womens0512.

Mayo Clinic. "Fitness Tips for Menopause: Why Fitness Counts." Accessed November 2012. www.mayoclinic.com/health/fitness-tips-for -menopause/MY00478.

Medline Plus. "Menopause." Accessed November 2012. www.nlm.nih.gov/medlineplus/ency/article/ 000894.htm.

Sunay, D., Ozdiken, M., Arslan, H., Seven, A., and Arai, Y. 2011. "The Effect of Acupuncture on Post-menopausal Symptoms and Reproductive Hormones: A Sham Controlled Clinical Trial." *Acupuncture in Medicine* 29:27–31. doi:10.1136/ aim.2010.003285.

PERK/TIP #84

Holt-Lunstad, J., Smith, T. B., and Bradley Layton, J. 2010. "Social Relationships and Mortality Risk: A Meta-Analytic Review." *PLoS Med* 7(7). e1000316. doi:10.1371/journal.pmed.1000316.

Spiegel, D. 2001. "Mind Matters: Coping and Cancer Progression." *Journal of Psychosomatic Research* 50:287–290.

Turner-Cobb, J. M., Sephton, S. E., Koopman, C., Blake-Mortimer, J., and Spiegel, D. 2000. "Social Support and Salivary Cortisol in Women with Metastatic Breast Cancer." *Psychosomatic Medicine,* 62:337–345.

Winzelberg, A. J., Classen, C., Alpers, G. W., Roberts, H., Koopman, C., Adams, R. E., and Taylor, C. B., 2003. "Evaluation of an Internet Support Group for Women with Primary Breast Cancer." *Cancer* 97:1164–1173.

PERK/TIP #85

Adluri, R. S., Zhan, L., Bagchi, M., Maulik, N., and Maulik, G., 2010. "Comparative Effects of a Novel Plant-Based Calcium Supplement with Two Common Calcium Salts on Proliferation and Mineralization in Human Osteoblast Cells." *Molecular Cell Biochemistry* 340:73–80. doi:10.1007/s11010-010-0402-0.

PERK/TIP #86

Dobson, Roger. November 11, 2008. "How Crying Can Make You Healthier." *The Independent.* Accessed September 2012. www.independent .co.uk/life-style/health-and-families/features/ how-crying-can-make-you-healthier-1009169 .html.

Frey II, W. H. 1985. *Crying: The Mystery of Tears.* Minneapolis: Winston Press.

Oroloff, J. July 27, 2010. "The Health Benefits of Tears." *Psychology Today.* Accessed September 2012. www.psychologytoday.com/blog/emotional-free dom/201007/the-health-benefits-tears.

Science IQ. "The Science of Tears." Accessed September 2012. www.scienceiq.com/Facts/Science OfTears.cfm.

PERK/TIP #87

American Academy of Sleep Medicine. "Sleeplessness May Impair the Brain's Inhibitory Control When Viewing High-Calorie Foods." Accessed September 2011. www.aasmnet.org/articles.aspx? id=2308.

American Heart Association. March 14, 2012. "Lack of Sleep May Increase Calorie Consumption." Accessed December 2012. http://news room.heart.org/pr/aha/lack-of-sleep-may-increase-calorie-230068.aspx.

BBC News Health. August 30, 2011. "Bad Sleep Ups Blood Pressure Risk." Accessed September 2011. www.bbc.co.uk/news/health-14681570.

Estroff Marano, H. July 01, 2003. "Bedfellows: Insomnia and Depression." *Psychology Today.* Accessed September 2011. www.psychologytoday

.com/articles/200307/bedfellows-insomnia-and
-depression.

Harvard University. 2007. "Study Shows Importance of Sleep for Optimal Memory Functioning." *Harvard Gazette.* Accessed September 2011. http://news.harvard.edu/gazette/story/2007/02/ study-shows-importance-of-sleep-for-optimal -memory-functioning/.

Laugsand, L. E., Vatten, L. J., Platou, C., and Janszky, I. 2011. "Insomnia and the Risk of Acute Myocardial Infarction: A Population Study." *Circulation* 124(19):2075–2081. doi:10.1161/CIRCU-LATIONAHA.111.025858.

Mayo Clinic. "Lack of Sleep: Can It Make You Sick?" Accessed September 2011. www.mayoclinic .com/health/lack-of-sleep/AN02065.

Pamidi, S., Aronsohn, R. S., and Tasali, E. 2010. "Obstructive Sleep Apnea: Role in the Risk and Severity of Diabetes." *Best Practice & Research: Clinical Endocrinology & Metabolism* 24:703–715. doi:10.1016/j.beem.2010.08.009.

University Hospitals Case Medical Center. August 2012. "Lack of Sleep Found to Be a New Risk Factor for Aggressive Breast Cancers." *ScienceDaily.* Accessed October 2012. www.sciencedaily.com/ releases/2012/08/120827113359.htm?utm_sourc e=feedburner&utm_medium=email&utm_cam paign=Feed%3A+sciencedaily%2Fhealth_medi cine%2Fbreast_cancer+%28ScienceDaily%3A+ Health+%26+Medicine+News+—+Breast+ Cancer%29.

PERK/TIP #89

Centers for Disease Control (CDC). "Fourth National Report on Human Exposure to Environmental Chemicals." Accessed August 2012. www .cdc.gov/exposurereport/pdf/FourthReport.pdf.

National Cancer Institute. "Cancer Trends Progress Report: 2011/2012 Update." Accessed August 2012. http://progressreport.cancer.gov/doc_detail.asp ?pid=1&did=2009&chid=91&coid=913&mid=# pesticides.

Pesticide Action Network. "Pesticides on Food." Accessed August 2012. www.panna.org/issues/ food-agriculture/pesticides-on-food.

U.S. Department of Health and Human Services. "2008–2009 Annual Report: Reducing Environmental Cancer Risk." Accessed August 2012. http://deainfo.nci.nih.gov/advisory/pcp/annual reports/pcp08-09rpt/PCP_Report_08-09_508.pdf.

PERK/TIP #90

American Psychological Association (APA). "Lying Less Linked to Better Health." Accessed October 2012. www.newswise.com/articles/lying -less-linked-to-better-health-new-research-finds.

PERK/TIP #91

American Cancer Society. "The Bottom Line on Soy and Cancer Risk." Accessed October 2012. www.cancer.org/cancer/news/expertvoices/post/2 012/08/02/the-bottom-line-on-soy-and-breast -cancer-risk.aspx.

American Institute for Cancer Research. "Soy Is Safe for Breast Cancer Survivors." Accessed November 2012. www.aicr.org/press/press-releases/soy-safe -breast-cancer-survivors.html.

Huffington Post. "Soy: Healthy or Harmful?" Accessed August 2012. www.huffingtonpost.com/ 2012/08/23/soy-healthy_n_1823052.html.

World Health Organization, "20 Questions on Genetically Modified Foods." Accessed September 2012. www.who.int/foodsafety/publications/ biotech/20questions/en/.

PERK/TIP #92

Ariga, T., and Seki, T. 2006. "Antithrombotic and Anticancer Effects of Garlic-Derived Sulfur Compounds: A Review." *Biofactors* 26:93–103.

Vaidya, V., Ingold, K. U., and Pratt, D. A. 2009. "Garlic: Source of the Ultimate Antioxidants—Sulfenic Acids." *Angewandte Chemie International Edition* 48:157–160.

PERK/TIP #94

American Cancer Society Guide to Quitting Smoking. Accessed November 2012. www.cancer.org/acs/groups/cid/documents/webcontent/002971-pdf.pdf.

Misaghi, N. September 9, 2012. E-mail to Susan Gonzalez. http://totalhealthnd.com.

PERK/TIP #95

Doobinin, P. August 31, 2012. E-mail to Susan Gonzalez. www.dnymc.org.

PERK/TIP #98

American Association of Pharmaceutical Scientists. "Study Reveals Vegetable-Derived Compounds Effective in Treating Triple Negative Breast Cancer." Accessed November 2012. www.aaps.org/News/Press_Room/Press_Releases/Study_Reveals_Vegetable-Derived_Compounds_Effective_in_Treating_Triple-Negative_Breast_Cancer/.

Oregon State University Linus Pauling Institute. "Isothiocyanates." Accessed September 2012. http://lpi.oregonstate.edu/infocenter/phytochemicals/isothio/.

Singh, S. V., Kim, S. H., Sehrawat, A., Arlotti, J. A., Hahm, E. R., Sakao, K., and Dhir, R.. 2012. "Biomarkers of Phenethyl Isothiocyanate-Mediated Mammary Cancer Chemoprevention in a Clinically Relevant Mouse Model." *Journal of the National Cancer Institute* 104(16):1228–1230. doi:10.1093/jnci/djs321.

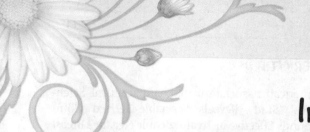

Index

About the Authors

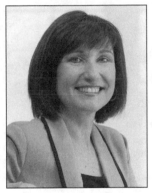

Florence Strang, B.A., B.Ed., M.Ed., is a registered psychologist with more than twenty years of experience in the fields of education and psychology. After being diagnosed with stage-3 breast cancer, she began to blog "The Perks of Having Cancer," as a way to help her stay positive through difficult cancer treatments. Her story is told in *Woman's World Magazine* (April 2012) and *Chicken Soup for the Soul: The Power of Positive* (2012). She lives in scenic Lewin's Cove, Newfoundland, with her daughter, Kaitlyn, and sons, Donovan and Ben.

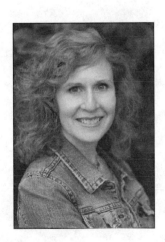

Susan Gonzalez, R.N., B.S.N., earned her nursing degree in New York in 1986. Diagnosed with cancer in 2005, Susan had a unique perspective on the disease, being a nurse in the patient's role. She took that knowledge and her passion for finding natural cures to fight disease and began a blog for those who wanted to make simple changes for healthy living with an emphasis on avoiding cancer. She currently lives in Atlanta, Georgia, with her husband and two daughters.